Clinical Cases in Endocrinology

Clinical Cases in Endocrinology

Editor: Noa Taylor

AMERICAN
MEDICAL PUBLISHERS
www.americanmedicalpublishers.com

AMERICAN
MEDICAL PUBLISHERS
www.americanmedicalpublishers.com

Cataloging-in-Publication Data

Clinical cases in endocrinology / edited by Noa Taylor.
p. cm.
Includes bibliographical references and index.
ISBN 979-8-88740-629-9
1. Endocrinology. 2. Endocrine glands--Diseases. I. Taylor, Noa.
RC648 .C55 2023
616.4--dc23

American Medical Publishers,
41 Flatbush Avenue,
1st Floor, New York,
NY 11217, USA

ISBN 979-8-88740-629-9 (Hardback)

Contents

Preface

The world is advancing at a fast pace like never before. Therefore, the need is to keep up with the latest developments. This book was an idea that came to fruition when the specialists in the area realized the need to coordinate together and document essential themes in the subject. That's when I was requested to be the editor. Editing this book has been an honour as it brings together diverse authors researching on different streams of the field. The book collates essential materials contributed by veterans in the area which can be utilized by students and researchers alike.

Endocrinology is a specialized field of medicine that focuses on the endocrine system, which includes glands that produce hormones to regulate various bodily functions. This field encompasses a wide range of disorders related to hormone imbalances and dysfunctions. These include thyroid disorders, polycystic ovary syndrome, and adrenal gland disorders. Thyroid disorders can involve either an overactive or underactive thyroid gland. Treatment options for these type of disorders may include medication to restore hormone balance, radioactive iodine therapy, or in some cases, surgical removal of the thyroid gland. Polycystic ovary syndrome is a hormonal disorder that affects women and can cause irregular menstrual periods, excess hair growth and fertility problems. The book aims to shed light on some of the unexplored aspects of endocrinology and the recent researches in this field. It will serve as a valuable source of reference for graduate and postgraduate students.

Each chapter is a sole-standing publication that reflects each author´s interpretation. Thus, the book displays a multi-facetted picture of our current understanding of application, resources and aspects of the field. I would like to thank the contributors of this book and my family for their endless support.

Editor

1

Hereditary Hypophosphatemic Rickets with Hypercalciuria (HHRH) Presenting with Genu Valgum Deformity: Treatment with Phosphate Supplementation and Surgical Correction

Juan M. Colazo,[1,2] Seth A. Reasoner,[2,3] Ginger Holt,[4] Marie C. M. Faugere,[5] and Kathryn M. Dahir[6]

[1]*Department of Biomedical Engineering, Vanderbilt University, Nashville, TN, USA*
[2]*Medical Scientist Training Program, Vanderbilt University School of Medicine, Nashville, TN, USA*
[3]*Department of Pathology, Microbiology and Immunology, Vanderbilt University Medical Center, Nashville, TN, USA*
[4]*Department of Orthopedics, Vanderbilt University Medical Center, Nashville, TN, USA*
[5]*Division of Nephrology, Bone and Mineral Metabolism, University of Kentucky, Albert B. Chandler Medical Center, Lexington, KY, USA*
[6]*Division of Diabetes, Endocrinology and Metabolism, Vanderbilt University Medical Center, Nashville, TN, USA*

Correspondence should be addressed to Juan M. Colazo; juan.m.colazo@vanderbilt.edu and Kathryn M. Dahir; kathryn.dahir@vumc.org

Academic Editor: J. Paul Frindik

We describe a case of hereditary hypophosphatemic rickets with hypercalciuria (HHRH) in a 32-year-old female with short stature, chronic pathologic genu valgum deformity, and knee pain who was referred to endocrinology clinic after previous inconclusive workups. We present imaging spanning 10 years of untreated disease. Biochemical studies showed hypophosphatemia with undetectable fibroblast growth factor 23 (FGF23.) Renal ultrasound revealed bilateral medullary nephrocalcinosis despite no apparent hypercalciuria. Due to concern for HHRH, genetic testing was performed that determined this patient to be homozygous in the *SLC34A3* gene for a previously described missense variant (c.1402C > T, p.Arg468Trp). There was no known family history of rickets. A bone biopsy with metabolic studies was performed for diagnostic and prognostic reasons. The histopathological findings along with tetracycline uptake studies were consistent with a diagnosis of HHRH. Treatment with phosphorous supplementation and surgical correction of her valgum deformity resulted in resolution of pain, but no change in bone histomorphometry.

1. Introduction

Hereditary hypophosphatemia rickets with hypercalciuria (HHRH) is an extraordinarily rare autosomal recessive disorder with an estimated prevalence of 1/250,000 [1]. Variants in the SLC34A3 gene encoding a sodium-dependent phosphate transporter (NaPi-IIc) have been implicated as responsible for this disease. The NaPi-IIc transporter is highly expressed in the nephron's proximal tubules, and its dysfunction results in phosphate wasting disorder.

Here, we report a case of HHRH presenting as a genu valgum deformity with pain in a 32-year-old female with no fracture history and unremarkable family history for metabolic bone disease. We review the pathophysiology, diagnosis, and treatment of HHRH and contrast HHRH and other phosphate wasting disorders.

2. Case Presentation

A 32-year-old Caucasian female presented to endocrinology clinic with severe left knee pain and a significant genu valgum deformity bilaterally. The patient reported being told that "she may have had rickets" at the age of 9 but was lost to follow-up. Ten years prior to this current presentation, she presented at the age of 22 with painful trochanteric bursitis. During this clinic appointment, X-ray images showed a significant genu valgum deformity at a Q- angle of 17° (Figure 1). Deformity correction was suggested at this time but was not performed. At that time, no endocrinologic workup was performed.

Now, at the age of 32, a complete medical history was obtained. She is currently taking over-the-counter vitamin D3, but no calcium supplementation. She is 155 cm (58.5 kg and BMI 23.79 kg/m^2), her mother is 173 cm, and her father is 188 cm. She has no siblings or children. She has no fracture or abnormal dentition history. There is no family history of rickets or other metabolic bone disease.

On physical examination, there is marked valgus alignment bilaterally, with left being significantly more prominent. Gait examination showed her left knee knocking into her right leg. X-ray scans were performed that showed a Q-angle of 23°, worsened from her presentation 10 years prior (Figure 1). Bone mineral density scans showed osteopenia of the left femoral head with normal lumbar spine density (Figure 2). Pertinent laboratory values displayed hypophosphatemia, elevated total vitamin D and 1,25-dihydroxyvitamin D, undetectable fibroblast growth factor 23 (FGF23), and low parathyroid hormone (Table 1). Twenty-four-hour urine showed inappropriately normal phosphate excretion and normal urine calcium. A renal ultrasound showed bilateral medullary nephrocalcinosis, without calculi (Figure 3). HHRH was suspected due to her described biochemistry and the presence of bilateral renal calcinosis. Thus, genetic testing was pursued, and this patient was determined to be homozygous in the *SLC34A3* gene for a previously described missense variant (c.1402C > T, p.Arg468Trp) (NM_080877.2) [2, 3]. Due to these findings, she was started on phosphorous supplementation (K-Phos Neutral 250 mg TID AC).

A right iliac crest bone biopsy was performed and sent for metabolic bone studies prior to the initiation of phosphorus. Histopathological findings included high porosity of the cortical bone, decreased cancellous bone, and decreased osteoid surface (Figure 4). Fluorescent light microscopy with tetracycline labelling showed a decrease in the mineralizing surface. Some double labels were seen in the subcortical bone. The distance between double labels was in the low-normal range. These results show previous weakly diffuse tetracycline deposition (Figures 4(e) and 4(f)), determined to be most likely due to her recent prescription of doxycycline for facial acne therapy which was stopped in advance of the biopsy. In summary, the metabolic bone biopsy showed low bone volume with reduced turnover of cancellous bone without evidence of osteomalacia.

Since the diagnosis of HHRH, she continued to receive phosphorous supplementation; meanwhile, vitamin D was stopped. Her abnormal laboratory values have resolved (Table 1). Her left knee pain has improved significantly. Six months after starting phosphorus supplementation, she underwent an uncomplicated left total knee arthroplasty (TKA) leading to gait correction (Figure 5). Biopsy at the time of surgery showed thin cortical bone and high porosity without evidence of osteomalacia, not significantly changed in comparison with her previous biopsy (Figure 6).

3. Discussion

The patient in this case initially presented at the age of 9 and received an ambiguous diagnosis of "rickets." She did not receive a definitive diagnosis and begin correct treatment until 20 years later. Like other cases in the literature, our case highlights the protracted diagnostic journey for many of these patients with incorrect or uncertain diagnoses along the way [4]. This patient had presented in childhood with leg pain and genu valgum deformity. To understand the differential diagnosis for deformities such as genu valgum or "knock knee," one must first understand the natural history of the alignment of the lower limbs [5]. In newborns and infants, "bowlegs" (bilateral genu varus) are physiologic. These become straight by around 18–24 months. By 2 or 3 years, "knock knee" (physiologic genu valgus) develops with an average Q-angle of about 12°. By 7 years, spontaneous correction usually occurs to the physiologic alignment of adult valgus (mean of about 7° in females and 5° in males) and anything >12° is considered pathological. If valgus is sustained past this point, it is considered pathological and can cause significant distress, referred pain, and pressure, causing trochanteric bursitis as seen in this case.

A correct workup for these deformities is essential. If a patient is misdiagnosed, surgical correction may fail and cause healing difficulties. The differentialdiagnosis for bilateral genu valgum includes physiologic, renal osteodystrophy (renal rickets), skeletal dysplasia, Morquio syndrome, spondyloepiphyseal dysplasia, chondroextodermal dysplasia, and metabolic disorders including HHRH. The differential diagnosis for unilateral genu valgum includes physeal injury from trauma, infection, or vascular insult, proximal metaphyseal tibia fracture, benign tumors (fibrous dysplasia, osteochondromas, and Ollier's disease), among others [6]. Our patient had bilateral valgus, with unilateral predominance. Thus, a metabolic bone disorder was most likely.

Tieder et al. were the first to describe the clinical phenotype of HHRH in a consanguineous Bedouin family [7]. Since then, case reports have been published from individuals from a variety of ethnicities, leading to the realization that HHRH is likely an underrecognized cause of rickets and osteomalacia [8]. In fact, patients misdiagnosed with osteoporosis have been later found to have HHRH [4]. Patients usually present in the first years of life with rickets, bone pain, short stature, and lower extremity deformities. Patients with this condition can also develop recurrent nephrolithiasis and/or medullary nephrocalcinosis. The classically published biochemical phenotype includes hypophosphatemia, phosphaturia, hypercalciuria, elevated 1,25-dihydroxyvitamin D levels, and suppressed PTH levels.

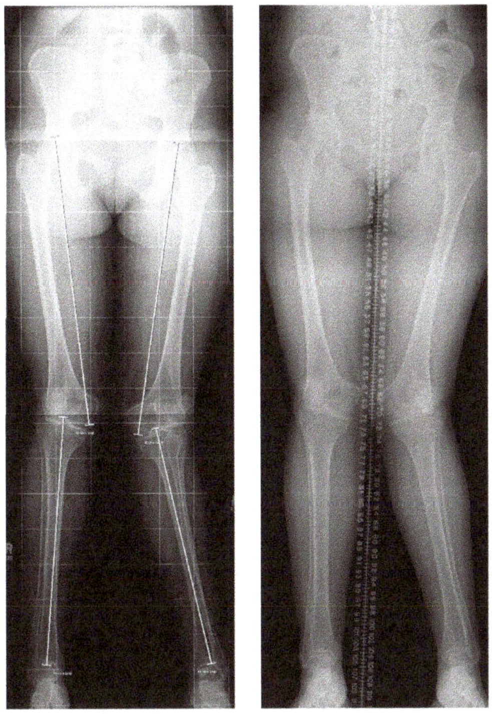

(a) (b)

Figure 1: Radiographs of lower extremity genu valgus. (a) At age 22, ten years prior to the current presentation, radiography displays genu valgum of the left knee measuring 17° with a hypoplastic lateral femoral condyle. (b) At current presentation, at age 32, redemonstration of genu valgum of the left knee measuring 23° with narrowing of the joint compartments at the knees and osteochondral irregularity of the talar dome on the right.

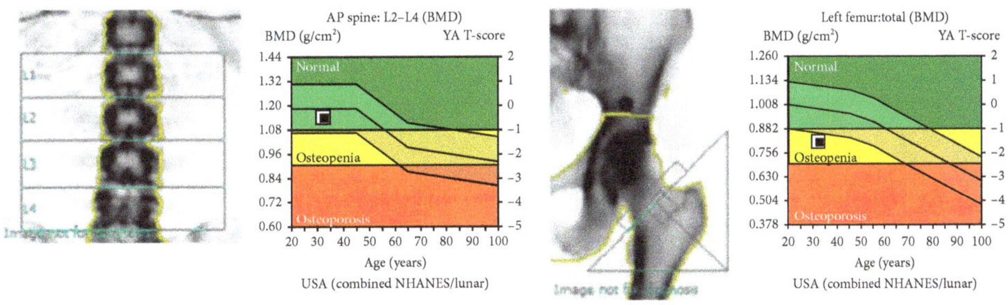

(a) (b)

Figure 2: Bone mineral density (BMD) scans (current presentation). (a) The BMD within the lumbar spine is 1.140 g/cm^2 which corresponds to a Z-score of −0.4. (b) The BMD within the left total hip is 0.807 g/cm^2 which corresponds a Z-score of −1.4. The BMD within the left femoral neck is 0.819 g/cm^2 which corresponds to a Z-score of −1.3.

We will discuss each of these electrolyte and endocrinologic abnormalities in more detail below.

HHRH is caused by variants in the *SLC34A3* gene which codes for the proximal tubular transporter NaPi-IIc. NaPi-IIc is one of three known phosphate transporters in the proximal tubule: NaPi-IIa, NaPi-IIc, and PiT_2 [9]. NaPi-IIc reabsorbs divalent phosphate (HPO_4^{2-}) from the filtrate in exchange of sodium ions. Variants in *SLC34A3*/NaPi-IIc lead to impaired phosphate reabsorption and thus phosphate wasting in the urine. At least 40 separate pathogenic variants in *SLC34A3* have been identified [1]. The inheritance pattern is autosomal recessive and often caused by compound heterozygotic variants. Interestingly, carriers of a single *SLC34A3* variant display an intermediate phenotype with increased frequency of renal calculi compared to the general population [10]. This patient's parents, presumed to be carriers, had no history of nephrolithiasis and were of normal stature.

Phosphate wasting in HHRH leads to elevation of 1,25-dihydroxyvitamin D levels, a key clue differentiating HHRH from other phosphate wasting disorders. Elevated 1,25-dihydroxyvitamin D levels in these patients cause increased calcium absorption from the gastrointestinal tract which results in transient hypercalcemia, suppressed PTH levels,

Table 1: Laboratory values.

Lab test (reference value)	At presentation	After 6 months of phosphorus supplementation
Phosphorus (2.3–4.7 mg/dL)	1.7	2.5
Calcium (8.5–10.5 mg/dL)	9.6	8.9
Creatinine (0.57–1.11 mg/dL)	0.82	0.83
Total vitamin D (25–80 ng/mL)	85	56
1,25-Dihydroxy vitamin D (19.9–79.3 pg/mL)	154	126
FGF23 (≤180)	<50	—
Bone-specific alkaline phosphate (premenopausal female: 4.5–16.9 μg/L)	12.1	12.7
Parathyroid hormone (16–77 pg/mL)	9	16
Urine phosphorus (400–1,300 mg/24 hr)	777*	—
Urine calcium (100–300 mg/24 hr)	155	—

*In patients with hypophosphatemia, urinary phosphate excretion above 100 mg/day or a fractional excretion, F_EPO_4, above 5 percent is indicative of renal phosphate wasting.

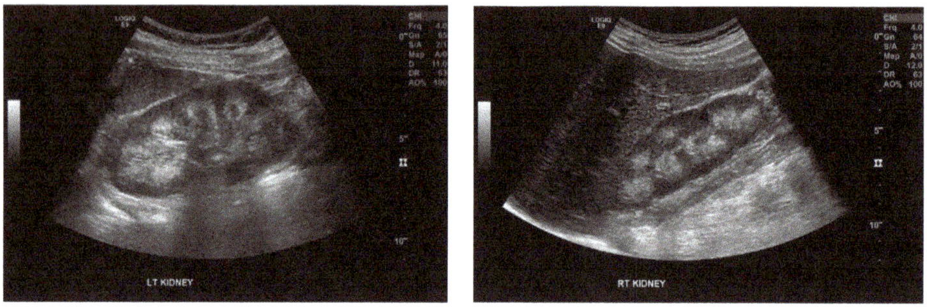

(a) (b)

Figure 3: Renal ultrasound (current presentation). (a) Left kidney measuring 11.7 cm in length. (b) Right kidney measuring 11.5 cm in length. Both kidneys have homogenous cortical echoes. The renal pyramids are hyperechoic consistent with bilateral medullar nephrocalcinosis.

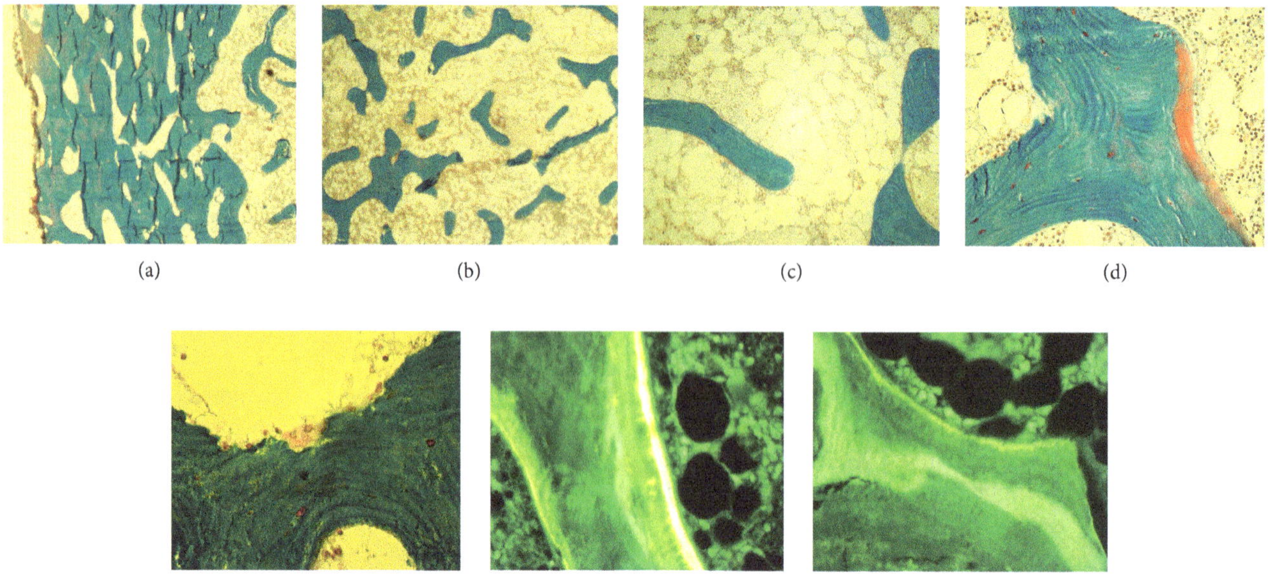

(e) (f) (g)

Figure 4: Iliac crest bone biopsy prior to phosphorus supplementation. Modified Masson–Goldner trichrome (a)–(e). High porosity of the cortical bone (a) and decreased cancellous bone volume (b). Low bone turnover and mild hypocellularity of bone marrow (c). Rare osteoid seam of normal thickness (d) and few osteoclasts (e). Fluorescent light microscopy: few tetracycline label (f) and evidence of a previous oxytetracycline label (g).

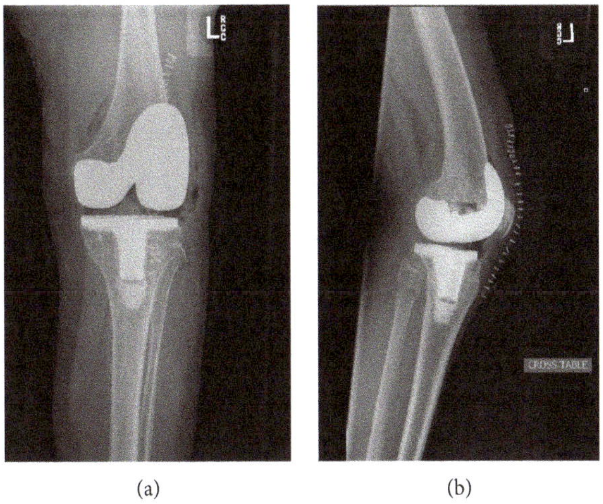

FIGURE 5: Postoperative radiographs. Postoperative imaging following corrective left total knee arthroplasty: anterior-posterior (a) and lateral views (b).

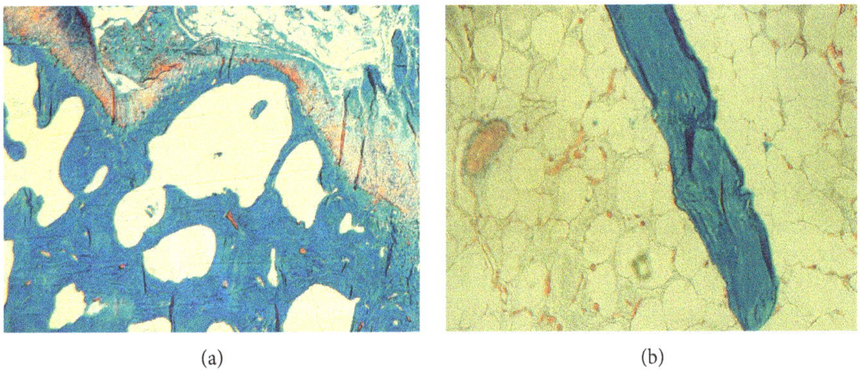

FIGURE 6: Intraoperative surgical biopsy after phosphorus supplementation. Modified Masson–Goldner trichrome of a femur specimen obtained at the time of knee arthroplasty displayed thin cortical bone and high porosity (a). Thin trabecula and adipose bone marrow (b). No significant change in comparison with her prior biopsy.

and a compensatory hypercalciuria [11]. Occasionally, an incidentally discovered hypercalcemia can trigger a diagnostic workup leading to the diagnosis of HHRH. The reduction in PTH-dependent calcium-reabsorption in the distal renal tubules ultimately leads to nephrolithiasis and/or nephrocalcinosis. Another differentiating feature between HHRH and other phosphate wasting disorders is the low levels of fibroblast growth factor 23 (FGF23) in HHRH. The normal physiologic function of FGF23 is the regulation of phosphate concentration in the blood. FGF23 is secreted by osteocytes when 1,25-dihydroxyvitamin D levels are elevated. FGF23 then acts on the kidneys by decreasing the expression of NaPi-IIc [12]. In turn, FGF23 decreases the reabsorption of phosphate, causing phosphate wasting. In addition, recent studies have shown that FGF23 may also suppress 1-alpha-hydroxylase, reducing its ability to activate vitamin D and therefore impairing calcium absorption and homeostasis [13].

In evaluating hypophosphatemia, the patient's levels of vitamin D, FGF23, and PTH are particularly useful. Vitamin D levels are elevated in HHRH, whereas they are low or inappropriately normal in conditions of FGF23 excess. Vitamin D deficiency, however, can mask laboratory features of HHRH and therefore must be assessed independently [8, 14, 15]. Hypophosphatemic disorders with FGF23 excess are more common than HHRH and are caused by variants directly affecting FGF23 and its metabolism. For example, X-linked hypophosphatemia is caused by variants in *PHEX* which is an inactivator of FGF23 and is approximately ten times more common than HHRH [16, 17].

Treatment of FGF23-mediated phosphate wasting involves phosphate and vitamin D supplementation. In conditions of FGF23 excess, an emerging treatment option is Burosumab, an anti-FGF23 IgG1 monoclonal antibody, which has been recently approved for use in X-linked hypophosphatemia [18]. Since HHRH is an FGF23-independent disorder, Burosumab would be ineffective. Currently, the only treatment for HHRH is long-term phosphorous supplementation which can singularly cause remission and rapid correction of bone mineralization capacity. Meanwhile, the addition of active vitamin D metabolites can cause symptom deterioration and worsening of hypercalciuria and nephrolithiasis [14, 19]. Ultimately, HHRH should be treated with phosphorus supplementation for at least 6 months before corrective surgery (e.g., osteotomy and TKA) is pursued to ensure that bone mineralization is no longer compromised. If not, poor bone healing and mineralization may occur, causing further deficits that may be irreversible. Ideally, identification of HHRH in childhood might prevent the need for surgical correction later in life. The variable clinical presentations of HHRH, however, may not be recognized until after childhood.

The constellation of symptoms in HHRH can be variable in their onset and severity. Patients presenting in childhood generally have rickets and/or nephrolithiasis. In adulthood, nephrolithiasis and bone pain are the most common presenting symptoms. The presence of renal calcifications is more uncommon and is often attributed to inappropriate treatment of HHRH with vitamin D. The variability in the age of presentation is due to incomplete penetrance from various variants and environmental factors [15]. Serum phosphate is sensitive to dietary intake of phosphate. And, in turn, the compensatory endocrinologic mechanisms lead to fluctuating laboratory values [19, 20]. In this case, the renal ultrasound demonstrating nephrocalcinosis was particularly pivotal in the diagnosis due to the equivocal urine calcium measurement. Given the lengthy differential diagnosis for phosphate wasting, genetic analysis is generally considered necessary for a conclusive diagnosis of HHRH.

4. Conclusions

Herein, we presented the first reported case of surgical correction of a genu valgus deformity caused by hereditary hypophosphatemic rickets with hypercalciuria (HHRH). HHRH is an underidentified cause of rickets and osteomalacia and may be misdiagnosed as osteoporosis. We reviewed phosphate wasting disorders and their distinguishing features.

Disclosure

The content in this report is solely the responsibility of the authors and does not necessarily represent the official views of the National Institutes of Health.

Authors' Contributions

JMC and SAR drafted the manuscript. MCMF supervised histopathological analysis. KMD and GH provided the medical and surgical care for the patient, respectively. KMD supervised the writing of this case report. All authors made effortful contributions to the final manuscript. Juan M. Colazo and Seth A. Reasoner contributed equally to this work.

Acknowledgments

JMC and SAR were supported by NIGMS of the National Institutes of Health under award number T32GM007347. MCMF was supported by Kentucky Nephrology Research Trust.

References

[1] C. Bergwitz and K.-I. Miyamoto, "Hereditary hypophosphatemic rickets with hypercalciuria: pathophysiology, clinical presentation, diagnosis and therapy," *Pflügers Archiv-European Journal of Physiology*, vol. 471, no. 1, pp. 149–163, 2019.

[2] C. Bergwitz, N. M. Roslin, M. Tieder et al., "SLC34A3 mutations in patients with hereditary hypophosphatemic rickets with hypercalciuria predict a key role for the sodium-phosphate cotransporter NaPi-IIc in maintaining phosphate homeostasis," *The American Journal of Human Genetics*, vol. 78, no. 2, pp. 179–192, 2006.

[3] S. Haito-Sugino, M. Ito, A. Ohi et al., "Processing and stability of type IIc sodium-dependent phosphate cotransporter mutations in patients with hereditary hypophosphatemic rickets with hypercalciuria," *American Journal of Physiology-Cell Physiology*, vol. 302, no. 9, pp. C1316–C1330, 2012.

[4] G. Dhir, D. Li, H. Hakonarson, and M. A. Levine, "Late-onset hereditary hypophosphatemic rickets with hypercalciuria (HHRH) due to mutation of SLC34A3/NPT2c," *Bone*, vol. 97, pp. 15–19, 2017.

[5] R. Espandar, S. M. J. Mortazavi, and T. Baghdadi, "Angular deformities of the lower limb in children," *Asian Journal of Sports Medicine*, vol. 1, no. 1, pp. 46–53, 2010.

[6] M. J. Lee, J. M. Perez-Rossello, and B. Weissman, "Pediatric developmental and chronic traumatic conditions, the osteochondroses, and childhood osteoporosis," in *Imaging of Arthritis and Metabolic Bone Disease*, B. Weissman, Ed., pp. 457–505, Mosby, Maryland Heights, MI, USA, 2009.

[7] M. Tieder, D. Modai, R. Samuel et al., "Hereditary hypophosphatemic rickets with hypercalciuria," *New England Journal of Medicine*, vol. 312, no. 10, pp. 611–617, 1985.

[8] A. L. Tencza, S. Ichikawa, A. Dang et al., "Hypophosphatemic rickets with hypercalciuria due to mutation inSLC34A3/type IIc sodium-phosphate cotransporter: presentation as hypercalciuria and nephrolithiasis," *The Journal of Clinical Endocrinology & Metabolism*, vol. 94, no. 11, pp. 4433–4438, 2009.

[9] C. A. Wagner, I. Rubio-Aliaga, and N. Hernando, "Renal phosphate handling and inherited disorders of phosphate reabsorption: an update," *Pediatric Nephrology*, vol. 34, no. 4, pp. 549–559, 2019.

[10] D. Dasgupta, M. J. Wee, M. Reyes et al., "Mutations in SLC34A3/NPT2c are associated with kidney stones and nephrocalcinosis," *Journal of the American Society of Nephrology*, vol. 25, no. 10, pp. 2366–2375, 2014.

[11] A. R. Tang, L. E. Hinz, A. Khan, and G. A. Kline, "Phosphate matters when investigating hypercalcemia: a mutation in SLC34A3 causing HHRH," *Endocrinol Diabetes Metab Case Reports*, vol. 2019, no. 1, 2019.

[12] X. Huang, Y. Jiang, and W. Xia, "FGF23 and phosphate wasting disorders," *Bone Research*, vol. 1, no. 2, pp. 120–132, 2013.

[13] F. Perwad, M. Y. H. Zhang, H. S. Tenenhouse, and A. A. Portale, "Fibroblast growth factor 23 impairs phos-

phorus and vitamin D metabolism in vivo and suppresses 25-hydroxyvitamin D-1α-hydroxylase expression in vitro," *American Journal of Physiology-Renal Physiology*, vol. 293, no. 5, pp. F1577–F1583, 2007.

[14] P. Phulwani, C. Bergwitz, G. Jaureguiberry, M. Rasoulpour, and E. Estrada, "Hereditary hypophosphatemic rickets with hypercalciuria and nephrolithiasis—identification of a novel SLC34A3/NaPi-IIc mutation," *Physiological Behaviours*, vol. 176, no. 5, pp. 139–148, 2011.

[15] B. Kremke, C. Bergwitz, W. Ahrens et al., "Hypophosphatemic rickets with hypercalciuria due to mutation in SLC34A3/NaPi-IIc can be masked by vitamin D deficiency and can be associated with renal calcifications," *Experimental and Clinical Endocrinology & Diabetes*, vol. 117, no. 2, pp. 49–56, 2009.

[16] S. S. Beck-Nielsen, Z. Mughal, D. Haffner et al., "FGF23 and its role in X-linked hypophosphatemia-related morbidity," *Orphanet Journal of Rare Diseases*, vol. 14, no. 1, pp. 1–25, 2019.

[17] M. E. Robinson, H. AlQuorain, M. Murshed, and F. Rauch, "Mineralized tissues in hypophosphatemic rickets," *Pediatric Nephrology*, 2019.

[18] T. O. Carpenter, M. P. Whyte, E. A. Imel et al., "Burosumab therapy in children with X-linked hypophosphatemia," *New England Journal of Medicine*, vol. 378, no. 21, pp. 1987–1998, 2018.

[19] H. Mualla, S. A. Bae, and A. Yaqub, "Autosomal dominant hypophosphatemic rickets presenting in a phenotypically normal adult female," *Case Reports in Endocrinology*, vol. 2019, Article ID 8917519, 5 pages, 2019.

[20] S. Amatschek, M. Haller, and R. Oberbauer, "Renal phosphate handling in human-what can we learn from hereditary hypophosphataemias?" *European Journal of Clinical Investigation*, vol. 40, no. 6, pp. 552–560, 2010.

2

Thyroid Eye Disease due to Immune Reconstitution Inflammatory Syndrome as a Consequence of Antiretroviral Therapy in the Setting of AIDS

Ravali Nallu,[1] Parvathy Madhavan,[1] Lisa Chirch,[2] and Pooja Luthra[1]

[1]*Department of Medicine, Division of Endocrinology and Metabolism, University of Connecticut, School of Medicine, Farmington, CT, USA*
[2]*Department of Medicine, Division of Infectious Diseases, University of Connecticut, School of Medicine, Farmington, CT, USA*

Correspondence should be addressed to Parvathy Madhavan; madhavan.parvathy@gmail.com

Academic Editor: Mihail A. Boyanov

We describe a case of worsening Graves' orbitopathy due to immune reconstitution inflammatory syndrome (IRIS) in a 38-year-old HIV-infected male after beginning ART (antiretroviral therapy). Two years after initiation of ART, the patient developed symptoms of hyperthyroidism and thyroid eye disease (TED) or Graves' orbitopathy (GO). Thyroid iodine uptake scan was consistent with Graves' disease. The CT scan of the orbits revealed minimal right-sided proptosis, consistent with GO. He was treated with methimazole and a short course of high-dose prednisone for GO. Thyroid function tests normalized, and eye symptoms eventually stabilized. This case demonstrates the importance of awareness and early recognition of IRIS in its many forms, as it has significant therapeutic implications.

1. Background

Antiretroviral therapy (ART) has dramatically improved the morbidity and mortality of patients infected with the human immunodeficiency virus (HIV), but it may also increase the risk of immune reconstitution inflammatory syndrome (IRIS). IRIS is characterized by a pathological inflammatory response to a pre-existing pathogen or antigen and paradoxical worsening of clinical status, after initiation of ART [1]. IRIS develops in 10–25% of patients with AIDS receiving ART [1]. Graves' disease (GD) occurs in 1-2% of patients with HIV as a late manifestation of IRIS [2]. GD is an autoimmune disease caused by production of IgG autoantibodies against the thyrotropin (TSH) receptor, binding and activating it and causing autonomous production of thyroid hormone [3]. Thyroid eye disease (TED) or Graves' orbitopathy (GO) occurs in about 25% of all patients with GD [1]. The incidence and prevalence of TED as a manifestation of IRIS is unknown. We discuss the rare occurrence of TED due to GD, as a result of IRIS, in a patient with AIDS.

2. Case

A 38-year-old male diagnosed with HIV-1 infection in 2014 was treated with ART. He did not have a prior history of thyroid disease although his sister had a history of hyperthyroidism. Physical examination was unremarkable. His baseline CD4+ T-cell count was very low at 32 cells/μl with a plasma HIV RNA of 213,000 copies/ml. The patient was started on ART with emtricitabine/rilpivirine/tenofovir disoproxil fumarate at an outside facility. On evaluation at our institution for a second opinion, he was transitioned to emtricitabine/tenofovir disoproxil fumarate, darunavir, ritonavir, and dolutegravir based on resistance testing that revealed reverse transcriptase mutations at the M184 and Y181 sites. This regimen resulted in complete suppression of HIV RNA within the first 12 weeks of therapy, accompanied by a significant rise of CD4+ T-cell count.

At presentation, the TSH level was normal at 1.34 mIU/l (0.27–4.20 mIU/l). Thyroid antibody levels were not available at that time.

Two years after initiation of ART (2016), the patient developed insomnia, palpitations, heat intolerance, unintentional 20 lbs weight loss, and bulging of the eyes. On exam, significant bilateral exophthalmos was noted, along with a prominent thyroid gland.

See Table 1 for laboratory data.

The thyroid iodine I-131 uptake scan showed diffuse increase in the uptake without evidence of hot or cold nodules.

The patient was diagnosed with GD with significant TED and started on antithyroid therapy with methimazole and a beta-blocker. The patient stopped the antithyroid medication after a few months and noticed further progression of eye symptoms. A CT scan of the orbits revealed minimal right-sided proptosis consistent with TED (Supplementary Materials available here). He was restarted on the methimazole and a short course of high-dose prednisone for TED. Thyroid function tests normalized, and eye symptoms eventually stabilized.

Table 1: Laboratory data.

	2014 (Pre-ART)	2016 (Post-ART)	2017	2018
TSH	1.34	<0.01	1.06	0.54
Free T4	N/A	2.38	0.99	N/A
TT3	N/A	526	139	128
TSI	N/A	>500%	N/A	N/A
CD4	32	396	343	344

TSH: 0.35–4.94 mIU/ml. Free T4:0.61–1.82 ng/dl. Total T3 (TT3): 48–178 ng/dl. Thyroid-stimulating immunoglobulins (TSI) < 122%. CD4+ T-cells, 430–1800 cells/μl; N/A, not available.

3. Discussion

HIV affects the immune system by specifically infecting the CD4+ T-cells, resulting in the development of a wide variety of opportunistic infections. Since the development and widespread use of highly active ART in the 1990s, there has been a significant reduction in the morbidity and mortality associated with the disease. However, a small subset of patients treated with ART, in particular those with very low nadir CD4+ T-cell counts, experience a paradoxical clinical deterioration associated with the recovery of the immune system. This has been described as an entity known as IRIS and is believed to affect about 10–40% of patients beginning ART [4]. This presentation is believed to be related to the recovery of immune function and restoration of the ability to mount an inflammatory response to both infectious and noninfectious agents. The exact mechanism is not completely understood. Resurgence of autoimmune conditions has most commonly been shown to occur in the later stages of AIDS [5].

GD as a consequence of IRIS after initiation of ART is well described [6]. It is thought to behave similarly to "conventional" GD and therefore should be treated in a similar manner. However, extrathyroidal manifestations of GD, such as TED, are not well characterized. TED is an inflammatory condition affecting the orbital tissue and occurs in about 25% of patients with GD [1]. It is characterized by lymphocytic infiltration of the extraocular muscles and orbital adipose tissue, orbital fibroblast proliferation and differentiation, deposition of hyaluronic acid and glycosaminoglycans, and de novo adipogenesis [7]. The pathogenesis of this condition is believed to be secondary to a complex interplay between genetic and lifestyle factors (e.g., cigarette smoking) leading to an inflammatory cascade, with involvement of autoantibodies such as TSH receptor (TSH-R) and insulin-like growth factor-1 (IGF-1) receptor [8].

TED has a spectrum of clinical manifestations and can range from mild disease to severe extraocular muscle dysfunction and vision loss due to exposure keratopathy or optic nerve compression [8]. ART treatment increases the CD4+ T-cell count in 2 phases: initial increase in the memory CD4+ T-cells that occurs in the first few months of therapy; and a slower and steady increase over many months to years, in the naive CD4+ T-cells, which originate from the thymus [9]. The CD4+ T-cells mature in the thymus, and cells which are capable of recognizing the major histocompatibility complex (MHC) molecules associated with foreign antigens enter the periphery, whereas those reacting with self-antigens undergo apoptosis [10]. However, initiation of ART causes intense regeneration of the thymus, resulting in an insufficient suppression of the autoreactive cells. This leads to the manifestation of a wide variety of autoimmune phenomenon including GD. Even though the functionality of the thymus is thought to decrease with age, recent reports have shown that it may remain active longer in HIV-infected individuals [11].

Another hypothesis for expansion of autoreactive T lymphocytes and their redistribution in IRIS is due to "molecular mimicry" due to homology between TSH-R and immunogenic HIV-related proteins [8]. Other predisposing factors associated with the development of IRIS include advanced immunodeficiency at baseline, more pronounced increase in CD4+ T lymphocytes, and genetic susceptibility [5].

In 2000, Jubault et al. [12] published a series of five patients, median age of 41 years, who developed GD after the initiation of ART. None of the patients had prior autoimmune conditions. In 2009, Vos et al. [13] described 3 similar cases and performed a literature review that revealed 13 reported cases of GD secondary to IRIS. Wong et al. [14] demonstrated a similar course in 13 HIV-infected patients of Chinese origin. In all of these studies, there was a direct relationship between the rise of the CD4+ T-cell count and corresponding suppression of the viral load, after beginning therapy with ART, and occurrence of GD. This was clearly demonstrated in our case as well. Chen et al. [15] published a cohort of 17 HIV-affected patients, predominantly African American, who developed autoimmune thyroid disease (AITD) as a late complication of IRIS, after treatment with ART.

Management of TED can be challenging in the presence of HIV infection. Patients with poorly controlled thyroid function have more severe manifestations of TED [16]. In addition, certain medications increase the possibility of thyroid dysfunction. In a large single-center cohort of HIV-infected patients, the prevalence of clinically apparent hyperthyroidism was 1.01%, most commonly associated with use of non-NRTI (NNRTI), particularly efavirenz [17]. On the other hand, there was a high prevalence of subclinical hypothyroidism, with the use of nucleoside reverse transcriptase inhibitor (NRTI), stavudine [18]. It is uncertain if these medications increase the severity of TED, but these associations should be kept in mind when choosing ART regimens. It is also important to consider interactions between ART and medications used in patients with TED. NNRTIs may induce cytochrome P450 (e.g., efavirenz), whereas ritonavir-boosted protease inhibitors (PI) inhibit cytochrome P450. Ritonavir and cobicistat (a pharmacologic booster) can significantly increase the concentration and effect of glucocorticoids, potentially leading to Cushing's syndrome [19]. It is important to closely monitor patients with HIV infection on high-risk medications for any manifestations of IRIS for prompt diagnosis and management.

4. Conclusion

Our case demonstrates the importance of being vigilant about the occurrence of various autoimmune conditions as manifestations of IRIS in patients receiving ART. These may occur even 1–3 years after initiation of therapy, as described in our case [10]. The management of GD and TED in the presence of HIV infection and ART appears to be equivalent to standard treatment with particular attention to potential drug interactions. Timely recognition and treatment may help to reduce the complications associated with these disorders.

Disclosure

This case report was presented in the 2018 Endocrine Society Meeting in Chicago.

References

[1] L. J. Haddow, P. J. Easterbrook, A. Mosam et al., "Defining immune reconstitution inflammatory syndrome: evaluation of expert opinion versus 2 case definitions in a South African cohort," *Clinical Infectious Diseases*, vol. 49, no. 9, pp. 1424–1432, 2009.

[2] K. Mayer, C. J. Hoffman, and T. T. Brown, "Thyroid function abnormalities in HIV infected patients," *Clinical Infectious Diseases*, vol. 45, no. 4, pp. 488–494, 2007.

[3] B. McIver and J. C. Morris, "The pathogenesis of Graves' disease," *Endocrinology and Metabolism Clinics of North America*, vol. 27, no. 1, pp. 73–89, 1998.

[4] M. A. French, P. Price, and S. F. Stone, "Immune restoration disease after antiretroviral therapy," *AIDS*, vol. 18, no. 12, pp. 1615–1627, 2004.

[5] L. E. Vega, "Espinoza LR HIV infection and its effects on the development of autoimmune disorders," *Pharmacological Research*, vol. 129, pp. 1–9, 2018.

[6] A. Weetman, "Immune reconstitution syndrome and the thyroid," *Best Practice & Research Clinical Endocrinology & Metabolism*, vol. 23, no. 6, pp. 693–702, 2009.

[7] R. Bahn, "Graves' ophthalmopathy," *New England Journal of Medicine*, vol. 362, no. 8, pp. 726–738, 2010.

[8] M. R. Edmunds, F. Mellington, R. L. Ford, B. Torlinska, K. Manavi, and K. Boelaert, "Clinical challenges of thyroid eye disease in HIV-positive patients on highly active antiretroviral therapy," *The Journal of Clinical Endocrinology & Metabolism*, vol. 100, no. 3, pp. 779–787, 2015.

[9] A. A. Parsa and A. Bhangoo, "HIV and thyroid dysfunction," *Reviews in Endocrine and Metabolic Disorders*, vol. 14, no. 2, pp. 127–131, 2013.

[10] B. Knysz, M. Bolanowski, M. Klimczak, K. Gladysz, and K. Zwolinska, "Graves' disease as an immune reconstitution syndrome in an HIV-1-positive patient commencing effective antiretroviral therapy: case report and literature review," *Viral Immunology*, vol. 19, no. 1, pp. 102–107, 2006.

[11] J. M. McCune, R. Loftus, D. K. Schmidt et al., "High prevalence of thymic tissue in adults with human immunodeficiency virus-1 infection," *Journal of Clinical Investigation*, vol. 101, no. 11, pp. 2301–2308, 1998.

[12] V. Jubault, A. Penfornis, F. Schillo et al., "Sequential occurrence of thyroid autoantibodies and Graves' disease after immune restoration in severely immunocompromised human immunodeficiency virus-1-infected patients," *Journal of Clinical Endocrinology & Metabolism*, vol. 85, no. 11, pp. 4254–4257, 2000.

[13] F. Vos, G. Pieters, M. Keuter, and A. van der Ven, "Graves' disease during immune reconstitution in HIV-infected patients treated with HAART," *Scandinavian Journal of Infectious Diseases*, vol. 38, no. 2, pp. 124–126, 2006.

[14] K. H. Wong, S. S. Chow, W. Lee, and S. S. Lee, "Clinical hyperthyroidism in Chinese patients with stable HIV disease," *Clinical Infectious Diseases*, vol. 39, no. 8, pp. 1257–1259, 2004.

[15] F. Chen, S. L. Day, R. A. Metcalfe et al., "Characteristics of autoimmune thyroid disease occurring as a late complication of immune reconstitution in patients with advanced human immunodeficiency virus (HIV) disease," *Medicine*, vol. 84, no. 2, pp. 98–106, 2005.

[16] M. F. Prummel, W. M. Wiersinga, M. P. Mourits, L. Koornneef, A. Berghout, and R. Van der Gaag, "Effect of abnormal thyroid function on the severity of Graves' ophthalmopathy," *Archives of Internal Medicine*, vol. 150, no. 5, pp. 1098–1101, 1990.

[17] S. Rasul, R. Delapenaha, F. Farhat, J. Gajjala, and S. M. Zahra, "Graves' disease as a manifestation of immune reconstitution in HIV-infected individuals after initiation of highly active antiretroviral therapy," *AIDS Research and Treatment*, vol. 2011, Article ID 743597, 4 pages, 2011.

[18] G. Madeddu, A. Spanu, F. Chessa et al., "Thyroid function in human immunodeficiency virus patients treated with highly active antiretroviral therapy (HAART): a longitudinal study," *Clinical Endocrinology*, vol. 64, no. 4, pp. 375–383, 2006.

[19] M. Foisy, E. Yakiwchuk, I. Chiu, and A. Singh, "Adrenal suppression and Cushing's syndrome secondary to an interaction between ritonavir and fluticasone: a review of the literature," *HIV Medicine*, vol. 9, no. 6, pp. 389–396, 2008.

3

Experimental Therapeutics for Challenging Clinical Care of a Patient with an Extremely Rare Homozygous *APOC2* Mutation

Masako Ueda,[1] Anna Wolska,[2] Frances M. Burke,[3] Maria Escobar,[1] Laura Walters,[1] Dusanka Lalic,[1] Robert A. Hegele,[4] Alan T. Remaley,[2] Daniel J. Rader,[1,3,5] and Richard L. Dunbar[1,6,7]

[1]*Department of Medicine, University of Pennsylvania, Philadelphia, PA, USA*
[2]*Lipoprotein Metabolism Laboratory, NHLBI, National Institutes of Health, Bethesda, MD, USA*
[3]*Division of Cardiovascular Medicine, Department of Medicine, University of Pennsylvania Health System, Philadelphia, PA, USA*
[4]*Department of Medicine, and Robarts Research Institute, Schulich School of Medicine and Dentistry, Western University, London, Ontario, Canada*
[5]*Translational Medicine and Human Genetics, Department of Medicine, University of Pennsylvania, Philadelphia, PA, USA*
[6]*Department of Medicine, Corporal Michael J. Crescenz VA Medical Center, Philadelphia, PA, USA*
[7]*Amarin Pharmaceuticals, Bedminster, NJ, USA*

Correspondence should be addressed to Masako Ueda; uedam19@gmail.com

Academic Editor: Eli Hershkovitz

Background. Among many causes of hypertriglyceridemia (HTG), familial chylomicronemia syndrome (FCS) is a rare monogenic disorder that manifests as severe HTG and acute pancreatitis. Among the known causal genes for FCS, mutations in *APOC2* only account for <2% of cases. Medical nutrition therapy is critical for FCS because usual triglyceride- (TG-) lowering medications are ineffective. Therapeutic plasma exchange (TPE) with fresh frozen plasma (FFP) is an option to urgently reduce TG and pancreatitis episodes. Several novel biologics are under development to treat HTG and may provide therapeutic options for FCS in the future. *Objective.* We present the challenging care of a 43-year-old man with FCS with apoC-II deficiency and the results of two types of TPE and of investigational TG-lowering biologic therapies. *Results.* The patient's lipid profile was consistent with FCS. A novel homozygous variant was identified in *APOC2*, and its pathogenicity was confirmed. Even on a fat-restricted diet, his care was tremendously complicated with unremitting bouts of pancreatitis. TPE with FFP replacement lowered TG >90% post-sessions and appeared to reduce pancreatitis episodes. Experimental ANGPTL3 and *APOC3* inhibitors each lowered TG by >50%. *Conclusions.* Our case demonstrates the importance of delineating and defining the underlying etiology of a rare disorder to optimize therapy and to minimize unfavorable outcomes.

1. Introduction

Hypertriglyceridemia (HTG) has numerous etiologies. It is often polygenic and multifactorial [1]. However, familial chylomicronemia syndrome (FCS) or type I hyperlipoproteinemia with severe HTG (OMIM: 238600) is a rare and often underdiagnosed monogenic disorder, with an estimated prevalence of 1/1,000,000. There are five known causal genes for FCS: lipoprotein lipase (*LPL*), apolipoprotein (apo) C-II (*APOC2*), apoA-V (*APOA5*), lipase maturation factor 1 (*LMF1*), and glycosylphosphatidylinositol-anchored high-density lipoprotein-binding protein 1 (*GPIHBP1*). Each gene product supports proper LPL synthesis or its function, namely, TG hydrolysis [2].

Abdominal pain of varying intensity due to acute pancreatitis is often the first manifestation of FCS, typically presenting in childhood or adolescence. Unfortunately, it is often disregarded as a childhood illness or can prompt an unnecessary exploratory procedure. Therefore, arriving at the correct diagnosis is often delayed. Pancreatitis is the most serious, potentially fatal, consequence of FCS. Other reversible clinical features include dermatological eruptive xanthomas, ophthalmological lipemia retinalis, and hepatosplenomegaly; however, not all features are present in every patient.

Fasting chylomicronemic plasma appears milky and viscous with TG > 1,000 mg/dL (11.3 mmol/L). Three pretreatment lipid findings may help distinguish FCS (Table 1) from polygenic or multifactorial chylomicronemia (type V hyperlipoproteinemia) [3]: (1) TG/total cholesterol (TC) ratio >5 (mg/dL)/(mg/dL) or >2.2 (mmol/L)/(mmol/L), (2) TG/apoB ratio >8.8 (mg/dL)/(mg/dL) or ≥10 (mmol/L)/(g/L), and (3) low apoB <75 mg/dL (0.75 g/L). ApoB is typically high in polygenic chylomicronemia [4].

Historically, the diagnosis of FCS relied on LPL functional analysis, but this is not standardized and is only offered at a few specialized centers [2]. Despite recent development of the FCS scoring system using clinical information to delineate FCS [5], definitive diagnosis by clinical criteria alone is still challenging due to overlapping features among chylomicronemias [1, 6, 7]. Nevertheless, characteristic clinical features and FCS scoring may be valuable in screening for FCS. Ultimately, in order to definitively diagnose FCS, molecular testing targeting FCS-associated genes is necessary and may be practical as genetic sequencing becomes more accessible due to declining cost and expanding availability [8, 9].

The most effective treatment for FCS is medical nutrition therapy with a fat-restricted diet with <15% of total calories as fats. FDA-approved TG-lowering medications are only marginally effective for FCS because they predominantly affect very-low-density lipoprotein (VLDL) metabolism more than the chylomicron metabolism and require "functional" LPL. Unresponsiveness to TG-lowering drugs could be an important clue to the diagnosis of FCS. Regardless, maintaining a long-term fat-restriction is very difficult.

Besides dietary management, therapeutic plasma exchange (TPE) with fresh frozen plasma (FFP) is sometimes used urgently to alleviate severe HTG and may curtail recurrent pancreatitis although it is cubersome chronically [10]. Several novel biologics suppressing the function of physiologic LPL inhibitors, such as angiopoietin-like 3 (ANGPTL3) and apoC-III, are under clinical development to treat HTG and may become treatment options for FCS in the future.

2. Objective

We present the challenging care of a 43-year-old man with FCS with a novel homozygous *APOC2* mutation and the effects of two types of TPE and of investigational TG-lowering biologics.

3. Method

The patient participated in an IRB-approved study investigating rare lipid disorders at the University of Pennsylvania and provided his consent for medical record review.

4. Case Presentation

A 43-year-old-man, originally from Sudan, presented to the Lipid Clinic, after being diagnosed with HTG during his first episode of pancreatitis at age 30. He had no physical stigmata of FCS. His fasting plasma appeared milky and turbid. His highest reported TG level was 7,112 mg/dL (80.3 mmol/L), TC 455 mg/dL (11.8 mmol/L), and high-density lipoprotein cholesterol (HDL-C) 12 mg/dL (0.31 mmol/L). His TG/TC ratio of 15.6 (mg/dL)/(mg/dL) (6.81 (mmol/L)/(mmol/L)) and profoundly low apoB of 13 mg/dL (<75 mg/dL) or 0.13 g/L, as well as TG/apoB ratio of 547 (mg/dL)/(mg/dL), 617 (mmol/L)/(g/L), were consistent with FCS. In addition, his FCS score of 10 provided further evidence that he was likely to have FCS [7].

Around the same time, he was also diagnosed with diabetes mellitus (DM), independent of pancreatitis. His family history was very suspicious for FCS with consanguinity on both sides of the family. Notably, his sister and one brother, as well as two maternal uncles had HTG with or without pancreatitis (Figure 1).

We identified a novel homozygous *APOC2* variant, c.215 G > C, p.R72 T [8], and proved its pathogenicity by demonstrating restored lipolytic activity after adding an apoC-II mimetic peptide (C-II-a) to the patient's plasma, reported elsewhere [11]. The variant, located in an amphipathic helical region of the protein, is predicted to disrupt its lipid-binding ability [12]. Therefore, we have definitively diagnosed the patient with FCS due to very rare apoC-II deficiency as an adult.

4.1. Management Challenges. His clinical course has been tumultuous with recurrent bouts of pancreatitis, ultimately developing chronic pancreatitis. Moreover, he suffered what appeared to be a transient ischemic attack (TIA) during a clinic visit. He became confused and could not stay standing. Fortunately, with fluid resuscitation, he recovered without residual sequelae. Hyperviscosity and its associated neurological deficits due to extremely high TG levels have been reported [13]. We suspected that plasma hyperviscosity resulting from dehydration after a prolonged travel excursion with the underlying FCS itself was likely to have contributed to this event.

Most of all, his dietary management proved problematic. In addition to a fat-restricted diet, limiting carbohydrate intake was required for his DM. Consequently, protein intake had to be maximized to fulfill his caloric needs. The patient often became confused about his dietary regimen, receiving conflicting advice from various healthcare providers who were unfamiliar with FCS. This did not improve until our nutritionist conferred with his other nutritionist to unify his management plan.

4.2. Chronological Report of Experimental Therapeutics. In early 2015, he participated in an IRB-approved TG-lowering study, testing the effectiveness of an experimental ANGPTL3 inhibitor. After a single dose, his TG fell ~50% from 3,437 mg/dL within 10 days (Figure 2(a)). The average reduction was ~40% during the first 80 days, and TG remained below baseline for 90 days post-dose.

Table 1: Typical characteristics of familial chylomicronemia syndrome.

General features of FCS	
Electrophoretic characteristic	Type I hyperlipoproteinemia
Genetics	Monogenic (biallelic, autosomal recessive)
Prevalence	1 in 100,000 to 1,000,000
Disease onset	Childhood/ adolescent > adulthood
Clinical manifestations	Abdominal pain Eruptive xanthoma Lipemia retinalis Pancreatitis Hepatosplenomegaly Lactescent plasma
Response to TG-lowering medications	None to marginal
Association with CVD	None to minimal risk
Lipoprotein features of FCS	
Major lipoproteins	Chylomicrons
Lipoprotein characteristics[1,2]	TG: >1,000 mg/dL; >11.3 mmol/L
	TG/TC ratio: >5 (mg/dL)/(mg/dL); >2 (mmol/L)/(mmol/L)
	TG/ApoB ratio: ≥8.8 (mg/dL)/(mg/dL); ≥10 (mmol/L)/(g/L)
	ApoB: <75 mg/dL; <0.75 g/L

FCS: familial chylomicronemia syndrome, CVD: cardiovascular disease, TG: triglyceride, TC: total cholesterol, and ApoB: apolipoprotein B.

Unfortunately, his unstable medical status with recurrent bouts of pancreatitis precluded him from participating in another therapy at that time. He had 7 hospital admissions during one year, of which 6 occurred within a 6-month period. Five hospitalizations were for acute pancreatitis, and two were for related complications: anorexia, anemia, and surgical intervention to relieve an intestinal obstruction caused by chronic pancreatitis. By this time, the majority of pancreas was replaced by multiloculated, fluid-filled cysts, compromising both exocrine and endocrine function and worsening his DM.

During the latter half of 2016, we prescribed TPE sessions to curtail pancreatitis episodes. Reportedly, his sister and brother often relied successfully on TPE to limit their recurrent pancreatitis. Initially, we prescribed TPE of 1 plasma volume (PV) exchange with FFP every few weeks. However, the patient received albumin replacements for the first three sessions as per their facility protocol. On albumin TPE, TG fell 70–85% to <1,000 mg/dL but rebounded to >2,000 mg/dL within 2 weeks of each session (Figure 2(b)). On FFP replacement, as originally planned, TG initially fell >95% to <150 mg/dL and even to <75 mg/dL post-sessions 2 and 3. Moreover, TG-rebound was gradual, maintaining <1,000 mg/dL between sessions and even one month after discharge from the hospital.

In late 2016, the patient elected to discontinue TPE in order to participate in another IRB-approved study of an experimental *APOC3* inhibitor. He received two doses of the biologic a week apart in 2017. About a week after the second dose, his TG fell by >60% and remained <1,000 mg/dL for 40 days post-dose 1. TGs did not rebound back to >2,000 mg/dL until 50 days post-dose (Figure 2(c)). Overall, these experiences with novel biologics were quite promising.

5. Discussion

Severe HTG is vastly heterogeneous, and identifying the underlying cause can reveal the most optimal therapy [14]. Once FCS is diagnosed, a low-fat diet should be prescribed as first-line treatment, and TG-lowering medications can be prescribed as adjuncts.

Compared to usual patients with FCS, our patient's management was tremendously challenging because of his concurrent DM. Moreover, other healthcare providers were not well-versed on the management principles of apoC-II deficiency. Unfortunately, reliance on their experience in treating typical HTG patients became a barrier for our patient's care, and we suspect that this practice has exacerbated our patient's clinical course.

Successful use of TPE for extreme HTG has been reported previously [10]. In one study, patients with medication-refractory HTG at risk for pancreatitis underwent TPE with albumin replacement. The average TG level of 1,929 mg/dL pre-TPE was reduced to 762 mg/dL post-TPE, ~60% reduction ($p \leq 0.0001$). Importantly, TPE was effective in preventing recurrent pancreatitis. We predicted that TPE with FFP replacement, which contains exogenous apoC-II, would outperform albumin replacement in our patient with apoC-II deficiency by supplying the very protein our patient lacked, and the results concurred with this expectation. Our results indicate that TPE with FFP can be used as a last resort when apoC-II deficiency has been diagnosed.

Frustratingly, recently developed TG-lowering medications are still not suitable for FCS. Novel omega-3s, which promise to improve dyslipidemia and even to improve cardiovascular outcomes [15, 16], newer formulations of fibrates [17], and niacin [18] are all not expected to have an appreciable TG-lowering effect in FCS. Off-label use of a novel microsomal triglyceride transfer protein inhibitor may lower TGs, but an unfavorable safety and drug interaction profile would preclude its long-term use [19]. Considering this bleak outlook, our patient's responses to both ANGPTL3 and *APOC3* biologic inhibitors were especially encouraging. In theory, enhancing residual LPL function is the main mechanism of TG-lowering, achieved by the suppression of ANGPTL3 protein or *APOC3* translation, thereby alleviating LPL inhibition. However, it was intriguing that inhibiting ANGPTL3 also had a positive effect in our patient who had no detectably functional apoC-II, the key cofactor for LPL function [11]. Therefore, the full scope of the effects of ANGPTL3 inhibition may still be unknown. We hope that such biologics would become available in the near future for treatment of FCS.

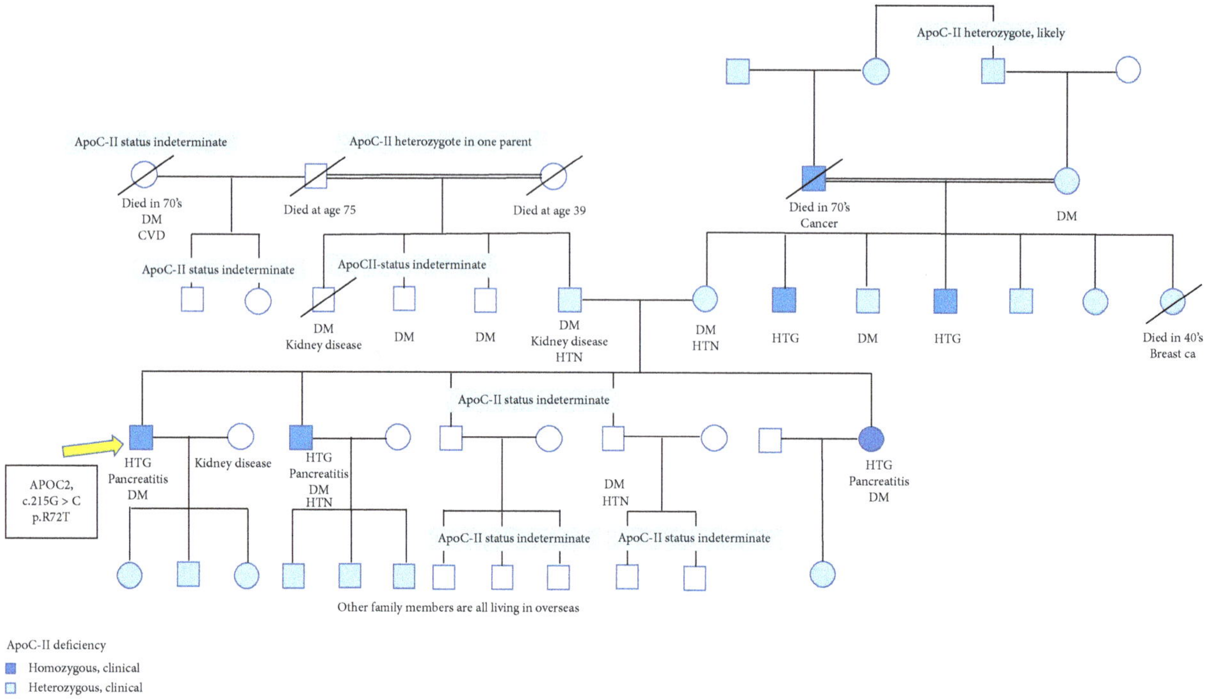

Figure 1: Patient's family pedigree. The patient is originally from Sudan, and many family members live overseas. Consanguinity is present on both sides. The patient's paternal and maternal grandparents are distantly related. The patient's sister and one brother have similar medical history with HTG and pancreatitis, as well as DM. His maternal uncles have HTG, and his maternal grandfather was known to have had HTG.

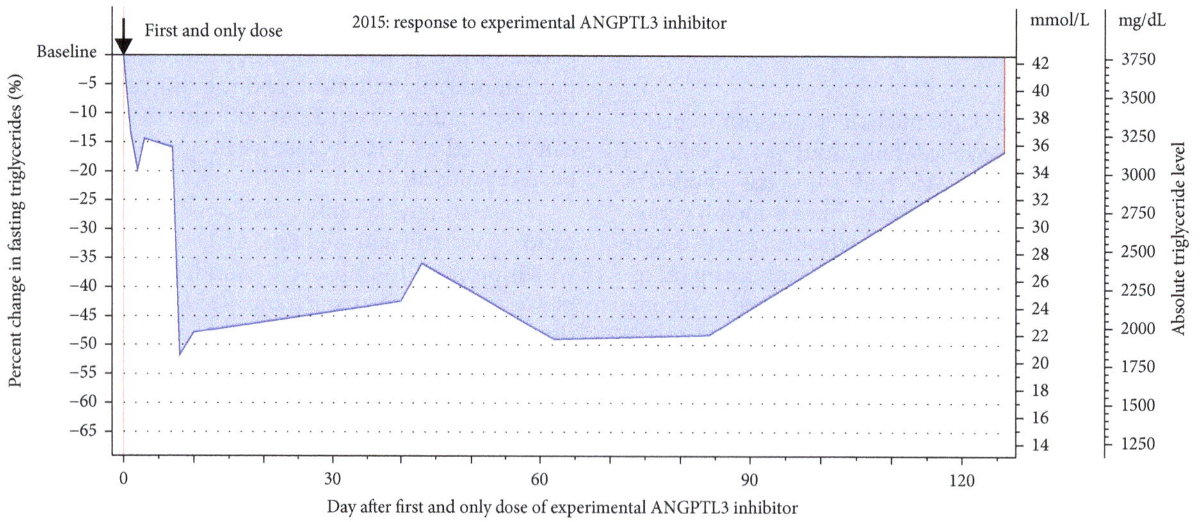

(a)

Figure 2: Continued.

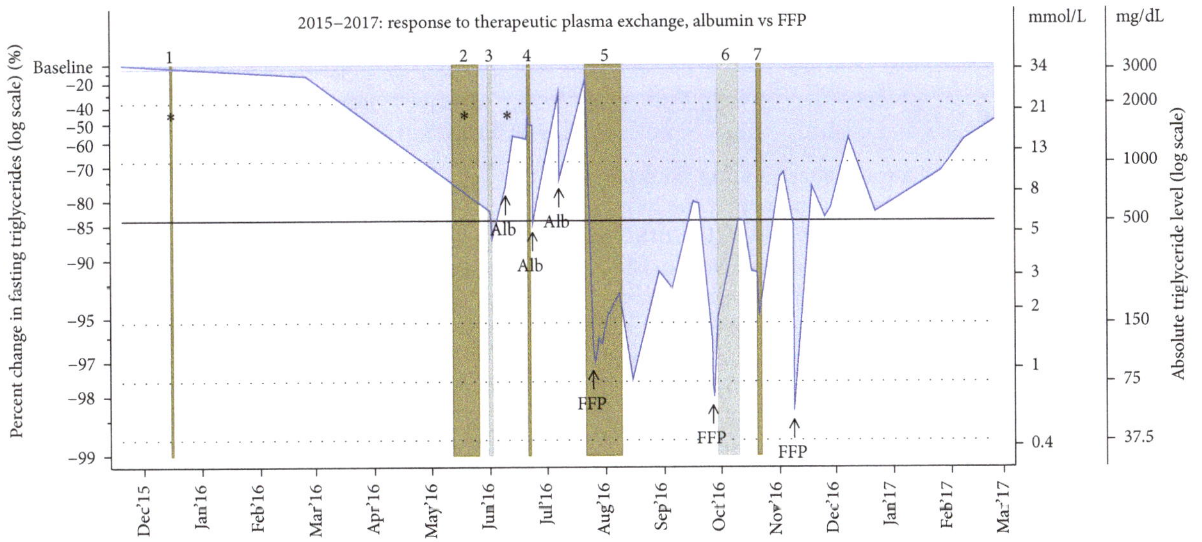

(b)

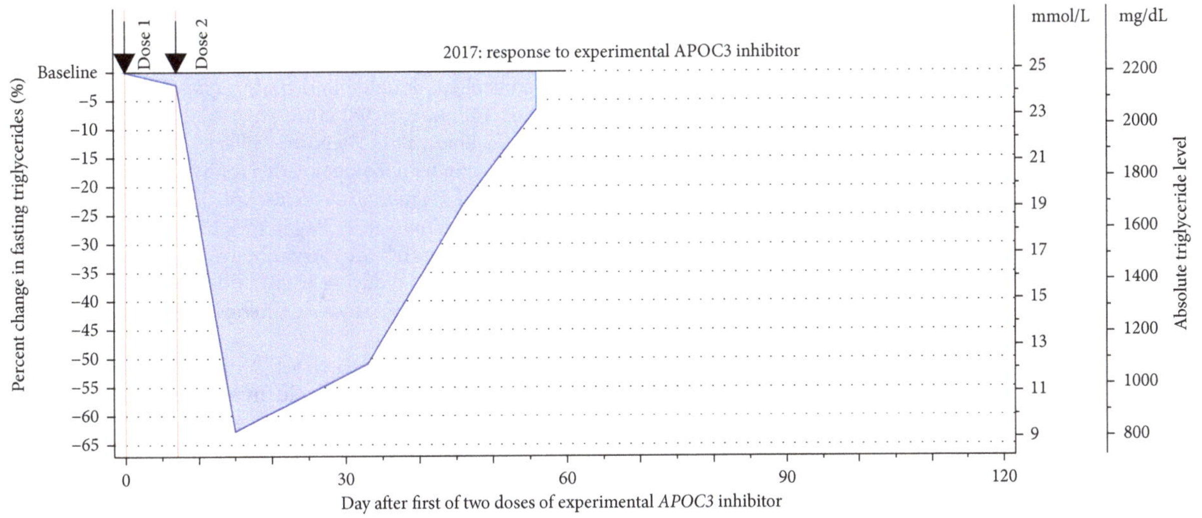

(c)

FIGURE 2: Fasting TG response to chronological therapeutic attempts. (a) The line represents our patient's TG response to a single dose of an experimental ANGPTL3 inhibitor. Within 10 days post-dose, TG fell >50%, remaining −50% to −35% below baseline for about 90 days afterwards. Overall, this effect lasted for about 120 days. (b) The line represents the patient's fasting TG in response to therapeutic plasma exchange (TPE) using two types of replacement infusions: albumin and fresh frozen plasma (FFP). The asterisks (∗) indicate times when TG data are unavailable. The vertical bars indicate 7 hospital admissions: admissions 1, 2, 4, 5, and 7 (brown) for pancreatitis, admission 3 (gray) for anorexia, weakness, and anemia, admission 6 (gray) for the management of duodenal obstruction for pancreatic cysts, receiving total parental nutrition before converting to jejunostomy feeding followed by slowly resuming oral intake after discharge. 5% albumin replacement only briefly lowered TG to about 500 to 1000 mg/dL after exchanging 1.0 plasma volume (PV). After switching, three sessions with FFP replacement were more effective in TG-lowering, with a sharp drop of TG to <150 mg/dL immediately post-infusion 1 and to <75 mg/dL post-infusions 2 and 3. His TG remained <1000 mg/dL for about a month even after the discharge from the hospital. (c) The line presents our patient's TG response to two doses of an experimental APOC3 inhibitor that were given a week apart. His baseline TG of 2,200 mg/dL fell >60% within about 15 days of the first dose. TG remained <1,000 mg/dL (<50%) until past 30 days, and <2,000 mg/dL for 55 days post-dose 1.

Lastly, apoC-II mimetic peptides effectively lowered TG in preclinical animal models of apoC-II deficiency [20]. In fact, adding one of these peptides normalized LPL activity in an *ex vivo* assay of our patient [11]. Ultimately, an apoC-II mimetic may become the most specific therapeutic option for apoC-II deficiency.

6. Conclusion

Our patient's case clearly illustrates the importance of carefully delineating the cause of a rare condition to manage appropriately and to minimize unfavorable outcomes. More importantly, all healthcare providers should be especially vigilant when caring for a patient with an unfamiliar disorder.

Conflicts of Interest

Masako Ueda, Maria Escobar, Laura Walters, and Dusanka Lalic have nothing to disclose. Anna Wolska reports she has a patent for apoC-II mimetic peptides (PCT/US2018/014532, 107102123) with royalties paid. Frances M. Burke reports personal fees from Akcea Therapeutics, outside the submitted work. Robert A. Hegele reports personal fees from Acasti, Akcea/Ionis, Amgen, HLS Therapeutics, and Sanofi during the conduct of the study. Alan T. Remaley reports he has a patent for apoC-II mimetic peptides (PCT/US2018/014532, 107102123) with royalties paid and a patent for 18A-CII mimetic peptide (#8,936,787) issued. Daniel J. Rader reports personal fees from Alnylam, Novartis, Pfizer, Ionis, and Akcea and grants from Regeneron, outside the submitted work. Richard L. Dunbar reports grants from Regeneron, grants and personal fees from Akcea, grants from Arizona Pharmaceuticals, grants from UniQure, grants from Astra-Zeneca, grants and others from Amarin, and others from ICON Clinical Services, outside the submitted work.

References

[1] R. A. Hegele, H. N. Ginsberg, M. J. Chapman et al., "The polygenic nature of hypertriglyceridaemia: implications for definition, diagnosis, and management," *The Lancet Diabetes & Endocrinology*, vol. 2, no. 8, pp. 655–666, 2014.

[2] A. J. Brahm and R. A. Hegele, "Chylomicronaemia-current diagnosis and future therapies," *Nature Reviews Endocrinology*, vol. 11, no. 6, pp. 352–362, 2015.

[3] T. Gotoda, K. Shirai, T. Ohta et al., "Diagnosis and management of type I and type V hyperlipoproteinemia," *Journal of Atherosclerosis and Thrombosis*, vol. 19, no. 1, pp. 1–12, 2012.

[4] J. de Graaf, P. Couture, and A. Sniderman, "A diagnostic algorithm for the atherogenic apolipoprotein B dyslipoproteinemias," *Nature Clinical Practice Endocrinology & Metabolism*, vol. 4, no. 11, pp. 608–618, 2008.

[5] P. Moulin, R. Dufour, M. Averna et al., "Identification and diagnosis of patients with familial chylomicronaemia syndrome (FCS): expert panel recommendations and proposal of an FCS score," *Atherosclerosis*, vol. 275, pp. 265–272, 2018.

[6] J. S. Dron, J. Wang, H. Cao et al., "Severe hypertriglyceridemia is primarily polygenic," *Journal of Clinical Lipidology*, vol. 13, no. 1, pp. 80–88, 2019.

[7] P. Moulin, R. Dufour, M. Averna et al., "Characterisation of patients with familial chylomicronaemia syndrome (FCS) and multifactorial chylomicronaemia syndrome (MCS): establishment of an FCS clinical diagnostic score," *Data in Brief*, vol. 21, pp. 1334–1336, 2018.

[8] C. T. Johansen, J. B. Dubé, M. N. Loyzer et al., "LipidSeq: a next-generation clinical resequencing panel for monogenic dyslipidemias," *Journal of Lipid Research*, vol. 55, no. 4, pp. 765–772, 2014.

[9] R. A. Hegele, A. J. Berberich, M. R. Ban et al., "Clinical and biochemical features of different molecular etiologies of familial chylomicronemia," *Journal of Clinical Lipidology*, vol. 12, no. 4, pp. 920–927, 2018.

[10] C. Stefanutti, S. Di Giacomo, A. Vivenzio et al., "Therapeutic plasma exchange in patients with severe hypertriglyceridemia: a multicenter study," *Artificial Organs*, vol. 33, no. 12, pp. 1096–1102, 2009.

[11] M. Ueda, R. L. Dunbar, A. Wolska et al., "A novel APOC2 missense mutation causing apolipoprotein C-II deficiency with severe triglyceridemia and pancreatitis," *The Journal of Clinical Endocrinology & Metabolism*, vol. 102, no. 5, pp. 1454–1457, 2017.

[12] A. Wolska, R. L. Dunbar, L. A. Freeman et al., "Apolipoprotein C-II: new findings related to genetics, biochemistry, and role in triglyceride metabolism," *Atherosclerosis*, vol. 267, pp. 49–60, 2017.

[13] R. Inokuchi, A. Matsumoto, R. Azihara et al., "Hypertriglyceridemia as a possible cause of coma: a case report," *Journal of Medical Case Reports*, vol. 6, no. 1, p. 412, 2012.

[14] R. L. Dunbar and D. J. Rader, "Demystifying triglycerides: a practical approach for the clinician," *Cleveland Clinic Journal of Medicine*, vol. 72, no. 8, pp. 661–666, 2005.

[15] R. L. Dunbar, S. J. Nicholls, K. C. Maki et al., "Effects of omega-3 carboxylic acids on lipoprotein particles and other cardiovascular risk markers in high-risk statin-treated patients with residual hypertriglyceridemia: a randomized, controlled, double-blind trial," *Lipids in Health and Disease*, vol. 14, no. 1, p. 98, 2015.

[16] D. L. Bhatt, P. G. Steg, M. Miller et al., "Cardiovascular risk reduction with icosapent ethyl for hypertriglyceridemia," *New England Journal of Medicine*, vol. 380, no. 1, pp. 11–22, 2019.

[17] A. D. Pradhan, N. P. Paynter, B. M. Everett et al., "Rationale and design of the pemafibrate to reduce cardiovascular outcomes by reducing triglycerides in patients with diabetes (PROMINENT) study," *American Heart Journal*, vol. 206, pp. 80–93, 2018.

[18] R. L. Dunbar and H. Goel, "Niacin alternatives for dyslipidemia: fool's gold or gold mine? Part I: alternative niacin regimens," *Current Atherosclerosis Reports*, vol. 18, no. 2, p. 11, 2016.

[19] S. Tuteja, D. Duffy, R. L. Dunbar et al., "Pharmacokinetic interactions of the microsomal triglyceride transfer protein inhibitor, lomitapide, with drugs commonly used in the management of hypercholesterolemia," *Pharmacotherapy: The Journal of Human Pharmacology and Drug Therapy*, vol. 34, no. 3, pp. 227–239, 2014.

[20] M. J. A. Amar, T. Sakurai, A. Sakurai-Ikuta et al., "A novel apolipoprotein C-II mimetic peptide that activates lipoprotein lipase and decreases serum triglycerides in apolipoprotein E-knockout mice," *Journal of Pharmacology and Experimental Therapeutics*, vol. 352, no. 2, pp. 227–235, 2015.

4

Functional Localization of Adult-Onset Idiopathic Nesidioblastosis

Jess C. Hercus,[1] **Pouneh Pasha,**[2] **Sadiq Al Lawati,**[3] **Peter Kim,**[4] **Andre Mattman**,[5] **Douglas Webber,**[5] **and David M. Thompson**[3]

[1]*Department of Biological Sciences, Simon Fraser University, Burnaby, British Columbia, Canada*
[2]*Division of Internal Medicine, Department of Medicine, University of British Columbia, 5913 1081 Burrard St., Vancouver, British Columbia V6Z 1Y6, Canada*
[3]*Division of Endocrinology, Department of Medicine, University of British Columbia, 2775 Laurel Street, 4th Floor, Vancouver, British Columbia V5Z 1M9, Canada*
[4]*Division of General Surgery, Department of Medicine, University of British Columbia, 2775 Laurel Street, 11th Floor, Vancouver, British Columbia V5Z 1M9, Canada*
[5]*Division of Pathology and Laboratory Medicine, Department of Medicine, University of British Columbia, G227-2211 Wesbrook Mall, Vancouver, British Columbia V6T 2B5, Canada*

Correspondence should be addressed to Jess C. Hercus; hercus@sfu.ca

Academic Editor: Toshihiro Kita

Nesidioblastosis is a rare pancreatic disorder involving enlarged beta cells throughout the pancreas, causing elevated insulin production. We present the case of a 53-year-old woman with the initial symptom of fasting hypoglycemia. No pancreatic lesions were indicated on computed tomography and magnetic resonance imaging scans, and an octreotide scan was negative for insulinoma. Selective arterial calcium stimulation (SACST) showed increased insulin production from the stimulation of 3 out of 5 arteries. The SACST results suggested a diagnosis of nesidioblastosis, which was confirmed by histopathology after a subtotal distal pancreatectomy. The patient has normal glucose tolerance after surgery with no further problems of hypoglycemia, indicating that this is a rare case of nesidioblastosis extending only partially through the pancreas.

1. Background

Nesidioblastosis is an extremely rare disorder; first described in infants in 1938 by Laidlaw [1], it was not found in adults until 1975 [2]. We present the first reported case of diffuse nesidioblastosis confined to the distal half of the pancreas. This case represents an intermediate form of nesidioblastosis, between highly localized focal nesidioblastosis and typical diffuse nesidioblastosis throughout the entire pancreas [3]. This distinction is clinically important as it will guide therapeutic decisions and likely prognosis for individual patients.

1.1. Case. A 53-year-old woman was referred to our clinic in 2017 with symptoms suggestive of hypoglycemia. An oral glucose tolerance test was normal. Fasting hypoglycemia was diagnosed after she underwent a 72-hour fast resulting in a low serum glucose of 3.1, with simultaneous inappropriately high insulin of 150 (NR < 95 pmol/L) and C-peptide at 1301 (NR: 325-1090). Imaging was then performed to try and determine the cause of her hypoglycemia. CT and MRI scans did not identify any pancreatic lesions or insulinomas, and an octreotide study did not show any areas of increased uptake. The patient's symptoms intensified, with nightly hypoglycemic symptoms that resulted in an inability to work. The patient's symptoms could not be controlled with medical management, so further investigations were undertaken in the hope of finding a lesion that could be surgically treated.

Selective arterial calcium stimulation (SACST) with hepatic venous sampling was performed, using the methods described by Thompson et al. [4]. There was a significant relative elevation in insulin levels following the stimulation of the superior mesenteric (SMA), gastroduodenal (GDA), and splenic arteries (SA), as shown in Table 1. No elevation was seen from the stimulation of the gastroepiploic (GEA) and hepatic arteries (HA). The maximal insulin concentration was seen in response to the stimulation of the SMA, at 235 pmol/L. The response from 3 arteries in SACST strongly suggested the presence of diffuse nesidioblastosis instead of a very small insulinoma [4], and the response from the SA suggested that the nesidioblastosis would be located around the tail of the pancreas [5]. However, the lack of response from 2 arteries suggested that the nesidioblastosis did not extend through the entire pancreas.

On the basis of the SACST results, a distal pancreatectomy was performed, removing the pancreatic tail region measuring 14.5 × 5.2 × 2.5 cm, and preserving the spleen and duodenum. The histopathology confirmed the presence of diffuse nesidioblastosis within the pancreatic tail, with increased numbers of islet cells (Figure 1), some of which had enlarged nuclei (Figure 2). Furthermore, when sectioned there was no evidence of discrete masses or lesions. This pathology was found to be uniformly distributed throughout all of the resected surgical specimens. While the remaining pancreas was not biopsied to prove the absence of pathological features of nesidioblastosis, we assume that there was no significant amount of remaining abnormality due to the elimination of hypoglycemia immediately postoperation.

The patient has done well postoperatively with no further hypoglycemia and normal fasting glucose tolerance for 34 months.

Table 1: Insulin concentrations (pmol/L) measured during SACST, at baseline levels, and then 20, 40, and 60 seconds after calcium gluconate injection.

	SMA	GDA	GEA	HA	SA
Baseline	28	28	24	29	24
20 sec.	26	83	27	40	30
40 sec.	235	85	33	33	73
60 sec.	156	71	31	32	58

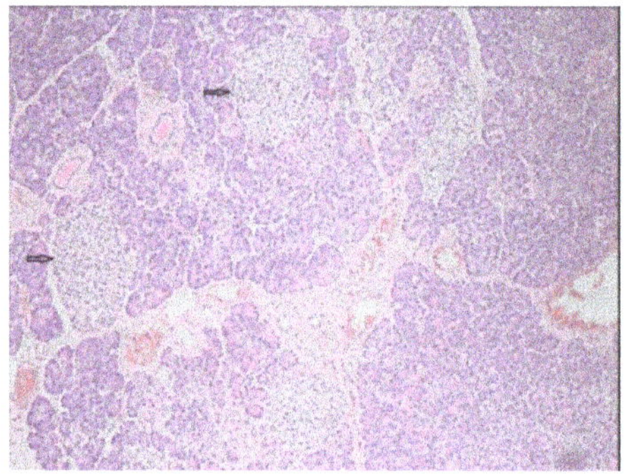

Figure 1: Pancreatic parenchyma at 100× magnification, with arrows indicating enlarged islets.

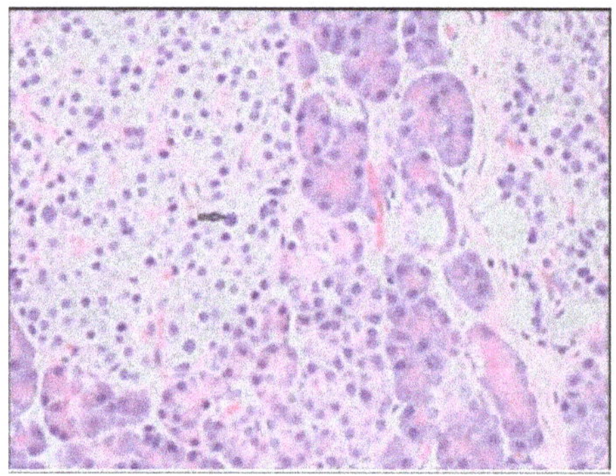

Figure 2: Islet cells at 200× magnification, with arrow indicating an enlarged nucleus.

2. Discussion

The differential diagnosis of endogenous hyperinsulinemic hypoglycemia in adults includes insulinoma and adult-onset nesidioblastosis. Insulinoma is significantly more common than nesidioblastosis, with approximately 1 to 3 cases per million [6]. Nesidioblastosis is estimated to account for 1% to 5% of cases of adult endogenous hyperinsulinemic hypoglycemia [7]. Clinically and biochemically, nesidioblastosis cannot be distinguished from insulinomas, and insulinomas smaller than 1 cm cannot be detected using imaging techniques [8], further complicating the differential diagnosis.

Selective arterial calcium stimulation can be used to aid in distinguishing between insulinoma and diffuse nesidioblastosis; if there is a significant relative elevation in insulin with the stimulation of 2 or more arteries, then nesidioblastosis is the probable diagnosis [4]. This is likely due to the diffuse nature of nesidioblastosis, whereas insulinomas are more localized and are more likely to respond only to stimulation of one artery. This also allows for some localization of nesidioblastosis, as in this case, where arterial stimulation aided in determining that the nesidioblastosis was primarily located in the pancreatic tail. However, there is some challenge due to individual variations in pancreatic arterial perfusion and anatomy that may produce problems when attempting to localize the abnormal cells [9].

Nesidioblastosis is characterized by the presence of many beta cells with enlarged nuclei and large amounts of clear cytoplasm, in most islets throughout the pancreas [10]. Typically, no abnormalities are seen in somatostatin, glucagon, and pancreatic polypeptide cells [7, 11]. Some patients have increased numbers of beta cells and islet hypertrophy, but this is not seen in all cases [12]. Peliosis-like vascular ectasia has been seen in some cases, often when other endocrinopathies are involved [13, 14]. Increased numbers of ductuloinsular complexes are seen occasionally, although most cases lack this feature [7]. Our case did show some beta cells with enlarged nuclei, and there were also an increased number of beta cells with islet hypertrophy.

Table 2: Selected previously reported cases of idiopathic nesidioblastosis with follow-up after surgery [7, 11, 19–27]. Distal pancreatectomy refers to the removal of the body and tail of the pancreas, typically no more than 60%. Subtotal pancreatectomy refers to removal of approximately 80% of the pancreas.

	Distal pancreatectomy	Subtotal pancreatectomy
Recurring hypoglycemia	12	3
No hypoglycemia	7	2

However, there was not an increase in ductuloinsular complexes, and no peliosis-like vascular ectasia was noted.

Diffuse nesidioblastosis is by far the most common form in adults [7]. Rare cases of adult focal nesidioblastosis have been reported [15–17], wherein exophytic lesions have been found on the pancreas containing cells characteristic of nesidioblastosis. Focal nesidioblastosis is much more common in neonates, making up roughly 40% of congenital nesidioblastosis cases [18].

In focal nesidioblastosis, abnormal beta cells are confined to exophytic lesions on the surface of the pancreas, whereas diffuse nesidioblastosis typically involves the entire pancreas [3].

We believe that our case represents a form of nesidioblastosis that is intermediate between focal and diffuse nesidioblastosis, as it was functionally localized to the tail region, but was clearly spread throughout the pancreas and was not exophytic. The localization is evidenced by our patient's lack of hypoglycemia after distal pancreatectomy, which is fairly rare when compared to other cases.

As shown in Table 2, most patients that undergo distal pancreatectomy for nesidioblastosis have further hypoglycemia, often requiring medication. This suggests that in their cases, the defective beta cells are spread throughout the entire pancreas. Even when subtotal pancreatectomy is considered, over half of patients still experience hypoglycemia. Furthermore, in cases where near-total or completion pancreatectomy was performed, nesidioblastosis was found throughout the entire pancreas [26].

We believe that we report the first case of adult nesidioblastosis that is diffuse in nature but limited to a specific region of the pancreas. It supports the value of using SACST in the diagnostic evaluation of patients with fasting hypoglycemia who do not have a mass visible on imaging. Knowledge of this condition will help plan the surgical approach and also provide physicians and patients a realistic expectation of the likelihood that partial pancreatic resection will reduce hypoglycemia to a meaningful degree.

References

[1] G. F. Laidlaw, "Nesidioblastoma, the islet tumor of the pancreas," *American Journal Of Pathology*, vol. 14, no. 2, pp. 125–134, 1938.

[2] R. Sandler, D. L. Horwitz, A. H. Rubenstein, and H. Kuzuya, "Hypoglycemia and endogenous hyperinsulinism complicating diabetes mellitus: application of the C-peptide assay to diagnosis and therapy," *The American Journal of Medicine*, vol. 59, no. 5, pp. 730–736, 1975.

[3] R. M. Witteles, F. H. Straus, S. L. Sugg, M. R. Koka, E. A. Costa, and E. L. Kaplan, "Adult-onset nesidioblastosis causing hypoglycemia," *Archives of Surgery*, vol. 136, no. 6, pp. 656–663, 2001.

[4] S. M. Thompson, A. Vella, G. B. Thompson et al., "Selective arterial calcium stimulation with hepatic venous sampling differentiates insulinoma from nesidioblastosis," *The Journal of Clinical Endocrinology & Metabolism*, vol. 100, no. 11, pp. 4189–4197, 2015.

[5] J. L. Doppman, R. Chang, D. L. Fraker et al., "Localization of insulinomas to regions of the pancreas by intra-arterial stimulation with calcium," *Annals of Internal Medicine*, vol. 123, no. 4, pp. 269–273, 1995.

[6] R. T. Jensen, G. Cadiot, M. L. Brandi et al., "ENETS consensus guidelines for the management of patients with digestive neuroendocrine neoplasms: functional pancreatic endocrine tumor syndromes," *Neuroendocrinology*, vol. 95, no. 2, pp. 98–119, 2012.

[7] M. Anlauf, D. Wieben, A. Perren et al., "Persistent hyperinsulinemic hypoglycemia in 15 adults with diffuse nesidioblastosis: diagnostic criteria, incidence, and characterization of beta-cell changes," *The American Journal of Surgical Pathology*, vol. 29, no. 4, pp. 524–533, 2005.

[8] M. Andreassen, E. Ilett, D. Wiese et al., "Surgical management, preoperative tumor localization, and histopathology of 80 patients operated on for insulinoma," *The Journal of Clinical Endocrinology & Metabolism*, vol. 104, no. 12, pp. 6129–6138, 2019.

[9] S. M. Thompson, A. Vella, F. J. Service, C. S. Grant, G. B. Thompson, and J. C. Andrews, "Impact of variant pancreatic arterial anatomy and overlap in regional perfusion on the interpretation of selective arterial calcium stimulation with hepatic venous sampling for preoperative localization of occult insulinoma," *Surgery*, vol. 158, no. 1, pp. 162–172, 2015.

[10] N. Albers, M. Lohr, U. Bogner, V. Loy, and G. Kloppel, "Nesidioblastosis of the pancreas in an adult with persistent hyperinsulinemic hypoglycemia," *American Journal of Clinical Pathology*, vol. 91, no. 3, pp. 336–340, 1989.

[11] A. Raffel, M. Krausch M, M. Anlauf et al., "Diffuse nesidioblastosis as a cause of hyperinsulinemic hypoglycemia in adults: a diagnostic and therapeutic challenge," *Surgery*, vol. 141, no. 2, pp. 179–184, 2007.

[12] G. Klöppel, M. Anlauf, A. Raffel, A. Perren, and W. T. Knoefel, "Adult diffuse nesidioblastosis: genetically or environmentally induced?" *Human Pathology*, vol. 39, no. 1, pp. 3–8, 2008.

[13] R. Chetty, M. Kennedy, S. Ezzat, and S. L. Asa, "Pancreatic endocrine pathology in von Hippel-Lindau disease: an expanding spectrum of lesions," *Endocrine Pathology*, vol. 15, no. 2, pp. 141–148, 2004.

[14] P. J. Pernicone and J. T. Lie, "Isolated peliosis of pancreatic islet cell adenoma," *Archives of Pathology & Laboratory Medicine*, vol. 111, no. 8, pp. 690-691, 1987.

[15] M. K. McElroy, A. M. Lowy, and N. Weidner, "Case report: focal nesidioblastosis ("nesidioblastoma") in an adult," *Human Pathology*, vol. 41, no. 3, pp. 447–451, 2010.

[16] S. T. Barbu, O. V. Fabian, I. Domsa et al., "Difficult diagnosis and localization of multi-focal nesidioblastosis in an adult: implications of near-infrared intraoperative imaging," *Pancreatology*, vol. 18, no. 4, pp. S83–S84, 2018.

[17] N. Shivathirthan, M. Joshi, and K. Patel, “Laparoscopic enucleation of focal nesidioblastosis of pancreas in an adult,” *International Hepato-Pancreato-Biliary Association*, vol. 21, no. S2, p. S515, 2019.

[18] C. Sempoux, Y. Guiot, F. Jaubert, and J. Rahier, “Focal and diffuse forms of congenital hyperinsulinism: the keys for differential diagnosis,” *Endocrine Pathology*, vol. 15, no. 3, pp. 241–246, 2004.

[19] V. Kalff, A. Iravani, T. Ackhurst et al., “Utility of 68 Ga-DOTA-Exendin-4 PET/CT imaging in distinguishing between insulinoma and nesidioblastosis in patients with confirmed endogenous hyperinsulinaemic hypoglycaemia,” *Internal Medicine Journal*, vol. 51, 2021.

[20] A. Dardano, G. Daniele, R. Lupi et al., “Nesidioblastosis and insulinoma: a rare coexistence and a therapeutic challenge,” *Frontiers in Endocrinology*, vol. 11, p. 10, 2020.

[21] M. Wong, L. Conway, C. Cooper, A. Sinha, and N. Nandi, “Nesidioblastosis in an adult with short gut syndrome and type 2 diabetes,” *AACE Clinical Case Reports*, vol. 5, no. 6, pp. e375–e379, 2019.

[22] E. Lozano-Melendez, M. Aguilar-Soto, L. E. Graniel-Palafox, L. E. Alfonso, Ceceña-Martínez, R. Valdez-Ortiz, and F. Solis-Jimenez, “Adult nesidioblastosis in chronic kidney disease,” *Case Reports in Endocrinology*, vol. 2019, Article ID 7640384, 6 pages, 2019.

[23] J. Martin-Grace, M. O’Tuathail, M. J. Hannon, N. Swan, D. O’Shea, and G. Tamagno, “Amlodipine for the medical treatment of adult-onset diffuse nesidioblastosis,” *Pancreas*, vol. 44, no. 7, pp. 1162–1164, 2015.

[24] C. Ferrario, D. Stoll, A. Boubaker, M. Matter, P. Yan, and J. J. Puder, “Diffuse nesidioblastosis with hypoglycemia mimicking an insulinoma: a case report,” *Journal of Medical Case Reports*, vol. 6, no. 1, p. 332, 2012.

[25] V. Schwetz, K. Horvath, P. Kump et al., “Successful medical treatment of adult nesidioblastosis with pasireotide over 3 years: a case report,” *Medicine*, vol. 95, no. 14, Article ID e3272, 2016.

[26] J. Ahn, S. E. Lee, E. S. Lee et al., “A case of nesidioblastosis causing hypoglycaemia after delivery,” *Diabetes Research and Clinical Practice*, vol. 83, no. 1, pp. e5–e7, 2009.

[27] R. D. Rinker, K. Friday, F. Aydin, B. M. Jaffe, and L. Lambiase, “Adult nesidioblastosis: a case report and review of the literature,” *Digestive Diseases and Sciences*, vol. 43, no. 8, pp. 1784–1790, 1998.

5

Abnormally Elevated Follicle-Stimulating Hormone (FSH) Level in an Infertile Woman

Aurore Catteau,[1] Kalyane Bach-Ngohou,[1,2] Justine Blin,[1,2] Paul Barrière,[2,3] Thomas Fréour,[2,3] and Damien Masson [1,2]

[1]*Laboratoire de biochimie, Institut de Biologie, CHU de Nantes, Nantes, France*
[2]*Faculté de médecine, Université de Nantes, Nantes, France*
[3]*Service de médecine et biologie du développement et de la reproduction, CHU de Nantes, Nantes, France*

Correspondence should be addressed to Damien Masson; damien.masson@chu-nantes.fr

Academic Editor: Mihail A. Boyanov

We report a case of 33-year-old woman with a 4-year primary infertility. A high isolated follicle-stimulating hormone (FSH) level was conflicting with the clinical situation and with other hormonal markers which were in favor of polycystic ovarian syndrome. We followed a strategy used to identify immune complexes involving FSH. The PEG precipitation test revealed that the high FSH level was almost exclusively due to the presence of autoimmune FSH immunoglobulin complex (macro-FSH). The profile obtained by gel filtration chromatography confirmed the presence of an FSH-immunoglobulin complex. Such immunological dysregulation could be explored in cases of unexplained infertility and recurrent IVF failure.

1. Introduction

The gonadotrophins, luteinizing hormone (LH) and follicle-stimulating hormone (FSH) are key regulators of the gonadal functions. Measurement of LH and FSH on day 3 of a spontaneous menstrual cycle, associated with E2 and AMH measurements, is essential to evaluate ovarian reserve in order to personalize ovarian stimulation protocol in women undergoing in vitro fertilization (IVF) [1]. Approximately 10%–20% of couples, which are unable to conceive, present an unexplained infertility with IVF failure [2]. In these cases, autoimmune mechanisms and production of autoantibodies can contribute to unexplained infertility. Elevated day 3 FSH levels can generally be observed in premature ovarian failure (POF) cases or gonadotrophin-secreting tumors. If the levels of FSH or LH are discordant with the clinical situation, the presence of anti-gonadotrophins should be evaluated by hormonal measurement after PEG precipitation and further confirmed by chromatography [3, 4]. This strategy and the procedures are equivalent to that used for the detection of a macroprolactin [4, 5].

2. Case Description

A 33-year-old woman was referred with her husband to the Department of Reproductive Medicine for a 4-year primary infertility. Both partners had no particular medical or surgical history, and physical examination was unremarkable. On the male side, sperm analysis was perfectly normal. On the female side, puberty started at 10 and menarche occurred at 16 years of age. Since then, this woman described major menstrual irregularity such as spaniomenorrhea or even amenorrhea. The antral follicle count (AFC) was high (approximately 40), strongly suggesting polycystic ovarian syndrome (PCOS) in accordance with Rotterdam criteria [6]. Overall hormonal assays performed are summarized in Table 1. Initial thyroid function tests revealed high thyroid-stimulating hormone (TSH) and normal free thyroxine level (T4L). Anti-thyroglobulin antibodies (AAT) were strongly positive. Serum estradiol (E2) and testosterone were found to be within normal ranges. Serum luteinizing hormone (LH) was moderately elevated. Serum anti-Müllerian hormone (AMH) level was remarkably high, in agreement with the PCOS diagnosis [7].

TABLE 1: Patients' results. (a) Serum hormonal concentrations on day 3 of a nonstimulated cycle. (b) Polyethylene Glycol precipitation (PEG) results.

Hormonal assays	Method	Patient	Normal reference range
(a) Day 3 of nonstimulated cycle			
LH (IU/L)	Elecsys® LH	18.6	2–11
FSH (IU/L)	Elecsys® FSH	112	1.5–13
E2 (pg/mL)	Cisbio estradiol	64.3	12–166
(pmol/L)	radioimmunoassay	236	44–609.2
hCG (IU/L)	Elecsys® hCG+β	<0.5	<5
AMH	Immunotech		
(ng/mL)	enzyme	9.4	2–6
(pmol/L)	immunoassay	67.1	14.3–42.8
TSH (mIU/L)	Elecsys® TSH	6.85	0.2–4
T4L (ng/L)	Elecsys® T4L	15.1	8.5–18
(pmol/L)		19.5	11–23.2
α-Subunit (IU/L)	Radioimmunoassay	0.19	0.02–0.90
AAT (U/ml)	Liaison® Anti-Tg	985	<100
Anti-ovarian Ab	Indirect immunofluorescence	Neg	Neg
Testosterone (ng/mL)	Cisbio testosterone radioimmunoassay	0.16	0.1–0.75
(nmol/L)		0.55	0.34–2.60
(b) After polyethylene glycol precipitation			
LH (IU/L)	Elecsys® LH	18.6	2–11
PEG unprecipitated LH (IU/L)		8.4	/
Recovery LH %		45.2	>40
FSH (IU/L)	Elecsys® FSH	112	1.5–13
PEG unprecipitated FSH (IU/L)		13.6	/
Recovery FSH %		12.1	>40

A remarkably high follicle-stimulating hormone (FSH) level was found (112 IU/L, normal range 1.5–13 IU/L), further confirmed in the next menstrual cycles with the same very elevated FSH value. Pituitary magnetic resonance imaging (MRI) was performed and was found normal. This very isolated FSH level was conflicting with the clinical situation and other hormonal markers which were in favor of PCOS.

For this patient, assay interference was suspected on the basis of discordance between the serum FSH and LH results and the clinical history. An interference in immunoassay is rare, but is very problematic because can drastically affect patient management. Endogenous immunoglobulins can be identified in this situation. Immunoglobulins can be directed against assay reagents or against analyte itself leading to the formation of macro-analyte corresponds to complex immunoglobulin-analyte. Interfering immunoglobulins can be identified by elimination with a polyethylene glycol precipitation and a specific identification. Like so, the analyte test is realized before and after treatment. If an interfering immunoglobulin is present, the recovery of analyte is reduced. A macro-analyte can be suspected if recoveries are normal (>40%) for others analytes [4].

In endocrinology, macro-hormone is frequently described for serum prolactin assays. If macro-prolactin is suspected, PEG precipitation is used to detect immunoglobulin interference [8]. Macroprolactin is biologically inactive but this presence is detected by all prolactin immunoassays and can lead to misdiagnosis. Collaboration between clinician and biologist can permit to suspect interference assays.

As this unexplained isolated high FSH level resembled macro-prolactin cases, we followed the same strategy in order to identify immune complexes involving FSH. Therefore, we measured FSH after polyethylene glycol (PEG) precipitation to screen for interference from autoimmune FSH immunoglobulin complex (macro-FSH). For this technique, 200 μL PEG 6000 solution (25%) was mixed with 200 μL sample, briefly vortex-mixed, and centrifuged for 15 min at 3000g at room temperature. FSH was then measured in the supernatant for recovery calculation. We used the same protocol to evaluate LH assays before and after PEG precipitation. The recovery rate of FSH was 12.1% and free-FSH (unprecipitated-FSH) level after PEG treatment was at the upper limit of the normal range (Table 1). LH assays have been also performed before and after PEG precipitation. Contrary to FSH, LH recovery following PEG precipitation was within normal ranges (>40%). No autoimmune LH immunoglobulin complex, macro-LH, was detected. This PEG precipitation test revealed that high FSH level in this patient was almost exclusively due to the presence of the high-molecular FSH form, the macro-FSH. The analysis of circulating FSH by gel filtration chromatography was subsequently performed using a column of Ultrogel® AcA 54. Serum was applied on the column and the fractions were collected for FSH determination.

The gel filtration profile in this patient is represented in Figure 1(a). A high molecular form of FSH immunoreactivity was detected. This elution profile differed significantly from the pattern obtained in a normal control subject (Figure 1(b)).

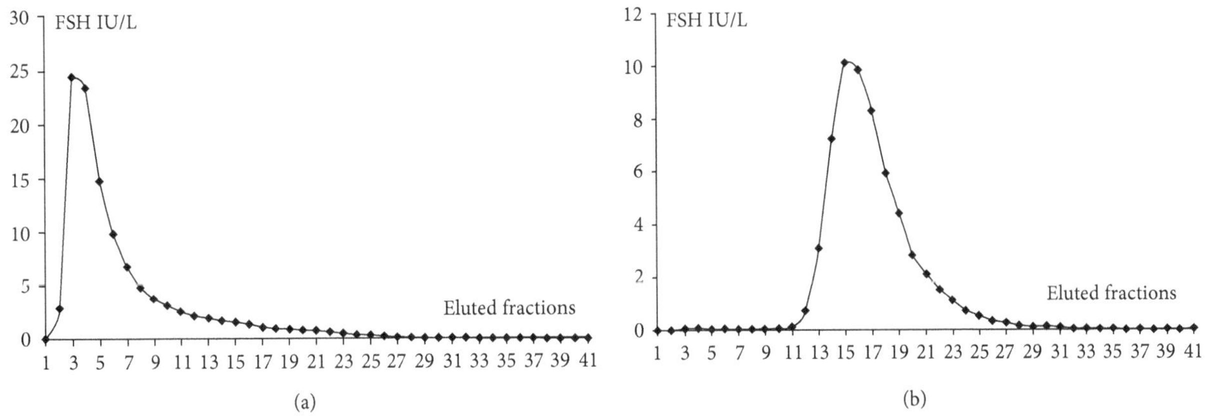

FIGURE 1: Gel filtration chromatography (GFC) elution profile. (a) Elution profile obtained with patient sample. (b) Elution profile obtained with normal control sample.

The high molecular mass peak corresponded to the molecular mass of an FSH-immunoglobulin complex. Additional analysis was performed. Serum was screened for ovarian autoantibodies by indirect immunofluorescence assay, but the result was negative. FSH is composed of two peptide subunits: alpha, common with LH, TSH, and hCG (human chorionic gonadotrophin), and beta that determines hormonal specificity. We wanted to evaluate if anti-FSH was directed against α or β subunit. An α-subunit assay and an hCG test by a β-subunit specific assay were realized (Table 1). The normal results indicated that these anti-FSH auto-antibodies were probably directed against β-subunit of FSH.

3. Discussion

We describe here a case of anti-FSH autoantibodies leading to persisting very high FSH serum levels in an infertile woman. FSH is a key regulator of the gonadal functions, along with LH. It is synthesized and released from the anterior pituitary gland as a heterodimeric glycoprotein of ~30 kDa molecular weight. It is composed of two peptide subunits: alpha, common with LH, TSH and hCG, and beta that determines hormonal specificity. Measurement of LH and FSH on day 3 of a spontaneous menstrual cycle, associated with E2 and AMH measurements, is essential to evaluate ovarian reserve in order to personalize ovarian stimulation protocol in women undergoing in vitro fertilization (IVF) [1]. Elevated day 3 FSH level can generally be observed in premature ovarian failure cases or gonadotrophin-secreting tumors [9, 10]. In this case, ovarian failure could be excluded because of elevated AFC and AMH levels. In our case, the description of menstrual irregularities such as spaniomenorrhea or even amenorrhea and an elevated AFC (approximately 40) are two Rotterdam criteria. The Rotterdam criteria define PCOS by the presence of at least two out of three criteria: oligo-anovulation, clinical and/ or biochemical hyperandrogenism, and polycystic ovaries ($\geq$12 follicles measuring 2–9 mm in diameter, or ovarian volume >10 ml in at least one ovary) [6]. A PCOS, a frequent endocrine disorder in women of reproductive age, is suspected for this patient. Moreover, AMH, a reliable marker of polycystic ovaries in PCOS, is here elevated [7, 11]. Furthermore pituitary MRI was normal, eliminating tumoral etiologies. Thus, premature ovarian failure and gonadotrophin-secreting tumor could be excluded. Therefore, another etiology was suspected for this isolated and persisting elevated FSH level.

Apart from PCOS, this patient presented a context of thyroid autoimmunity. This is frequent in women of reproductive age, and can be associated with female infertility and even negatively affect IVF outcome [12]. Furthermore, some studies have also suggested a connection between autoimmune thyroiditis and PCOS [13]. Several studies have described association between premature ovarian failure and autoimmune diseases such as adrenal autoimmunity, Hashimoto thyroiditis, diabetes mellitus, and rheumatoid arthritis. Among all autoimmune diseases associated with POF, thyroid disorders are the most common [14]. It has been proposed that reduced fertility might be associated with the dysregulation of immune system reactions resulting in enhancement of autoantibody production [15]. This autoimmunity increases miscarriage risks, reduces female fecundity and infertility treatment success. In case of an autoimmune disease, such as thyroid disorders, presence of anti-gonadotrophins (anti-LH, anti-FSH) is described in infertile women [14].

These antibodies have been identified in poor responders [14] and in cases of repeated implantation failure [15]. These observations suggested that these antibodies could inhibit either FSH or LH effects on folliculogenesis and ovulation *in vivo*, by interrupting the hormone-receptor binding or by increasing their clearance. An immunization against exogenous gonadotropins has been suggested to explain the presence of anti-FSH or anti-LH antibodies in women undergoing IVF, and may increase with repeated IVF cycles [16]. However, no exogenous FSH had been given to our patient before infertility work-up, ruling out this hypothesis. Consequently, anti-gonadotrophin autoimmunity may represent an interesting pathophysiological mechanism in POF.

Concerning anti-FSH, majority of these autoantibodies are directed against β-subunit of follicle-stimulating hormone [3]. These antibodies predominantly recognized a region of 16 amino-acids, probably representing the immunodominant epitope [17]. The β-subunit plays a role in FSH receptor binding. Therefore, the presence of anti-FSH directed against

β-subunit can explain the infertility cases. In our patient, analyses were in favor of autoantibodies directed against β-subunit [18].

These autoantibodies deeply affect basal hormonal status and compel assisted reproductive technology (ART) specialists to adapt treatment strategies. Long term oestroprogestative contraceptive pill treatment has been suggested in order to suppress gonadotrophin secretion and consequently autoantibody production. Others advise an immune-modulating therapy such as glucocorticoid treatment for women with autoimmune diseases, anti-ovarian or anti-gonadotrophin antibodies in order to recover a satisfactory ovarian function and ultimately improve IVF outcome [15, 19]. However, these strategies have not been proven to be relevant yet in such cases, and the best protocol remains to be identified. In the case reported here, the couple was informed of these options and finally decided not to try these treatment. Concerning PCOS, eating right, exercising, and not smoking were very much suggested. In absence of hyperandrogenism, antiandrogen prescription was not necessary. Ovulation induction with clomiphene was proposed but the couple finally decided not to perform medically assisted procreation [20]. Treatment by L-thyroxine was started.

From an analytical point of view, anti-gonadotrophin antibodies can interfere with immunoassays via the formation of circulating hormone—immunoglobulin complexes [4]. The presence of heterophilic antibodies directed against antibodies of different animal species present in immunoassay [21], found in cases of rheumatoid arthritis for example, can also lead to falsely high or falsely low results in commonly used immunoassays such as FSH, LH, hCG or AMH. Important analytical steps should be followed when the presence of anti-gonadotrophins is suspected. Firstly, the same sample should be reanalyzed with the same assay, as the presence of antibody interference can give varying results when repeating the test. Secondly, hormonal measurement should be performed with an alternative assay. Indeed, the use of different antibodies in various immunoassays can lead to different sensitivity to analytical interference. Another strategy is to perform several dilutions. Serial dilutions of serum will differentiate true analyte from cross reactivity due to heterophile antibodies. Serial dilution of serum assays were made by dilution of the sample using the manufacturers' diluents. A nonlinear relationship is often obtained for serial dilutions in the presence of heterophile antibodies. However, it is possible to observe linear relationship in the serial dilutions in samples containing heterophile antibodies [22]. The presence of heterophilic antibodies can then be confirmed by adding irrelevant animal immunoglobulin to the sample prior to reassay, which may neutralize interfering antibodies. Finally, the presence of anti-gonadotrophins should be evaluated by hormonal measurement after PEG precipitation and further confirmed by chromatography. This strategy and the procedures are equivalent to those used for the detection of a macroprolactin [8].

Anti-FSH autoantibodies were identified in this patient referred for infertility workup and presenting with unexplained elevated isolated FSH levels. Such immunological dysregulation could be explored in cases of unexplained infertility and recurrent IVF failure. As anti-gonadotrophins can interfere with immunoassays, the dialog between biologist and clinician is obviously crucial to prevent from clinical misdiagnosis.

4. Conclusion

Isolated high basal FSH level can occur in a limited number of clinical situations, such as ovarian failure and gonadotrophin-secreting tumor. To identify the presence of anti-FSH autoantibodies, FSH measurement after PEG precipitation is recommended and should be confirmed by gel filtration chromatography. Anti-gonadotrophins were found in some infertile women and these antibodies could inhibit hormone activity in vivo and diminish efficacy of ovarian stimulation treatment. These autoantibodies must be screened in order to adapt treatment strategies and improve chances of pregnancy. The communication between the laboratory specialist and clinician is crucial to avoid clinical misdiagnosis.

Abbreviations

PCOS: Polycystic ovarian syndrome
TSH: Thyroid-stimulating hormone
T4L: Free thyroxine
AAT: Anti-thyroglobulin antibodies
E2: Estradiol
LH: Luteinizing hormone
AMH: Anti-Müllerian hormone
FSH: Follicle-stimulating hormone
MRI: Magnetic resonance imaging
PEG: Polyethylene glycol
macro-FSH: Autoimmune FSH immunoglobulin complex
hCG: Human chorionic gonadotrophin
IVF: Undergoing in vitro fertilization
POF: Premature ovarian failure.

Acknowledgments

The authors would like to acknowledge Najiba Lahlou (Laboratoire de Biologie Hormonale – Hôpital Cochin, Paris, France) for her participation in the experiments (Gel filtration chromatography).

References

[1] E. S. Sills, M. M. Alper, and A. P. H. Walsh, "Ovarian reserve screening in infertility: practical applications and theoretical directions for research," *European Journal of Obstetrics and Gynecology and Reproductive Biology*, vol. 146, no. 1, pp. 30–36, 2009.

[2] W. S. Vitek, O. Galárraga, P. C. Klatsky, J. C. Robins, S. A. Carson, and A. S. Blazar, "Management of the first in vitro fertilization cycle for unexplained infertility: a cost-effectiveness analysis of split in vitro fertilization-intracytoplasmic sperm injection," *Fertility and Sterility*, vol. 100, no. 5, pp. 1381–1388, 2013.

[3] K. Haller-Kikkatalo, A. Salumets, and R. Uibo, "Review on

autoimmune reactions in female infertility: antibodies to follicle stimulating hormone," *Clinical and Developmental Immunology*, vol. 2012, Article ID 762541, 15 pages, 2012.

[4] R. Webster, M. Fahie-Wilson, P. Barker, V. K. Chatterjee, and D. J. Halsall, "Immunoglobulin interference in serum follicle-stimulating hormone assays: autoimmune and heterophilic antibody interference," *Annals of Clinical Biochemistry*, vol. 47, no. 4, pp. 386–389, 2010.

[5] M. N. Fahie-Wilson, R. John, and A. R. Ellis, "Macroprolactin; high molecular mass forms of circulating prolactin," *Annals of Clinical Biochemistry*, vol. 42, no. 3, pp. 175–192, 2005.

[6] Rotterdam ESHRE/ASRM-Sponsored PCOS consensus workshop group, "Revised 2003 consensus on diagnostic criteria and long-term health risks related to polycystic ovary syndrome (PCOS)," *Human Reproduction*, vol. 19, no. 1, pp. 41–47, 2004.

[7] P. Pigny, E. Gorisse, A. Ghulam et al., "Comparative assessment of five serum antimüllerian hormone assays for the diagnosis of polycystic ovary syndrome," *Fertility and Sterility*, vol. 105, no. 4, pp. 1063–1069, 2016.

[8] L. Beltran, M. N. Fahie-Wilson, T. J. McKenna, L. Kavanagh, and T. P. Smith, "Serum total prolactin and monomeric prolactin reference intervals determined by precipitation with polyethylene glycol: evaluation and validation on common immunoassay platforms," *Clinical Chemistry*, vol. 54, no. 10, pp. 1673–1681, 2008.

[9] L. Katznelson, J. M. Alexander, H. A. Bikkal, J. L. Jameson, D. W. Hsu, and A. Klibanski, "Imbalanced follicle-stimulating hormone beta-subunit hormone biosynthesis in human pituitary adenomas," *The Journal of Clinical Endocrinology and Metabolim*, vol. 74, no. 6, pp. 1343–1351, 1992.

[10] S. Christin-Maitre and R. Braham, "General mechanisms of premature ovarian failure and clinical check-up," *Gynecology Obstetrics and Fertility*, vol. 36, no. 9, pp. 857–861, 2008.

[11] M. P. Lauritsen, J. G. Bentzen, A. Pinborg et al., "The prevalence of polycystic ovary syndrome in a normal population according to the Rotterdam criteria versus revised criteria including anti-Mullerian hormone," *Human Reproduction*, vol. 29, no. 4, pp. 791–801, 2014.

[12] A. Busnelli, A. Paffoni, L. Fedele, and E. Somigliana, "The impact of thyroid autoimmunity on IVF/ICSI outcome: a systematic review and meta-analysis," *Human Reproduction Update*, vol. 22, no. 6, pp. 793–794, 2016.

[13] N. Gleicher, A. Weghofer, and D. H. Barad, "Cutting edge assessment of the impact of autoimmunity on female reproductive success," *Journal of Autoimmunity*, vol. 38, no. 2–3, pp. J74–J80, 2012.

[14] T. Forges, P. Monnier-Barbarino, G. C. Faure, and M. C. Béné, "Autoimmunity and antigenic targets in ovarian pathology," *Human Reproduction Update*, vol. 10, no. 2, pp. 163–175, 2004.

[15] V. Muller, K. Ob'edkova, I. Krikheli et al., "Successful pregnancy outcome in women with recurrent IVF failure and anti-hCG autoimmunity: a report of three cases," *Case Reports in Immunology*, vol. 2016, Article ID 4391537, 5 pages, 2016.

[16] K. Haller, A. Salumets, M. Grigorova et al., "Putative predictors of antibodies against follicle-stimulating hormone in female infertility: a study based on in vitro fertilization patients," *American Journal of Reproductive Immunology*, vol. 57, no. 3, pp. 193–200, 2007.

[17] B. Gobert, C. Jolivet-Reynaud, P. Dalbon et al., "An immunoreactive peptide of the FSH involved in autoimmune infertility," *Biochemical and Biophysical Research Communications*, vol. 289, no. 4, pp. 819–824, 2001.

[18] K. M. Fox, J. A. Dias, and P. Van Roey, "Three-dimensional structure of human follicle-stimulating hormone," *Molecular Endocrinology*, vol. 15, no. 3, pp. 378–389, 2001.

[19] T. Forges, P. Monnier-Barbarino, F. Guillet-May, G. C. Faure, and M. C. Béné, "Corticosteroids in patients with antiovarian antibodies undergoing in vitro fertilization: a prospective pilot study," *European Journal of Clinical Pharmacology*, vol. 62, no. 9, pp. 699–705, 2006.

[20] A. Badawy and A. Elnashar, "Treatment options for polycystic ovary syndrome," *International Journal of Women's Health*, vol. 3, pp. 25–35, 2011.

[21] H. Cappy, P. Pigny, M. Leroy-Billiard, D. Dewailly, and S. Catteau-Jonard, "Falsely elevated serum antimüllerian hormone level in a context of heterophilic interference," *Fertility and Sterility*, vol. 99, no. 6, pp. 1729–1732, 2013.

[22] E. García-González, M. Aramendía, D. Álvarez-Ballano, P. Trincado, and L. Rello, "Serum sample containing endogenous antibodies interfering with multiple hormone immunoassays. Laboratory strategies to detect interference," *Practical Laboratory Medicine*, vol. 4, pp. 1–10, 2016.

6

Adrenal Myelolipoma Masquerading as an Adrenal Malignancy

Davida A. Robinson,[1] Margaret Kemeny,[1] Juliana E. Muchinyi,[1] Madiha Yasin,[2] Nilda I. Montes,[1] Sandeep Tuli,[3] Radhika Jaiswal,[2] Amanda Carter,[2] Michal-Ann Derezil,[2] Hanna Jang,[1] and David Reich[4]

[1]*Icahn School of Medicine at Mount Sinai, Queens Hospital Center, Department of Surgery, 82-68 164th Street, New York, NY 11432, USA*
[2]*Zucker School of Medicine at Hofstra and Northwell, Northwell Health-North Shore University Hospital, Department of Medicine, Division of Endocrinology, 500 Hofstra University Hempstead, New York, NY 11549, USA*
[3]*Ichahn School of Medicine at Mount Sinai- Queens Hospital Center, Department of Radiology, 82-68 164th Street, New York, NewYork 11432, USA*
[4]*Ichahn School of Medicine at Mount Sinai- Queens Hospital Center, Department of Medicine, Division of Endocrinology, 82-68 164th Street, New York, NewYork 11432, USA*

Correspondence should be addressed to David Reich; reichd@nychhc.org

Academic Editor: Wayne V. Moore

An adrenal myelolipoma presenting with suspicious features may pose a diagnostic challenge to surgeons and endocrinologists. In this case report of an adult patient with undiagnosed congenital adrenal hyperplasia presenting with bilateral adrenal masses, we review his radiographic and clinical findings which were highly suspicious for adrenal malignancy. Features of adrenal myelolipoma that may resemble malignant lesions are reviewed. This case report highlights important features of adrenal myelolipoma that the surgeon and endocrinologist should be aware of. The importance of avoiding overtreating adrenal myelolipomas presenting as tumors of uncertain malignant potential is crucial.

1. Introduction

Adrenal myelolipoma (AML) is most commonly asymptomatic and diagnosed incidentally on imaging studies obtained for other indications unrelated to the adrenal mass [1]. The majority of adrenal incidentalomas are benign adrenocortical adenomas, with only a 1.9% incidence of cancer [1]. Myelolipomas generally are benign tumors occurring in the adrenal gland and rarely in extra-adrenal locations that are characterized by mature adipose tissue intermixed with hematopoietic elements [2–4]. Likewise, AMLs are most commonly incidental findings, accounting for up to 15% of adrenal incidentalomas [2, 5, 6]. The exact pathophysiology and histogenesis of AML are not well understood; however, a possible mechanism involves adrenocortical metaplasia of capillary reticuloendothelial cells in response to pathologic stimuli (e.g., trauma and infection) or long-term ACTH stimulation, which in turn results in cellular differentiation of mesenchymal stem cells into myeloid and adipose tissues [5].

AMLs have characteristic radiographic and microscopic features, yet diagnosis of AML is not always straightforward and may present diagnostic challenges to the clinician. We present a case of a large AML masquerading as an invasive adrenal malignancy in a patient with previously undiagnosed (and therefore untreated) congenital adrenal hyperplasia (CAH) due to 21-hydroxylase deficiency (21-OHD) diagnosed in adulthood.

2. Case Presentation

A 48-year-old male presented to the surgical oncology clinic for follow-up of bilateral adrenal masses detected incidentally on computed tomography (CT) scan of the abdomen and pelvis obtained for unrelated indications. The patient had no significant medical history. On exam, he was noted to have short stature at 139.7 cm but was otherwise normally developed. Blood pressure was 115/76 mmHg and pulse was 76 beats per minute. No abdominal masses, lymphadenopathy, or peripheral edema were present. Contrast-enhanced CT of the abdomen and pelvis revealed an 8.4 cm × 6.2 cm × 7.5 cm complex, multilobulated, fat containing left adrenal mass that also contained a more solid component with calcification that appeared to abut or possibly invade the pancreatic tail. This raised the suspicion for malignancy (Figures 1 and 2). There was also a 1.6 x 2 × 2.5 cm and 1.7 × 1.5 × 1.8 cm nodule in the right adrenal gland (Figures 1, 2). A CT of the abdomen and pelvis with and without contrast with a washout protocol was subsequently obtained. The macroscopic fat on the left adrenal mass had a Hounsfield units (HU) density of < -40. The soft tissue component with calcified portions had a precontrast density of 24 HU, a postcontrast density of 110 HU, and a delayed phase density of 86 HU. The absolute washout was 28%, and the relative washout was 22%. This is consistent with an indeterminant lesion and not adenoma. The left adrenal mass remained stable in size, and the suspected invasion of the pancreatic tail was again demonstrated. Pre, post, and delayed density characteristics of the right adrenal nodules were 29 HU precontrast, 104 HU postcontrast, and 50 HU on delayed images for the larger nodule in right adrenal and 33 HU, 139 HU, and 62 HU for the smaller right adrenal nodule. They both had an absolute and relative washout percentages of 72% and 52%, respectively, for the larger nodule and 73% and 55%, respectively, for the smaller right adrenal nodule. They were consistent with lipid-poor adenomas. A positron emission tomography (PET) scan revealed heterogeneous fluorodeoxyglucose (FDG) avidity localizing to the left adrenal mass. The nonfatty components in the left adrenal mass demonstrated a maximal standard uptake value (SUVmax) ranging from 5.6 to 6.3. The right adrenal gland, including the nodules, was also FDG avid with a maximal SUV of 5.8 (Figure 3). The fatty regions of the left adrenal mass were not metabolically active. The solid component in the left adrenal mass had an uptake on PET scan that was greater than the hepatic background. This can be seen with the adenomatous or hematopoietic components of myelolipoma but may also occur in malignant conditions. Benign adrenal lesions typically demonstrate SUV uptake values that are equivalent to or less than the hepatic background activity. Mildly avid foci in the mediastinum and right hilum were also identified, which were nonspecific and believed to represent subcentimeter reactive inflammatory nodes. There was no evidence for FDG avid nodal metastasis on the PET/CT. Staging CT of the chest was also negative for intrathoracic metastatic disease.

A complete biochemical laboratory evaluation was performed (Table 1). Blood tests revealed elevated aldosterone. However, plasma renin activity was normal (3.911 ng/mL/h), and serum potassium was 5.3 mmol/L, effectively ruling out primary aldosteronism. Plasma normetanephrine was borderline elevated; however, 24-hour urine total metanephrines were within normal limits, and the patient lacked any symptomatology characteristic of pheochromocytoma. Steroid precursors, dehydroepiandrosterone

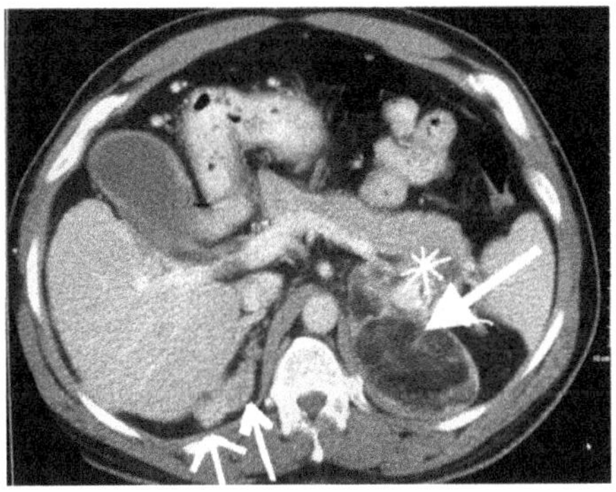

Figure 1: A contrast-enhanced computed tomography (CT) image demonstrating two nodules in the right adrenal gland (small arrows) and a large, left adrenal mass with calcifications (large arrow) and suspected invasion of the left adrenal mass into the tail of the pancreas (asterisk).

sulfate (DHEAS), and 17-hydroxyprogesterone were elevated, which raised the suspicion of malignancy. The constellation of this patient's clinical, laboratory, and radiographic features, namely, short stature with concomitant elevation in ACTH and steroid precursors, dehydroepiandrosterone sulfate (DHEAS), and 17-hydroxyprogesterone, in addition to bilateral adrenal lesions, also raised the suspicion of CAH due to 21-OHD. Thyroid function tests were consistent with subclinical hypothyroidism (elevated TSH, with normal free T4), which was treated; thyroid peroxidase antibodies were very high, consistent with Hashimoto's thyroiditis. Baseline cortisol level was low, and ACTH was markedly elevated at 160 pg/mL.

The decision was made to proceed with surgical resection of the left adrenal gland secondary to inability to exclude adrenal malignancy due to large size, apparent invasion into the tail of the pancreas, indeterminate (nonadenoma) washout characteristics, and FDG avidity. The patient underwent exploratory laparotomy with left adrenalectomy and distal pancreatectomy. Hydrocortisone 50 mg IV was given preoperatively and continued every 6 hours in the perioperative period. The left adrenal mass extended high into the retroperitoneum, abutting but not involving the splenic hilum and upper pole of the left kidney, with fibrinous attachments to the tail of the pancreas anteriorly. There was no lymphadenopathy or other signs of metastatic disease present on exploration. Frozen section of the adrenal mass was positive for myelolipoma. Final pathology documented a 10.0 cm × 8.2 cm × 6.5 cm adrenal gland weighing 175 g, with the left adrenal mass positive for AML, and one adrenal cortical adenoma. The tail of the pancreas contained one microscopic, well differentiated 2 mm neuroendocrine tumor, with a Ki67 labeling index of <3% and a low mitotic rate.

The patient was continued on hydrocortisone and levothyroxine postoperatively and discharged home on postoperative day 5 after an uneventful hospital course. Given the significant elevation of the serum 17-hydroxyprogesterone level, his short stature was reportedly lower than his biological paternal and maternal heights (72 inches

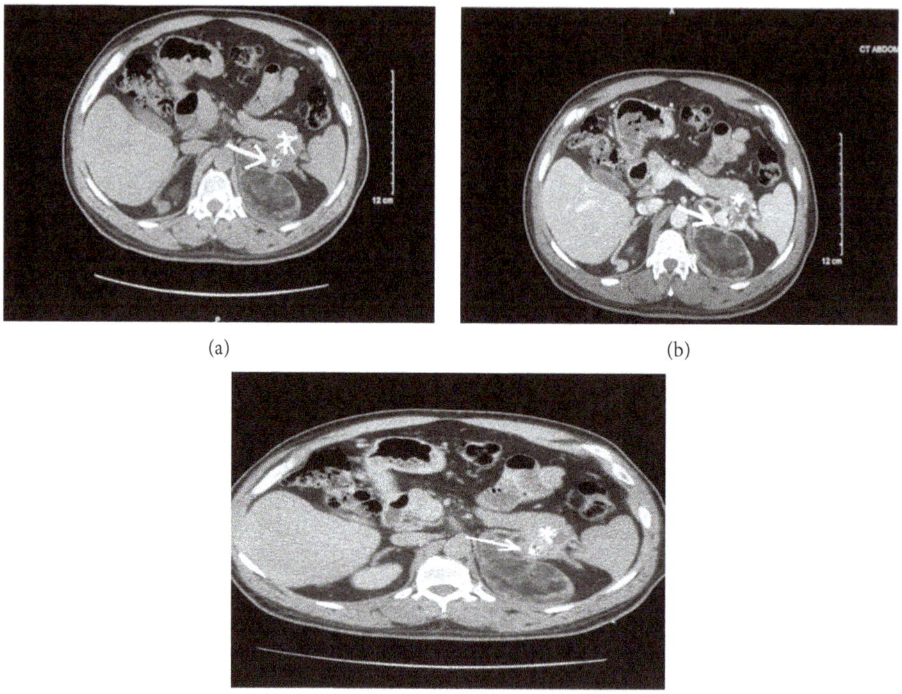

(a) (b) (c)

FIGURE 2: A multiphase CT with noncontrast (a), contrast (b), and delayed (c) images demonstrating the enhancing solid component of the left adrenal mass (arrow) and the region of questioned pancreatic invasion (asterisk).

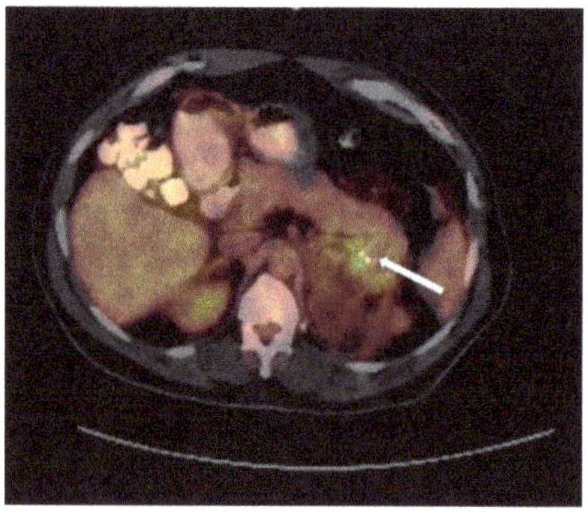

FIGURE 3: A positron emission tomography (PET) scan demonstrating metabolic uptake with focality localizing to the enhancing solid component of the left adrenal mass seen on the multiphase CT study.

and 64 inches, respectively), and on the presence of myelolipoma on final pathology, the diagnosis of CAH due to 21-OHD was highly suspected. Full gene analysis sequencing for the CYP21A2 gene was performed to evaluate for suspected CAH due to 21-OHD. The results revealed that both copies of the CYP21A2 gene carry the pathogenic variant c.293–13C > G, supporting diagnosis of CAH due to 21-OHD. Testicular ultrasound was also performed to rule out adrenal rest tumors. No adrenal rest tumors were seen, although testicular size was somewhat small bilaterally, with maximum dimension of the right and left testicle at 3.0 cm. Hydrocortisone therapy will be continued indefinitely to potentially prevent further growth of the remaining contralateral adrenal gland. The patient's plasma renin activity was somewhat elevated when measured following hospital discharge, and fludrocortisone 0.1 mg daily was added to the hydrocortisone 10 mg twice daily dose.

3. Discussion

AML was initially most commonly discovered on autopsy; however, as diagnostic imaging has become more sophisticated, it is most commonly diagnosed incidentally on imaging studies obtained for other indications [1]. Although the exact pathophysiological mechanism in tumor formation remains unclear, elevated ACTH levels and persistent stimulation by ACTH, as in both CAH and Cushing's disease, have been implicated to play a role in the development of AML [7–11]. In fact, in patients with untreated CAH, the incidence of both adrenal hyperplasia and adrenal neoplasms increases with increased severity of the enzymatic defect, especially in myelolipomas occurring within an adenoma [8, 9]. In a systematic review of 420 cases of AML, 10% of cases were associated with CAH [12]. Similarly, Falhannar et al. reported that 45% of genetically proven CAH carriers had adrenal incidentalomas, and of these, greater than 50% had bilateral adrenal lesions [13].

CAH is an autosomal recessive disorder that is most commonly due to 21-OHD due to mutation in the CYP21A2 gene [10, 14, 15]. Less commonly, CAH may occur secondary to 17-hydroxylase deficiency and 11-hydroxylase deficiency [11]. 21-OHD, in turn, results in impaired production of cortisol and elevated adrenocorticotropic hormone (ACTH), which enhances adrenal

Table 1: Endocrinologic laboratory tests.

Lab test	Patient value	Reference range
Gastrin	177 pg/mL	<100 pg/mL
Renin activity, Pl	6.683 ng/mL/h	0.167–5.380 ng/mL/h
Aldosterone	41.8 ng/dL	</ = 23.2 ng/dL
Plasma normetanephrine, Pl	147.6 pg/mL	0.0–125.8 pg/mL
Plasma metanephrine, Pl	25.2 pg/mL	0.0–88.0 pg/mL
Cortisol AM*	0.7 ug/dL	6.0–18.4 ug/dL
Cortisol AM	4.6 ug/dL	6.0–18.4 ug/dL
DHEAS*	299 ug/dL	95.0–530.0 ug/dL
DHEAS	598 ug/dL	95.0–530.0 ug/dL
24 hours urine metanephrine	63 mcg/24 h	44–261 mcg/24 h
24 hours urine normetanephrine	169 mcg/24 h	119–451 mcg/24 h
24 hours total urine metanephrine	232 mcg/24 h	211–646 mcg/24 h
Fractionated 24-hour urine epinephrine	4 ug/24 h	0–20 ug/24 h
Fractionated 24-hour urine norepinephrine	23 ug/24 h	0–135 ug/24 h
Fractionated 24-hour dopamine	276 ug/24 h	0–510 ug/24 h
Testosterone	447.0 ng/dL	249.0–836.0 ng/dL
17-Hydroxyprogesterone	6078 ng/dL	27–199 ng/dL
11-Heoxycortisol	40 ng/dL	</ = 76 ng/dL
TSH	7.85 uIU/mL	0.27–4.20 uIU/mL
Free T4	0.9 ng/dL	0.9–1.8 ng/dL
Thyroid peroxidase antibody	1608.0 IU/mL	</ = 34.9 IU/mL
Thyroglobulin antibodies	<20.0	</ = 40.0 IU/mL
ACTH	160.0 pg/mL	7.2–63.3 pg/mL
21-Hydroxylase antibodies	Negative	Negative

*Status post 1 mg dexamethasone suppression test.

androgen secretion. Increased stimulation by ACTH is considered the pathophysiological mechanism behind adrenal hyperplasia, but whether ACTH hypersecretion also causes tumor growth is unclear [11]. Many patients with CAH who are diagnosed with AMLs are either untreated or their condition is poorly controlled with chronic elevations in ACTH [11]. CAH due to 21-OHD has been categorized as classical and nonclassical forms. The classical form is traditionally thought to manifest as the simple virilizing or salt wasting forms. However, in contemporary teaching, the distinction between purely "salt wasting" and purely "simple virilizing" subtypes of classical CAH should be discouraged [16], and CYP21A2 allelic variants and their phenotypic manifestations are believed to occur on a continuum. In nonclassical 21-OHD, in which there is a partial hydroxylase enzyme deficiency, 20–50% of normal enzyme function is present, sufficient to adequately suppress ACTH over secretion [15]. In patients with milder enzymatic defects or with nonclassic, attenuated form of 21-OHD, postnatal virilization, menstrual irregularities, and short stature are sometimes present [7]. At birth, patients with nonclassical adrenal hyperplasia have normal genitalia with normal baseline 17-OH progesterone levels. Growth may eventually be arrested in these patients due to early epiphyseal fusion compromising final height [15]. Suchartlikitwong et al. presented a case of a 39-year-old male with untreated CAH presenting with acute adrenal insufficiency and severe virilization as noted by short stature, skin hyperpigmentation, micropenis, and no palpable testes, who was found to have bilateral AMLs [17]. Overall, the frequency of germ cell mutation in CYP21A2 was 21% in patients with bilateral incidentalomas [11].

All incidentally diagnosed adrenal masses should undergo hormonal evaluation to determine the presence of a functional tumor. It is estimated that 10–20% of AMLs have been associated with some endocrine disorders, 85% of which involve the pituitary-adrenal axis, including Cushing syndrome, congenital adrenal hypoplasia with 21-OHD or 17-hydroxylase deficiency, Conn syndrome, and androgenital syndrome due to primary aldosteronism [6, 7, 18]. AMLs have also been associated with increased catecholamine production and pheochromocytoma [18, 19]. In some cases, the endocrine disorder is due to myelolipomatous metaplasia within a functioning cortical neoplasm, most commonly adrenocortical adenoma; however, there have been cases reported in which myelolipoma itself has been associated with hyperfunctioning of the adrenal cortex without a recognizable adrenocortical lesion [7]. Thus, myelolipomatous adrenal lesions, whether true AMLs or adrenocortical neoplasms with myelolipomatous elements, may lead to hyperfunction of either the adrenal cortex or the adrenal medulla [6, 7, 18, 19].

The key diagnostic feature of AML is the presence of adipose tissue within an adrenal mass. However, in some instances, as in our patient, diagnosing AML based on radiological imaging features is not straightforward, especially as AMLs may occur synchronously with other benign or malignant adrenal lesions [2, 6]. In addition, adrenal tumors may be of uncertain malignant potential when tumor characteristics lack major criteria for malignancy such as high mitotic activity, atypical mitosis, or vascular invasion, but demonstrate minor criteria, such as large size, tumor necrosis, capsular invasion, or moderate FDG avidity on PET scan [20, 21]. In the presence of bilateral disease, presence of systemic disease, including metastatic neoplasms, should be considered [5]. Differential diagnoses and suspected preoperative diagnoses of liposarcoma, retroperitoneal sarcoma, adrenal metastatic lesion, and adrenocortical carcinoma have been reported in the literature for adrenal masses later proven to be benign AMLs [2, 5, 22]. AMLs with hemorrhage and necrosis, especially when occurring within an adrenal adenoma, as reported by Al-Brahim et al. may erroneously suggest a diagnosis of adrenocortical carcinoma on radiologic imaging [2]. Lastly, AML may be associated with a false positive 18F-FDG PET scan due to possible FDG uptake related to the trophic adrenal effect of ACTH [1, 23], as in our case which demonstrated 18-FDG avidity. Similarly, Kocak et al. reported a case of a 46-year-old male with benign, bilateral AML secondary to CAH confirmed on pathology following bilateral adrenalectomy, which demonstrated unilateral hypermetabolic activity of the right mass on preoperative PET scan with a maximum SUV of 11.8 [24]. Malignant transformation or metastatic spread of AML has not been reported.

The presence of macroscopic fat tissue in an adrenal lesion does not automatically rule out the possibility of a malignant lesion, which was another reason why we ultimately sent our patient to surgery. It is imperative for clinicians to be mindful of this when evaluating patients with this important radiographic feature. Macroscopic fat in an adrenal lesion has been described in adrenocortical carcinomas, adrenal oncocytic neoplasms, which are very rare adrenal neoplasms that can sometimes behave in a malignant fashion, and collision tumors, which are tumors composed of two different adjacent histologies, such as myelolipoma with coexisting adrenocortical carcinoma or myelolipoma with a metastatic lesion from a separate extra-adrenal primary malignancy [25–28].

Management of AML is dependent on size of the lesion, clinical presentation, and inability to exclude cancer. Surgery is typically reserved for lesions that are symptomatic, large (>6-7 cm), increasing in size on serial imaging, or with indeterminant malignant potential [19, 24, 29, 30]. While AMLs are most commonly clinically quiescent and diagnosed incidentally, rarely they come to clinical attention due to symptomatology. Abdominal and/or flank pain due to mass effect or tumor necrosis, vomiting, hematuria, rupture, and life-threatening hemorrhage have been described in the literature [6]. In the case of bilateral AML, which most frequently occurs in individuals with CAH, monolateral symptoms are the most commonly reported clinical feature. Monolateral adrenalectomy is recommended for the symptomatic tumor, leaving the contralateral adrenal gland in place in order to preserve some adrenal hormone function. Bilateral adrenalectomy is reserved for symptomatic tumors or tumors >7 cm. With proper medical management, the remaining AML will hopefully remain stable (though this is not guaranteed), as in the case reported by Zattoni et al., in which a patient with bilateral AML (17 cm × 12 cm (−20 HU) on the right and 2.3 cm × 2.5 cm (−5 HU) on the left) underwent an open right adrenalectomy with radiological surveillance demonstrating no recurrence on the right side and a left lesion that remained stable over time [30]. The presence of bilateral adrenal lesions should raise the suspicion for a systemic condition, including infection or metastasis from an extra-adrenal primary tumor, as well as conditions of ACTH excess, including CAH or a hereditary pheochromocytoma syndrome [5]. In cases where the diagnosis of adrenal malignancy is uncertain, particularly in instances where the adrenal incidentaloma demonstrates imaging characteristics that are suspicious for malignancy and/or the patient has a known primary malignancy, there may be a diagnostic role for percutaneous fine needle aspiration of the mass; however, this carries an associated potential risk of bleeding, tumor rupture, and subsequent tumor dissemination [31].

In terms of our case, based on CT washout data, the right adrenal lesion was most consistent with benign, lipid-poor adenoma. The larger left adrenal lesion was probably myelolipoma, but a superimposed malignancy could not be ruled out based on the foci of FDG avidity, greater than the hepatic background, within the solid component of the left adrenal mass. Our patient underwent surgical resection due to the large size of the left adrenal lesion and an overall clinical picture that was highly suspicious for a malignant process, including radiographic evidence of possible involvement of the pancreatic tail. He was subsequently diagnosed with AML in association with CAH, classic type, secondary to 21-OHD. The patient is doing well and remains on steroid replacement therapy consisting of hydroxycortisone 10 mg twice daily and fludrocortisone 0.1 mg once daily in addition to levothyroxine 50 mcg daily for treatment of subclinical hypothyroidism. Although our patient did not have overt aldosterone deficiency, fludrocortisone 0.1 mg daily, in addition to hydrocortisone 10 mg twice daily, dose steroid therapy was initiated, in compliance with the current recommendations that suggest that most nonhypertensive adults with classic CAH benefit from continued fludrocortisone treatment. Also, in patients with 21-hydroxylase deficiency-induced CAH, mineralocorticoid replacement may permit dose reduction of daily glucocorticoid requirements, which in turn may reduce the risk of iatrogenic Cushing syndrome due to overreplacement of glucocorticoids [16, 32]. Depending on subsequent androstenedione and testosterone levels, with a goal ratio in CAH of <2 (normal is < 0.5), the hydrocortisone dose can be adjusted [32]. The initial dose of hydrocortisone given to the patient on discharge after surgery was 10 mg thrice daily, but this was reduced to 10 mg twice daily when outpatient labs revealed a testosterone level of 73.6 ng/dL and a serum androstenedione level of 17 ng/dL (normal: 40–150 ng/dL). It is possible that steroid therapy will help prevent further growth of the remaining adrenal gland, obviating the need for a future right adrenalectomy. Although our patient will be maintained on hydrocortisone and fludrocortisone indefinitely, had his remaining adrenal gland been resected, he would be glucocorticoid and mineralocorticoid dependent with daily steroid replacement required for survival, a far more potentially dangerous clinical scenario than he is currently in. Regularly scheduled serial clinical monitoring and imaging surveillance to assess for tumor growth will be conducted. Periodic monitoring for adrenal rest tumors via testicular ultrasound will also be performed.

4. Conclusion

AML may represent a diagnostic dilemma for surgeons and endocrinologists, particularly when occurring synchronously with other benign or malignant adrenal lesions, lesions in nearby structures, and in lesions with associated tumor rupture or necrosis, which may give a radiographic appearance of heterogeneity, suggesting a radiologic diagnosis of adrenocortical carcinoma. This is especially true for AMLs occurring within an adrenal adenoma, in which there is a radiologic appearance of a suspicious heterogeneous lesion with a rim of normal appearing adrenal tissue. In addition, large size and FDG avidity on PET scan may occur in AML, which may also resemble a malignant lesion. Surgeons should be aware of these findings associated with AMLs to avoid diagnostic pitfalls which may result in over diagnosing malignancy and over treating a benign disease.

Abbreviations

AML: Adrenal myelolipoma
CAH: Congenital adrenal hyperplasia
CT: Computed tomography
FDG: Fluorodeoxyglucose
HU: Hounsfield units
PET: Positron emission tomography
SUV: Standard uptake value
21-OHD: 21-Hydroxylase deficiency.

Acknowledgments

The authors would like to thank Mr. Robert Lee for his assistance in obtaining articles for review.

References

[1] M. Tzanela, D. A. Vassiliadi, and S. Tsagarakis, *Endocrinology in Clinical Practice*pp. 203–222, CRC Press, New York, NY, USA, 2nd ed. edition, 2014.
[2] N. Al-Brahim and S. Asa, "Myelolipoma with adrenocortical adenoma: an unusual combination that can resemble carcinoma," *Endocrine Pathology*, vol. 18, no. 2, pp. 103–105, 2007.
[3] A. Bhansail, R. J. Dash, S. K. Singh, A. Behra, P. Singh, and B. D. Radotra, "Adrenal myelolipoma: profile of six patients with a brief review of literature," *International Journal of Endocrinology and Metabolism*, vol. 1, pp. 33–40, 2003.
[4] L. D. Thompson and J. R. Goldblum, Eds., *Endocrine Pathology: A Volume in Foundation Diagnostic Pathology Series*, pp. 227–230, Churchill Livingstone, Philadelphia, PA, USSA, 2006.
[5] W. Polamaung, N. Wisedopas, P. Vasinanukorn, P. Pak-art, and T. Snabboon, "Asymptomatic bilateral giant adrenal myelolipomas: case Report and review of literature," *Endocrine Practice*, vol. 13, no. 6, pp. 667–671, 2007.
[6] A. Kodzo-Grey Venyo, "Myelolipoma of the adrenal gland: a review and update of the literature," *Pulsus J Surg Res*, vol. 2, pp. 50–63, 2018.
[7] M. B. Umpierrez, S. Fackler, G. E. Umpierrez, and J. Rubin, "Adrenal myelolipoma associated with endocrine dysfunction: review of the literature," *The American Journal of the Medical Sciences*, vol. 314, no. 5, pp. 338–341, 1997.
[8] S. Jaresh, E. Kornely, H. K. Kley, and R. Schlaghecke, "Adrenal incidentaloma and patients with homozygous or heterozygous congenital adrenal hyperplasia," *Journal of Clinical Endocrinology & Metabolism*, vol. 74, pp. 685–689, 1992.
[9] T. Matsuda, H. Abe, M. Takase et al., "Case of combined adrenal cortical adenoma and myelolipoma," *Pathology International*, vol. 54, no. 9, pp. 725–729, 2004.
[10] I. Nermoen, J. Rørvik, S. H. Holmedal et al., "High frequency of adrenal myelolipomas and testicular adrenal rest tumours in adult Norwegian patients with classical congenital adrenal hyperplasia because of 21-hydroxylase deficiency," *Clinical Endocrinology*, vol. 75, no. 6, pp. 753–759, 2011.
[11] E. German-Mena, G. B. Zibari, and S. N. Levine, "Adrenal myelolipomas in patients with congenital adrenal hyperplasia: review of the literature and a case report," *Endocrine Practice*, vol. 17, no. 3, pp. 441–447, 2011.
[12] Á. Decmann, P. Perge, M. Tóth, and P. Igaz, "Adrenal myelolipoma: a comprehensive review," *Endocrine*, vol. 59, no. 1, pp. 7–15, 2018.
[13] H. Falhannar and D. J. Torpy, "Congenital adrenal hyperplasia due to 21-hydroxylase deficiency presenting as adrenal incidentaloma, A systematic review and metaanalysis," *Endocrine Practice*, vol. 22, pp. 736–752, 2016.
[14] D. P. Merke and R. J. Auchus, "Congenital adrenal hypoplasia due to 21-hydroxylase deficiency," *New England Journal of Medicine*, vol. 383, pp. 1258–1261, 2020.
[15] A. A. Parsa and M. I. New, "Steroid 21-hydroxylase deficiency in congenital adrenal hyperplasia," *The Journal of Steroid Biochemistry and Molecular Biology*, vol. 165, pp. 2–11, 2017.
[16] R. J. Auchus and L. K. Nieman, *Treatment of Classic Congenital Adrenal Hyperplasia Due To 21 Hydroxylase Deficiency in Adults*Up to Date, Waltham, MA, USA, 2015, http://www.uptodate.com/contents/treatment-of-classic-congenital-adrenal-hyperplasia-due-to-21-hydroxylase-deficiency-in-adults.
[17] S. Suchartlikitwong, R. Jasti, J. Lado-Abeal, and A. M. Rivas Mejia, "Bilateral adrenal myelolipomas presenting as acute adrenal insufficiency in an adult with congenital adrenal hyperplasia," *BMJ Case Reports*, vol. 12, Article ID e226826, 2019.
[18] M. Han, A. L. Burnett, E. K. Fishman, and F. F. Marshall, "The natural history and treatment of adrenal myelolipoma," *The Journal of Urology*, vol. 157, no. 4, pp. 1213–1216, 1997.
[19] K. T. Montone, M. Rosen, E. S. Siegelman, F. Fogt, and V. A. LiVolsi, "Adrenocortical neoplasms with myelolipomatous and lipomatous metaplasia: report of 3 cases," *Endocrine Practice*, vol. 15, no. 2, pp. 128–133, 2009.
[20] M. Bisceglia, O. Ludovico, A. Di Mattia et al., "Adrenocortical oncocytic tumors: report of 10 cases and review of the literature," *International Journal of Surgical Pathology*, vol. 12, no. 3, pp. 231–243, 2004.
[21] L. Jeffrey Medeiros and L. M. Weiss, "New developments in the pathologic diagnosis of adrenal cortical neoplasms: a review," *American Journal of Clinical Pathology*, vol. 97, no. 1, pp. 73–83, 1992.
[22] H. Akamatsu, M. Koseki, H. Nakaba et al., "Giant adrenal myelolipoma: report of a case," *Surgery Today*, vol. 34, no. 3, pp. 283–285, 2004.
[23] S. Leboulleux, D. Deandreis, C. Escourrou et al., "Fluorodesoxyglucose uptake in the remaining adrenal glands during the follow-up of patients with adrenocortical carci-

noma: do not consider it as malignancy," *European Journal of Endocrinology*, vol. 164, no. 1, pp. 89–94, 2011.
[24] K. Kocak, I. Nuhoglu, S. Mungan, P. Duman, H. Coskun, and S. Turkyilmaz, "Bilateral adrenal myelolipomas secondary to congenital adrenal hyperplasia: a rare case of typical asymmetrical 18F-FDG AVID," *Acta Endocrinologica*, vol. 12, pp. 491-492, 2010.
[25] N. Egbert, K. M. Elsayes, S. Azar, and E. M. Caoili, "Computed tomography of adrenocortical carcinoma containing macroscopic fat," *Cancer Imaging*, vol. 10, no. 1, pp. 198–200, 2010.
[26] D. S. Ranathunga, L. A. Cherpak, N. Schieda, T. A. Flood, and M. D. F. McInnes, "Macroscopic fat in adrenocortical carcinoma: a systematic review," *American Journal of Roentgenology*, vol. 214, no. 2, pp. 390–394, 2020.
[27] A. Balasubramanian, J. Scovell, A. E. Dowell, and W. Mayer, "Adrenocortical neoplasm of uncertain malignant potential with a myelolipomatous component," *BMJ Case Reports*, vol. 13, no. 6, Article ID e234591, 2020.
[28] M. G. Pakalniskis, K. Ishigami, B. L. Pakalniskis, and N. Fujita, "Adrenal collision tumour comprised of adrenocortical carcinoma and myelolipoma in a patient with congenital adrenal hyperplasia," *Journal of Medical Imaging and Radiation Oncology*, vol. 64, no. 1, pp. 67-68, 2020.
[29] O. Ioannidis, S. Papaemmanouil, S. Chatzopoulos et al., "Giant bilateral symptomatic adrenal myelolipomas associated with congenital adrenal hyperplasia," *Pathology and Oncology Research*, vol. 17, no. 3, pp. 775–778, 2011.
[30] D. Zattoni, R. Balzarotti, and R. Rosso, "The management of bilateral myelolipoma: case report and review of the literature," *International Journal of Surgery Case Reports*, vol. 12, pp. 31–36, 2015.
[31] E. Belezini, D. Daskalopoulou, and S. Markidou, "Fine needle aspiration of adrenal myelolipoma: a case report," *Cytopathology*, vol. 3, no. 1, pp. 31–34, 1992.
[32] P. W. Speiser, W. Arlt, R. J. Auchus et al., "Congenital adrenal hyperplasia due to steroid 21-hydroxylase deficiency: an endocrine society clinical practice guideline," *Journal of Clinical Endocrinology & Metabolism*, vol. 103, no. 11, pp. 4043–4088, 2018.

7

A Rare and Potentially Fatal Etiology of Hypercalcemia in an Infant

Ambreen Sonawalla,[1] Vildan Tas,[2] Manish Raisingani,[3] and Emir Tas[3]

[1] *Pediatric Residency Program, University of Arkansas for Medical Sciences, Little Rock, AR, USA*
[2] *Department of Pediatrics, University of Arkansas for Medical Sciences, Little Rock, AR, USA*
[3] *Department of Pediatrics, Division of Endocrinology and Diabetes, University of Arkansas for Medical Sciences, Little Rock, AR, USA*

Correspondence should be addressed to Emir Tas; etas@uams.edu

Academic Editor: Lucy Mastrandrea

Hypercalcemia is an uncommon finding in children. Hypercalcemia has various etiologies including parathyroid dependent and independent mechanisms. Increased activity of the 1-alpha-hydroxylase enzyme in granulomatous diseases is a well-defined but an extremely rare cause of hypercalcemia in pediatric patients, particularly in infants. We describe the case of an infant who presented with failure to thrive, hepatosplenomegaly, and hypercalcemia who was initially treated with steroids but was later diagnosed with disseminated histoplasmosis in the absence of an underlying immunodeficiency. Extra caution should be used before considering steroids for the treatment of hypercalcemia and, whenever possible, steroids should not be initiated until a definite etiology is identified.

1. Introduction

Serum calcium level is tightly regulated as calcium is important for numerous cellular functions including cell membrane integrity, muscle contraction, and neuronal excitability [1]. Calcium regulation involves a very-well orchestrated interplay between parathyroid hormone, 1,25-dihydroxy vitamin D, phosphorus, and multiple organ systems including the gut, kidneys, skin, and liver.

Hypercalcemia is an infrequently encountered biochemical abnormality in the pediatric age group [2]. The most common causes, unlike in adults, are parathyroid hormone independent processes. Among them, granulomatous diseases, such as fungal infections, are an uncommon but recognized cause of hypercalcemia [3]. Granulomatous diseases lead to increased activity of the 1alpha-hydroxylase enzyme which converts 25-hydroxy vitamin D to 1,25-dihydroxy vitamin D, the biologically active form.

Hypercalcemia of any cause is initially treated symptomatically, with the ultimate treatment decided by the underlying cause. Steroids have typically been used in the treatment of hypercalcemia when it is secondary to excess vitamin D ingestion or increased 1alpha-hydroxylase activity such as in granulomatous disorders [4].

2. Case Presentation

A 7-month-old ex-30-week preterm female infant presented to the emergency department of our hospital with a two-month history of worsening intermittent vomiting and failure to thrive despite nutritional optimization and trial of different infant formulas. Past medical history was notable for prolonged NICU stay mainly due to delays in oral feeding. She had no pulmonary, cardiac, or intestinal complications of prematurity. She did not require any surgical procedure or hospital admission following NICU discharge at around 6 weeks of age. History is also negative for recent fevers or recurrent infections.

On presentation, she was in no acute distress and had normal vital signs. Weight and height were both below the first percentile. Physical examination was significant for the presence of hepatosplenomegaly. Laboratory workup was notable for elevated transaminases and significant hypercalcemia (4.47 mmol/L; Normal Range: 2.12-2.74mmol/L).

Table 1: Calcium metabolism markers at each of the hospital admissions.

	Initial presentation (Baseline)	Second admission (+7 weeks)	Third admission (+15 weeks)
Total calcium (RR: 2.12-2.74 mmol/L)	4.47	3.37	2.47
Ionized calcium (RR: 1.1-1.3 mmol/L)	2.43	1.83	1.35
25 hydroxy vit D (RR: 20-200 nmol/L)	153		50.2
1,25 dihydroxy vit D (RR: 49.7-197.9 pmol/L)	364		92.9
Parathyroid hormone (RR: 12-65 ng/L)	5.3		
Phosphorus (RR: 1.39-2.39 mmol/L)	1.55		1.1
Albumin (RR: 3.5 – 4.5 g/L)	4.4	4.1	2.4
Urine Ca:Cr ratio	1.85		

Baseline phosphorus level was normal and the parathyroid hormone level was appropriately suppressed as seen in Table 1. She was admitted to hospital for management and further workup.

Aggressive intravascular fluid resuscitation with normal saline only partially improved serum calcium levels. Furosemide and calcitonin were used in succession, but they also failed to have a noticeable impact on serum calcium levels. Two doses of pamidronate, 0.5 mg/kg each two days apart, were eventually successful in restoring normal calcium levels. She also switched to low calcium infant formula, Calcilo- XD.

An extensive workup for viral and fungal etiologies was negative, as was the evaluation for metabolic, genetic, and oncologic causes of hypercalcemia. The skeletal survey did not show any lytic lesions; CT scan of the chest, abdomen, and pelvis was negative for the presence of lymphadenopathy or pulmonary lesions. Hepatosplenomegaly was confirmed with a CT scan; however, the underlying pathology was not revealed until a liver biopsy was performed for persistently elevated liver enzymes and massive hepatomegaly. Liver biopsy showed lobular histiocytic infiltrate with well-formed granulomas, hemophagocytosis, and increased portal/periportal and pericellular fibrosis with bridging indicating chronicity, with no further evidence to indicate an underlying etiology of the granulomas.

She was discharged home after 3 weeks of hospitalization once adequate weight gain and normal and stable calcium levels were achieved. Liver enzymes were improved but remained elevated. She had required readmission after one month for the recurrence of vomiting and poor weight. She had no fevers. Workup on this admission showed leukopenia and return of hypercalcemia (Table 1). Chronic granulomatous disease, immunodeficiency, tuberculosis, and hemophagocytic lymphohistiocytosis (HLH) were considered in the differential; however, screening was negative. HLH genotyping showed only a single allele mutation on UNC13 gene, but this variant did not explain her findings. Despite the lack of a standard definition of infantile sarcoidosis, this disease was considered due to elevated levels of angiotensin-converting enzyme (ACE) at 108 U/L (18-90). In the light of negative results for a possible underlying immunodeficiency and malignancy, she was placed on prednisolone 1 mg/kg/day for hypercalcemia. She remained afebrile and was discharged home in stable condition with prednisolone.

After 5 weeks of prednisolone treatment, she presented with daily emesis and low-grade fevers. Complete blood count showed pancytopenia, peripheral smear showed fungal elements. She was admitted to the intensive care unit for disseminated fungal infection. Urine Histoplasma antigen was found to be positive. Systemic antifungal treatment was started. Of note, serum calcium and liver enzyme levels were normal during the third admission (Table 1). Because of disseminated fungal infection, prednisolone was discontinued and a hydrocortisone taper was initiated. She had an excellent response to antifungal treatment. Hepatosplenomegaly resolved and all other serum markers have improved. She remained on systemic antifungal treatment for 9 months. She made full-recovery and caught up with growth and development.

3. Discussion

Hypercalcemia results when there is increased bone resorption, excessive intestinal absorption, or decreased renal excretion of calcium, or a combination of these processes. It may be asymptomatic or present with hypotonia, poor feeding, vomiting, failure to thrive (FTT), constipation, polyuria, dehydration, seizures, or, even psychiatric symptoms depending on the age of the patient [5]. Establishing the etiology requires concomitant evaluation of serum total and ionized calcium, phosphorus, magnesium, intact parathyroid hormone, 25-hydroxy vitamin D ($25(OH)D_3$), and 1,25-dihydroxy vitamin D ($1,25(OH)_2D_3$) concentrations, as well as renal function and urinary calcium excretion [4]. Unlike in adults, hypercalcemia in children is most commonly secondary to parathyroid hormone independent processes. These include hypervitaminosis D and A, medications, malignancies, granulomatous disorders, endocrinopathies, renal tubular disorders, chronic inflammatory disorders, and infections [5].

Hypervitaminosis D may be from elevated levels of $25(OH)D_3$ concentrations, which is usually due to excess ingestion of vitamin D, or from elevated levels of $1,25(OH)_2D_3$ which may be from malignancy, granulomatous diseases, subcutaneous fat necrosis of the newborn, or idiopathic infantile hypercalcemia [5].

Granulomatous diseases, including fungal infections, are a rare but well-established cause of hypercalcemia [6]. The mechanism is extra-renal production of $1,25(OH)_2D_3$ by 1alpha hydroxylase in activated macrophages within the granulomas, best described in sarcoidosis [7]. The elevated level of the active vitamin D metabolite causes hypercalcemia by a combination of increased intestinal absorption and reduced bone resorption of calcium, as well as increased renal tubular reabsorption. These macrophages are not responsive to negative feedback from elevated levels of $1,25(OH)_2D_3$ but respond to steroids.

Initial management of hypercalcemia depends on the presence of symptoms and degree of elevation of serum calcium, but ultimate treatment depends on the underlying cause. Symptomatic patients are treated with hydration and furosemide. If hypercalcemia persists, calcitonin and bisphosphonates may be used. The latter is effective especially when the primary cause of the hypercalcemia is increased mobilization of bone calcium. Our patient's severe, symptomatic hypercalcemia (Table 1) did not respond to any of the first line treatments. She had a temporary response to IV bisphosphonates but returned with hypercalcemia after only 4 weeks of the infusion therapy as the bisphosphonate did not target the underlying etiology. The role of steroids in the treatment of hypercalcemia in granulomatous diseases is well-established [3, 5]. Steroids exert their action by suppressing the excess 1alpha-hydroxylase activity and decreasing extra-renal production of $1,25(OH)_2D_3$ [8]. Prednisone or prednisolone at a dose of 1 mg/kg/day divided into two doses is the recommended treatment regimen [4]. Our patient's calcium level remained normal and stable following initiation of the steroid treatment.

Histoplasmosis, a granulomatous fungal infection, is the most common endemic fungus in the United States. Most patients remain asymptomatic and have a self-limited illness [9]. Fever, respiratory symptoms, lymphadenopathy, splenomegaly, and poor weight gain are among the most common signs and symptoms, but hypercalcemia is a rare manifestation. None of the 40 infants described by Odio et al. had hypercalcemia as a finding of disseminated histoplasmosis [10]. Surprisingly, our patient had an atypical presentation for fungal infection and did not present with any of the classic symptoms.

The literature is scarce on hypercalcemia in children and adults with histoplasmosis. Steele et al. [11] described a 10-month-old infant with disseminated histoplasmosis who presented with FTT, vomiting, hepatosplenomegaly, and hypercalcemia. Hypercalcemia in this infant was successfully managed with dietary calcium restriction alone; however, it is not clear whether the timing of antifungal treatment in the course of the fungal infection had prevented worsening hypercalcemia. Surprisingly, the infant had to be maintained on a low calcium diet even at 3-year follow up. This is in contrast to our patient who, though was initially placed on a low calcium and vitamin D formula, did not continue to require it when the underlying cause of the hypercalcemia, the fungal infection, had been controlled. Two adult cases with histoplasmosis related hypercalcemia were initially diagnosed with sarcoidosis based on the presenting clinical and laboratory data. One of the patients was found to have histoplasmosis soon after steroid treatment was begun for presumed sarcoidosis [12]. Hypercalcemia in this case resolved with the treatment of the fungal infection. The patient described by Walker et al. [13], however, presented with prolonged malaise, fever, nausea, vomiting, and weight loss. He was readmitted to the hospital after initiation of steroids, with recurrent fever and died from widespread organ disease and cardiac arrest. A postmortem examination found evidence of disseminated histoplasmosis.

Our patient was also initially placed on steroid treatment due to presumed sarcoidosis. Although there are no well-established diagnostic criteria for infantile sarcoidosis, the constellation of her signs and symptoms along with laboratory data including elevated angiotensin-converting enzyme activity in the absence of other explanation for hypercalcemia was the reason of this decision. The correct diagnosis was reached when she presented with pancytopenia, a few weeks into prednisone treatment.

4. Conclusion

Hypercalcemia is an uncommon biochemical abnormality in the pediatric age group. Disseminated fungal infections such as histoplasmosis are also uncommon in an otherwise healthy infant, and hypercalcemia is a rare presenting symptom in such patients. However, even in the absence of classic signs of fungal infections, as was the case in our patient, it is important to consider fungal causes in hypercalcemia with granulomas and evidence of hypervitaminosis D.

Steroids are a well-established treatment for hypercalcemia in granulomatous diseases. Although steroids may resolve several of the overlapping symptoms, they can also unmask the fungal infection and have potentially lethal consequences. It is therefore important to exclude infectious granulomatous etiologies prior to initiating steroid therapy for hypercalcemia.

Disclosure

The abstract of this case was presented as a poster at the 101st Annual Meeting of the Endocrine Society, 2019, New Orleans, LA; and abstract was published in the supplemental issue of the *Journal of the Endocrine Society* (JES).

References

[1] D. Goltzman, *Pediatric Endocrinology 5th edition*, Fima Lifshitz, Ed., vol. 2, Disorders of Calcium and Mineral Metabolism, 2016, Section IV , Chapter 23, page 539.

[2] J. D. McNeilly, R. Boal, M. G. Shaikh, and S. F. Ahmed, "Frequency and aetiology of hypercalcaemia," *Archives of Disease in Childhood*, vol. 101, no. 4, pp. 344–347, 2016.

[3] P. J. Tebben, R. J. Singh, and R. Kumar, "Vitamin D-mediated hypercalcemia: mechanisms, diagnosis, and treatment," *Endocrine Reviews*, vol. 37, no. 5, pp. 521–547, 2016.

[4] F. Lifshitz, "Pediatric endocrinology: growth, adrenal, sexual, thyroid, calcium, and fluid balance disorders," 2019, https://www.barnesandnoble.com/p/pediatric-endocrinology-fifth-edition-volume-2-fima-lifshitz/1112253732/2678657265790?st=PLA&sid=BNB_New+Marketplace+Shopping+Books&sourceId=PLAGoNA&dpid=tdtve346c&2sid=Google_c&gclid=EAIaIQobChMIia-Ynbzu4AIVmrrACh1XzgFvEAYYAiABEgInS_D_BwE.

[5] V. J. Stokes, M. F. Nielsen, F. M. Hannan, and R. V. Thakker, "Hypercalcemic disorders in children," *Journal of Bone and Mineral Research*, vol. 32, no. 11, pp. 2157–2170, 2017.

[6] T. P. Jacobs and J. P. Bilezikian, "Clinical review: rare causes of hypercalcemia," *The Journal of Clinical Endocrinology & Metabolism*, vol. 90, no. 11, pp. 6316–6322, 2005.

[7] R. S. Mason, T. Frankel, Y. L. Chan, D. Lissner, and S. Posen, "Vitamin D conversion by sarcoid lymph node homogenate," *Annals of Internal Medicine*, vol. 100, no. 1, pp. 59–61, 1984.

[8] L. M. Sandler, C. G. Winearls, L. J. Fraher, T. L. Clemens, R. Smith, and J. L. O'Riordan, "Studies of the hypercalcaemia of sarcoidosis: effect of steroids and exogenous vitamin D3 on the circulating concentrations of 1, 25-dihydroxy vitamin D3," *The Quarterly Journal of Medicine*, vol. 53, no. 210, pp. 165–180, 1984.

[9] L. J. Wheat, M. M. Azar, N. C. Bahr, A. Spec, R. F. Relich, and C. Hage, "Histoplasmosis," *Infectious Disease Clinics of North America*, vol. 30, no. 1, pp. 207–227, 2016.

[10] C. M. Odio, M. Navarrete, J. M. Carrillo, L. Mora, and A. Carranza, "Disseminated histoplasmosis in infants," *The Pediatric Infectious Disease Journal*, vol. 18, no. 12, pp. 1065–1068, 1999.

[11] C. J. Steele and M. B. Kleiman, "Disseminated histoplasmosis, hypercalcemia and failure to thrive," *The Pediatric Infectious Disease Journal*, vol. 13, no. 5, pp. 421-422, 1994.

[12] K. V. Liang, J. H. Ryu, and E. L. Matteson, "Histoplasmosis with tenosynovitis of the hand and hypercalcemia mimicking sarcoidosis," *JCR: Journal of Clinical Rheumatology*, vol. 10, no. 3, pp. 138–142, 2004.

[13] J. V. Walker, D. Baran, N. Yakub, and R. B. Freeman, "Histoplasmosis with hypercalcemia, renal failure, and papillary necrosis. Confusion with sarcoidosis," *Journal of the American Medical Association*, vol. 237, no. 13, pp. 1350–1352, 1977.

8

From ACTH-Dependent to ACTH-Independent Cushing's Syndrome from a Malignant Mixed Corticomedullary Adrenal Tumor: Potential Role of Embryonic Stem Cells

Claudia Ramírez-Rentería,[1,2] Ana Laura Espinosa-De-Los-Monteros,[1] Espinosa-Cardenas Etual,[1] Daniel Marrero-Rodríguez,[2,3] Guillermo Castellanos,[4] Rocio Arreola-Rosales,[4] Guillermo Montoya-Martinez,[5] Keiko Taniguchi-Ponciano,[6] Paola Briseño-Díaz,[7] Mayte Lizeth Padilla-Cristerna,[7] María del Pilar Figueroa-Corona,[7] and Mercado Moises[1,2]

[1]*Endocrinology Service, UIM Enfermedades Endocrinas, Hospital de Especialidades, Centro Médico Nacional, S.XXI, Instituto Mexicano del Seguro Social, Av Cuauhtemoc 330, Col. Doctores, CP 06720, Mexico City, Mexico*
[2]*UIM Enfermedades Endocrinas, Hospital de Especialidades, 23 Centro Médico Nacional, S.XXI, Instituto Mexicano del Seguro Social, Mexico City, Mexico*
[3]*Molecular Biomedicine Department, Center for Research and Advanced Studies, Instituto Politécnico Nacional, Av Cuauhtemoc 330, Col. Doctores, CP 06720, Mexico City, Mexico*
[4]*Pathology Department, Hospital de Especialidades, Centro Médico Nacional, S.XXI, Instituto Mexicano del Seguro Social, City. Av Cuauhtemoc 330, Col. Doctores, CP 06720, Mexico City, Mexico*
[5]*Urology Department, Hospital de Especialidades, Centro Médico Nacional, S.XXI, Instituto Mexicano del Seguro Social, Av Cuauhtémoc 330, Col. Doctores, CP 06720, Mexico City, Mexico*
[6]*Laboratorio de Neuroendocrinología Comparada, Departamento de Ecología y Recursos Naturales, Biología, Facultad de Ciencias, Universidad Nacional Autónoma de México, Exterior Circuit S / N, C.U. Coyoacán 04510, Mexico City, Mexico*
[7]*Departamento de Biomedicina Molecular Centro de Investigacion y 49 Estudios Avanzados, Av Instituto Politécnico Nacional 2508, San Pedro Zacatenco, Gustavo A. Madero, 07360 Ciudad de México, Mexico City, Mexico*

Correspondence should be addressed to Mercado Moises; moises.mercado@endocrinologia.org.mx

Academic Editor: Hidetoshi Ikeda

Context. Truly, mixed corticomedullary adrenal tumors (MCATs) may not come from colliding tumors but from a single stem cell. *Objective.* To report the immunohistochemical and molecular evaluation of a patient with ectopic ACTH syndrome (EAS) from a MCAT which has single cells with features of both 96 medullary and cortical differentiation. *Case Description and Methods.* A 16-year-old woman presented with severe EAS and a large right MCAT composed of ACTH-secreting cells resembling pheochromocytoma and another lineage similar to adrenal carcinoma. Immunohistochemistry (IHC) showed positivity for medullary (ACTH, chromogranin A, synaptophysin, and PS-100) and epithelial components (inhibin, melan-A, and calretinin). Embryonic stem cell markers were evaluated using RT/PCR and immunofluorescence. After initial surgery, the tumor recurred shifting to rapidly progressive ACTH-independent liver metastasis. *Results.* Histopathology and IHC revealed two distinct and intermingled cellular patterns, while some cells immunostained for both medullary and cortical markers. Demonstration of all stem cell biomarkers by RT/PCR and immunofluorescence was predominantly localized to the nucleus, whereas SOX2 immunoreactivity was evident in the cytoplasm as well. *Conclusion.* The expression of cancer stem cell biomarkers points towards the involvement of primitive embryonic cells as the origin of this neoplasm and maybe to the clinically aggressive and biochemically changing behavior.

1. Introduction

Mixed corticomedullary adrenal tumors (MCATs) are very rare and present as a single heterogeneous mass composed of intimately admixed adrenocortical and medullary cells [1–9]. The medullary component usually consists of pheochromocytes, whereas the cortical component is usually an adrenocortical adenoma or less frequently an adrenocortical carcinoma [1–9]. Clinical and/or biochemical evidence of cortisol hypersecretion, putatively by the cortical component, has been documented in about half of the reported cases of mixed corticomedullary adrenal tumors [1–9]. These tumors are especially rare in young patients. On the contrary, catecholamine hypersecretion by the pheochromocytoma component appears to be less frequent [1–9]. A significant proportion of MCAT is clinically and biochemically nonfunctioning lesions. Although pheochromocytomas have been reported to be the source of ectopic ACTH secretion (EAS) [10], there are no published cases where EAS has been demonstrated in the context of a MCAT. Also, most EAS-associated tumors tend to be well-differentiated tumors that can be treated with surgery and/or coadjuvant therapies over several years, while in mixed tumors, the most aggressive pathology usually determines prognosis. Persistence or recurrence of MCAT has not been extensively studied due to lack of complete biological and clinical testing on most of these tumors due to lack of awareness and multidisciplinary teams. Ectopic sources of hormones may be silent before the tumor reaches a critical mass or if treatments are controlling hormonal secretion, but we are unaware of other cases where a tumor shifts from EAS primary tumor to ACTH-independent metastasis. We herein describe the case of a young woman with ectopic ACTH syndrome due to a MCAT with an unusual biological behavior once it became metastatic.

2. Case Summary

A previously healthy 16-year-old woman presented with a 4-month history of progressive 12 kg weight gain, fatigue, and muscle weakness to the point of being mostly bedridden and incapable of walking without assistance. Her menstrual periods had been absent for almost a year, and just two months prior to consultation, she developed easy bruising, facial plethora, acne, and hirsutism, as well as severe depression. The patient is a high school student who does not smoke, consume alcohol, or use any recreational drugs. Her family history is unremarkable, negative for diabetes, thyroid conditions, and cancer. On physical exam, her weight was 77 Kg, height 1.48 (BMI 35.1 Kg/m^2), blood pressure 150/100 mmHg, pulse 95 and regular, and temperature 37°C. She had marked facial plethora with moon facies, truncal obesity, and severe muscle atrophy in upper and lower extremities, as well as inflammatory acne and terminal hair growth over her chin, arms, and chest (Ferriman–Gallwey score of 8). Her abdomen, upper arms, and thighs were covered by multiple purple striae up to 5 cm wide and 20 cm long.

General laboratory evaluation revealed a serum glucose of 100 mg/dL (normal 70–99), mild hyponatremia of 134 mEq/L (normal 135 a 145), and hypokalemia of 3.2 mEq/L (normal 3.5–5.0) and a normal corrected calcium with mild hypoalbuminemia, normal renal function tests, and mildly elevated liver enzymes. The cell blood count revealed relative lymphopenia and normocytic anemia. Hormonal work up showed normal thyroid function tests, a low-normal estradiol level with suppressed gonadotropins and a serum total testosterone of 42 μg/dL (normal < 40 in females), and dehydroepiandrosterone sulphate (DHEA-S) of 379 μg/dL (normal 61–493). Morning serum cortisol was 43 μg/dL (normal 4.5–24) suppressing to 38 μg/dL after 1 mg of dexamethasone administered the night before (normal suppression < 1.8); urinary free cortisol (UFC) was 2798 μg/day (normal 12.8–82.5), and plasma corticotrophin (ACTH) 36 pg/mL (normal 10–50, ACTH >15 in the context of Cushing's syndrome is considered to be ACTH dependent and <5 is ACTH independent). Her serum cortisol was basically unchanged after an 8 mg, overnight dexamethasone suppression test. Inferior petrosal sinus venous sampling revealed a central-to-peripheral ACTH gradient of 1.3 after the administration of desmopressin. Other hormonal tests included a calcitonin <2 pg/mL (normal < 5) and a chromogranin A of 19 pg/mL (normal < 15), as well as normal serum and urinary catecholamines and 5-hydroxiindolacetic acid. Pituitary magnetic resonance imaging (MRI) was normal, but a thoracoabdominal, high-resolution, contrast CT scan disclosed a heterogeneous, mostly hypodense, 9.3 × 7.6 × 10.4 cm lesion arising from the right adrenal gland (27–61 HU); the left adrenal gland looked atrophied (Figure 1(a)). Metaiodobenzylguanidine (MIBG) scintigraphy did not show any adrenal uptake. A 99Tc-HYNIC scan revealed mild uptake in the right adrenal gland.

She was started on spironolactone, losartan, and amlodipine for blood pressure control, as well as potassium replacement. Two days after admission, she developed hyperglycemia with a fasting serum glucose level up to 650 mg/dL that was treated with an infusion of regular insulin. She underwent open resection of the right adrenal mass without complications. Postoperatively, she presented clinical and biochemical hypocortisolism, with serum cortisol levels below 2 μg/dL (normal 5–20). Over the ensuing few weeks, her clinical condition improved remarkably, losing 15 Kg, serum potassium remained normal without the need for specific replacement, and she began walking without assistance. She was discharged home with normal blood pressure, serum potassium, and serum glucose. Since we have no mitotane available, she completed 31 sessions of external beam radiotherapy to a total dose of 55.8 Gy. She was able to come off glucocorticoid replacement 5 months after the surgical removal of the adrenal tumor, and her UFC remained normal. Three months after surgery, control imaging and laboratory tests did not show any tumor activity. Tumor pathology showed a mixed adrenal pathology with a Ki-67 of 40%. All details on microscopy and molecular findings are detailed in the methods section. Sixteen

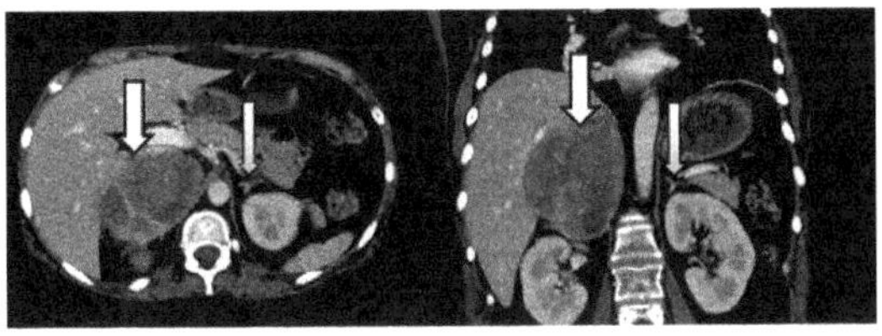

(a)

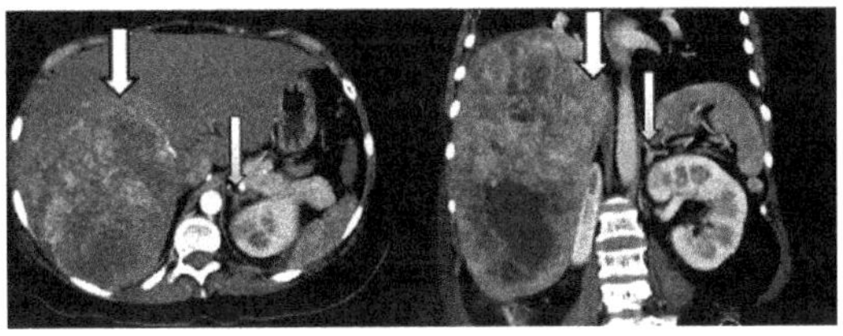

(b)

FIGURE 1: High-resolution, contrast abdominal CT scan, at diagnosis (a) and 16 months after right adrenalectomy (b). (a) Axial and coronal views showing a large, heterogeneous right adrenal mass and an atrophic left adrenal gland. (b)Axial and coronal views showing a large, heterogeneous hepatic mass and a somewhat hypoplastic left adrenal gland.

months after surgery, her UFC started to increase again. Symptoms, signs, and comorbidities of hypercortisolism eventually reappeared, including weight gain, easy bruising, a few purple striae, hair loss, and fatigue, and she developed fasting hyperglycemia. At this point, her UFC rose to 849 mcg/day, but her plasma ACTH remained suppressed (2.35 pg/mL), and therefore, endogenous hypercortisolism was again diagnosed but in this occasion, considered to be ACTH-independent; the testosterone level rose to 88.5 ng/dL, but her DHEA-S remained within normal limits (normal ranges and laboratory history in Table 1). This change in the biochemical and clinical behavior of the tumor prompted additional molecular and medical tests. A control CT scan of her abdomen revealed two large, metastatic liver lesions, measuring 6.4 and 8 cm, respectively, as well as a 7.6 cm peritoneal implant (Figure 2(b)). She declined biopsy of the liver metastases. She was started on palliative chemotherapy with paclitaxel and carboplatinum, without any biochemical or clinical response. The patient stopped visiting the hospital 4 months after the initial chemotherapy due to symptom progression and deteriorating functional status.

3. Methods

The patient and her legal guardian signed the appropriate informed consent and confidentiality agreement for the case review and publication after careful explanations. All investigations were performed on the excised tumoral tissues as well as on peripheral blood and urine samples obtained before and after surgery.

3.1. Endocrine Evaluation. Hormonal determinations were performed using commercially available immunoassays as follows: serum cortisol was measured by means of the Liaison assay (REF 313261, DiaSorin, Italy), with a sensibility of 0.16 μg/dL, and inter- and intra-assay coefficients of variation (CV) of 4.8% and 5.0%, respectively. For urine cortisol, we used the same immunoassay after methylene chloride extraction. ACTH was measured by a chemiluminescent immunoassay (REF 313221, DiaSorin, Italy) with a detection limit of 1.6 pg/mL and inter- and intra-assay CVs of 5.5% and 2.6%, respectively. Chromogranin A (CgA) was measured by an immunochemiluminimetric assay with a sensitivity of 1.5 μg/mL (Quest Diagnostics, San Juan Capistrano, CA). For metanephrines, normetanephrines, epinephrine, norepinephrine, and dopamine, we used enzymatic immunoassays (TriCat TM ELISA, IBL International GMBH, Germany). The same assays were used during the whole follow-up and repeated twice for quality control.

3.2. Pathology and Immunohistochemistry. The surgical specimen was fixed overnight in a phosphate-buffered, 10% formalin solution and later on, paraffin embedded and sliced. Routine hematoxylin-eosin (HE) staining was performed on 3 μm sections of the paraffin blocks. Immunohistochemistry (IHC) was carried out on 2 μm tissue sections using the following specific monoclonal antibodies (all purchased from DAKO Corp): corticotropin (ACTH, 1 : 50 dilution), chromogranin A (CgA, 1 : 50 dilution), synaptophysin (SNP, 1 : 50 dilution), PS-100 (1 : 400 dilution), CD56 (1 : 50 dilution), melan-A (1 : 50 dilution), calretinin (1 : 50 dilution), inhibin (1 : 50 dilution), p53 (1 : 50), steroidogenic factor-1 (SF-1, 1 : 50 dilution), and Ki67 (1 : 50 dilution). Double-labelling IHC was performed with two different chromogenes, horseradish peroxidase and alkaline phosphatase, each linked to monoclonal antibodies against CgA (to identify medullary cells) and inhibin (to identify cortical cells), respectively, using the same antibody dilutions and incubation times. All immunostains were standardized using appropriate controls.

3.3. SOX-2, NANOG, and OCT4 mRNA and Protein Expression. Total RNA was extracted and purified from frozen tumor tissue using the RNeasy tissue Mini Kit (Qiagen Inc., USA). After verifying integrity by means of Agilent Bioanalyzer 2100 (manufacturer), 1 μg of purified RNA was retrotranscribed using the SuperScript VILO Master Mix (Applied Biosystems, CA, USA). The resulting cDNA was used to amplify SOX-2, NANOG, and OCT4 transcripts using specific forward and reverse primers, which are depicted in Table 2, along with the expected size of PCR products. End point PCR was carried out according to the following protocol: an initial, 5°minute, long denaturing step at 95°C followed by 40 cycles of 30 seconds at 95°C, 30 seconds at 60°C, and 30 seconds at 72°C, ending with a final 5°minute, final extension step. The gene encoding ribosomal protein subunit 18 (RPS18) was concomitantly amplified and used as an internal constitutive control. PCR products were visualized on 2%, ethidium bromide-stained agarose gel electrophoresis and their identity verified with the aid of molecular weight markers.

Table 1: Hormonal evaluation at diagnosis and at 3 and 16 months after right adrenalectomy.

	At diagnosis	3 months PO	16 months PO	Normal range
LH (mIU/mL)	<0.1	13.47	0.9	2–7
FSH (mIU/mL)	<0.1	5.16	<0.1	2–7
Estradiol (pg/mL)	62.5	16.52	10	50–200
Total testosterone (μg/dL)	42.4	19.25	24.3	<40
DHEA-s (μg/dL)	379	25.6	77.2	61–493
ACTH (pg/mL)	38.6	12.27	2.35	10–50
Urinary free cortisol (μg/day)	2798	20.23	849	12.8–82.5
Aldosterone (pg/mL)	140.3	—	—	12–157
PRA (ng/mL/h)	17.1	—	—	0.2–2.8
CgA, x upper limit of normal	1.26	0.33	—	1

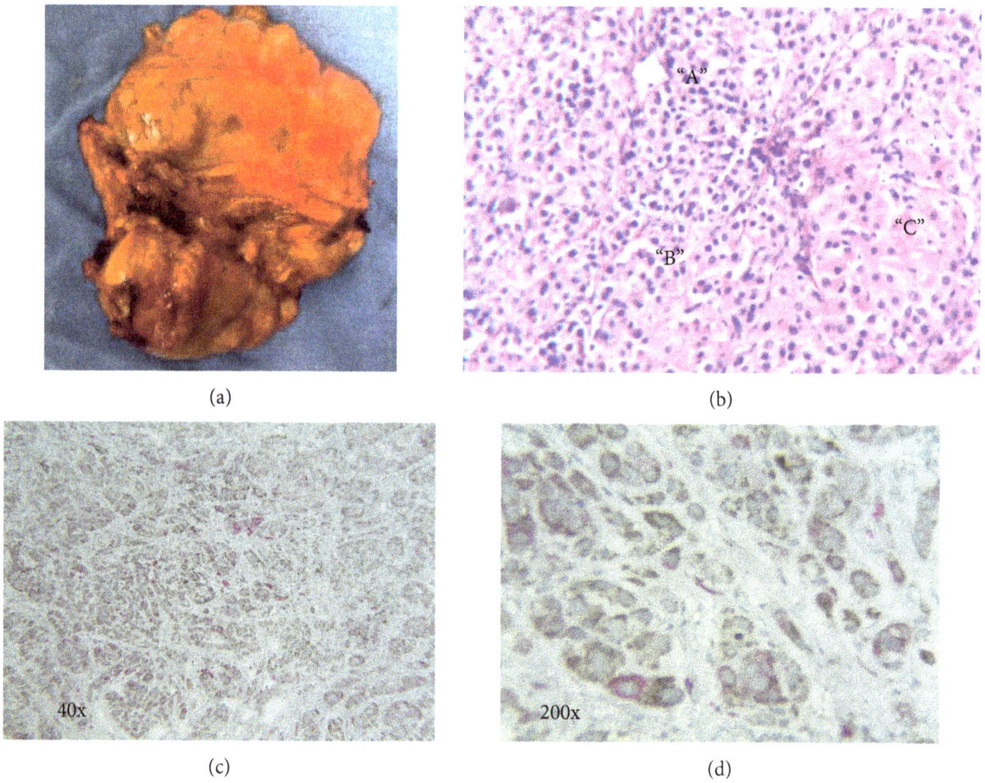

Figure 2: (a) Macroscopic view of the excised tumor. (b) Hematoxylin and eosin stain of the tumor (10x) showing three cellular patterns: "A" corresponds to the medullary neuroendocrine component, "C" corresponds to the cortical component, and "B" shows cells of an intermediate phenotype. (c, d) Double-label immunohistochemistry, with antibodies to CgA linked to horseradish peroxidase (brown) and antibodies against inhibin linked to alkaline phosphatase (red).

Table 2: Primer sequences and expected PCR product sizes.

	Sequence	Product size (bp)
SOX2 forward	ACACCAATCCCATCCACACT	224
SOX2 reverse	GCAAACTTCCTGCAAAGCTC	
NANOG forward	TGCAAATGTCTTCTGCTGAGAT	287
NANOG reverse	GTTCAGGATGTTGGAGAGTTC	
OCT4 forward	CGTGAAGCTGGAGAAGGAGAAGCTG	246
OCT4 reverse	AAGGGCCGCAGCTTACACATGTTC	
RPS18 forward	AATCCACGCCAGTACAAGATCCCA	240
RPS18 reverse	TTTCTTCTTGGACACACCCACGGT	

Immunofluorescence was performed on paraffin-embedded tumor tissues. They were first deparaffinized at 67°C by 30 min in xylene and subsequently hydrated with alcohol and distilled water. For epitope unmasking, the tissue sample was immersed in a 10 mM EDTA buffer at pH 8.05, autoclaved for 10 minutes, and washed with phosphate buffer (PBS) at pH 7.4. Autofluorescence was minimized by immersing the sample in 0.05 M NH4Cl for 30 minutes, and later on, cross sections were blocked with 3% bovine serum albumin (BSA) for 2 hours. The tissue sample was incubated with primary antibodies against SOX-2 (GTX627405-GeneTex), OCT-4 (GTX627419-GeneTex), and NANOG (GTX627421-GeneTex) diluted 1 : 100 in PBS containing 1% BSA for one hour and later on, with the Cy3-conjugated goat antibody against mouse IgG (81–6515, Invitrogen) for 30 minutes. Finally, the specimen was mounted on VECTASHIELD-DAPI mounting medium, and images were captured with a confocal microscope (Leica SP8, Barcelona, Spain).

The same assays were used for all the similar evaluations and repeated for quality control.

4. Results

4.1. Histopathology Evaluation. The excised tumor was a 330 g, 12 cm heterogeneous, tan-brown mass with bright yellow areas surrounded by a thin fibrous capsule (Figure 2(a)). The cut surface was soft and lobulated by fibrous septa with intermixed light gray-brown zones and granular necrotic mantles.

Histopathology of the tumor was complex. On HE, two different, yet, intermixed cellular patterns vaguely separated from each other were evident, designated from now on as patterns *A* and *C* with purely descriptive purposes (Figure 2(b)). Pattern *A* consisted of distinctly nested, medium-sized cells with scant to moderate cytoplasm, ill-defined cell membrane, oval nuclei with coarsely granular chromatin, and occasional inconspicuous nucleoli. Pattern *C* consisted of mantles and trabeculae of large polygonal cells with a well-defined cell membrane, abundant clear to eosinophilic granular cytoplasm, round to oval nuclei with small nucleoli, and finely dispersed chromatin. A third mixed pattern, pattern *B*, was observed in which the cells adopted to a variable degree, an intermediate or transitional phenotype between patterns *A* and *B*. Mitotic figures were numerous (up to 6 per high-power field) and randomly distributed. Mantles of ischemic necrosis constituted approximately 30% of the tumor volume.

4.2. Immunohistochemistry. Pattern *A* cells expressed a neuroendocrine immunophenotype as they positively stained for CgA, SNP, and CD56, as well as focally for ACTH. Interestingly, the cell nests of pattern *A* were rimmed by a discrete network of fusiform cells with slender cytoplasm and elongated nuclei with dense chromatin that immunostained for PS-100. Pattern *C* cells expressed an adrenocortical phenotype characterized by positive immunostaining for SF-1, inhibin, calretinin, and melan-A. Immunohistochemical studies confirmed our impression upon H&E staining that the two cellular patterns were intermingled, without clear limits between them, and frequently exhibiting transitional areas (i.e., pattern *B*). Proliferative index assessed by Ki-67 immunostaining was 40%, preferentially expressed by pattern "C" cell type, although not restricted to it. Double-labelling IHC confirmed the coexistence of medullary (anti-CgA antibodies) and cortical (anti-inhibin antibodies) cells within the tumor, with the former somewhat predominating over the latter (Figures 2(c) and 2(d)). Interestingly, a few of the cells clearly showed reactivity to both antibodies.

4.3. SOX-2, NANOG, and OCT4 mRNA and Protein Expression. RT/PCR using specific primers for SOX-1, NANOG, and OCT4 confirmed the expression of the corresponding transcripts of the expected molecular weight as shown in Figure 3.

Immunofluorescence using specific antibodies against stem cell antigens revealed predominantly nuclear NANOG and OCT4 reactivity, whereas SOX_2 immunoreactivity was localized to both the nucleus and the cytoplasm (Figure 4).

5. Discussion

The differential diagnosis of Cushing's syndrome represents one of the major challenges that clinical endocrinologists face. A sequential work up, usually starting with screening tests aimed to confirming the existence of endogenous hypercortisolism followed by the establishment of ACTH dependency or independency and ending with biochemical tests and imaging techniques aimed at localizing the original source of the condition, is essential for an accurate diagnosis and thus for the establishment of an effective therapeutic plan [11]. In the vast majority of cases, adrenal Cushing's syndrome is due to cortical adenomas and more rarely carcinomas, which are ACTH-independent conditions [12, 13]. Patients with ACTH-dependent Cushing's syndrome have either a pituitary ACTH-producing adenoma (Cushing's disease) or ectopic ACTH production associated to a neuroendocrine neoplasm that is more commonly located in the thymus, lungs, or endocrine pancreas [11, 13]. Over 80% of patients with Cushing's syndrome have an ACTH-secreting corticotroph adenoma, whereas ectopic 30 ACTH syndrome (EAS) accounts for 20% of all adult cases [11, 13]. Overall, EAS is very rare and has an incidence of 1–4 new cases per 10 million inhabitants per year and is extremely rare in young or pediatric populations [14, 15].

We present a very young patient, with severe clinical and biochemical ACTH-dependent Cushing's syndrome. The lack of cortisol suppression with the administration of 8 mg of DXM, the absence of a pituitary adenoma upon MRI, and the lack of a petrosal-to peripheral ACTH gradient pointed to an ectopic ACTH source. CT scanning of the chest and abdomen did not reveal any bronchial, thymic, or pancreatic lesions; instead and somewhat to our surprise given the patient's ACTH levels, we found a large heterogeneous right adrenal mass. Although urinary metanephrines and catecholamines were within normal limits and the adrenal mass

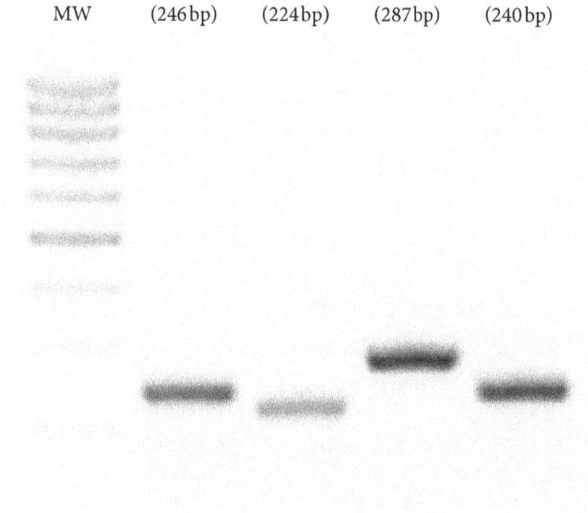

FIGURE 3: Ethidium bromide-stained agarose gel electrophoresis of RT/PCR products showing clearly defined bands corresponding to NANOG, OCT4, and SOX_2 amplicons of the expected size (RPS18: ribosomal protein S18).

did not take up MIBG, we entertained the possibility of a pheochromocytoma as the actual source of ectopic ACTH, being the only previous adrenal EAS-related tumors reported so far. The patient underwent surgical resection of the adrenal mass, which proved to be a mixed corticomedullary tumor, consisting of two distinct but intermingled populations of cells: the classical medullary cells with "zellballen" appearance arranged in nests, surrounded by sustentacular cells, and an adrenocortical component with a different phenotype and a third population showing both characteristics. It must be pointed out that our patient harbored a single primary tumor with different cell populations and not different tumors that grew enough to collide with each other, also called colliding tumors, which may be found in all sorts of publications regarding mixed tumors, and that may have different origins, pathophysiology, and outcomes. As in previously reported cases of truly MCAT tumors, the medullary component immunostained positively for the usual chromaffin markers (SNP, CgA, S-100, and CD56), and it had a clearly positive ACTH immunohistochemistry (which is a requirement to diagnose ectopic sources of ACTH). The adrenocortical carcinoma component was positive for epithelial markers such as melan-A, inhibin, and calretinin with a very high Ki-67 proliferative index of 40%, which reflects the malignant potential of the lesion. Most neuroendocrine neoplasias are well-differentiated tumors that usually report Ki-67 immunostainings of <2% and very rarely show Ki-67% over 20%. High Ki-67 and a poorly differentiated morphology classify the tumor as a grade 3 neuroendocrine carcinoma, which predicts a poor prognosis right from the beginning. On the contrary, Ki-67 values in adrenal carcinomas are quite variable, ranging from 2 to 80%, but a mitotic index of >10% is considered to be of poor prognosis factor. The proper cutoff for mitotic indexes for all endocrine tumors is still a matter of debate, but by any definition, this tumor showed an atypical behavior that could not be ignored and warranted close follow-up with laboratory and imaging even if the patient had no clinical signs of tumor recurrence. We should clarify that the patient showed biochemical recurrence a few weeks before the clinical symptoms recurred. There were no clear signs of tumor recurrence in the previous imaging study despite the frequency with which they were done, stating the fast growth and aggressiveness of the metastasis. This should remind all the interdisciplinary team members that we need more than one test to detect tumor growth and that full-blown clinical syndromes may be related to advanced disease.

We considered the possibility of the presence of a stem cell origin due to the atypical tumor pathology and behavior as well as the reports of higher frequencies of stem cell tumors in the pediatric population. The adrenocortical niche is complex, and some aspects of its development have been studied recently. Alterations in these mechanisms are associated with pediatric adrenal tumors, including stem cells. Pediatric adrenal tumors are usually detected in the first few years of life, but this patient would still be considered as a teenager or a young adult. She may be old for the classical pediatric tumor, but she is considerably young for the classical adult presentation which is over 50 years of age. Guidelines for many neoplasias, including endocrine neoplasias, consider the existence of "atypical tumors," which may warrant further suspicion and evaluations. They may be defined as atypical if they are large, multihormonal, multicentric, or without classical risk factors for their presentation. The definition may change for every organ and pathology. This definition includes most mixed pathology tumors.

Mixed corticomedullary tumors are extremely rare, including the present one, and there are only 26 cases reported in the English literature since its initial description in 1969 by Mathison et al. [16]. However, the medullary component has usually been reported as a benign pheochromocytoma [17], and the adrenocortical component can be either an adenoma [1–3, 6, 7, 9] or a carcinoma [4, 5, 8]. There have been only 3 previously reported cases of malignant, mixed adrenocortical tumors [4, 5, 8]. In one of these cases [4], the medullary and cortical tum or cells appeared to collide with each other, whereas in the other two patients [5, 8], like in our case, the two cell populations do not collide but are intermingled instead. Interestingly, none of these three patients presented with clinical signs or symptoms of hypercortisolism, in contrast to our patient who had severe clinical and biochemical, ACTH-dependent Cushing syndrome.

The coexistence of cortical and medullary cells was demonstrated by double-labeling IHC using antibodies against CgA and inhibin. Interestingly, a few of these cells positively immunostained for both markers, which prompted us to hypothesize that this mixed tumor may have arisen from a common pluripotential stem cell. After confirming that the tumor expressed its mRNAs by means of RT/PCR, we performed immunofluorescence studies using antibodies against OCT4, NANOG, and SOX2. The tumor immunostained for these three antigens which are considered to be cancer stem cell biomarkers, since they are critical regulators of self-renewal and pluripotency of embryonic

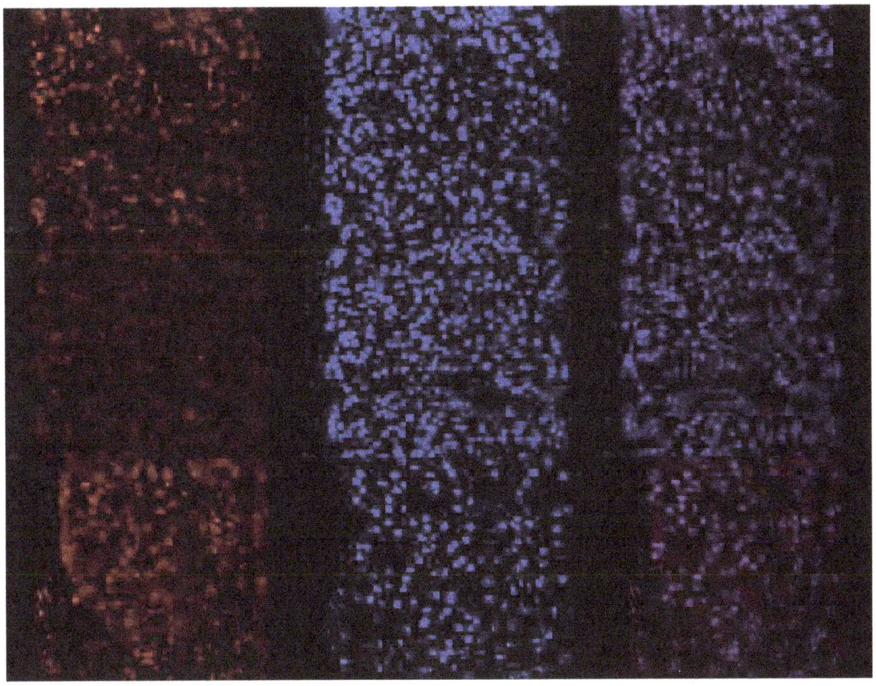

FIGURE 4: Immunofluorescence staining showing NANOG nuclear reactivity; OCT4 reactivity is predominantly nuclear and scant in the cytoplasm; SOX_2 immunoreactivity is localized to both nucleus and cytoplasm (Cy3: cyanine dye; DAPI: 4',6-diamidino-2-fenilindol).

stem cells, and thus can regulate proliferation and differentiation [18, 19]. OCT4 is a POU domain transcription factor that promotes epithelial-mesenchymal transition and inhibits apoptosis through the regulation of miR125B-BAK1 pathways [19]. SOX_2 is involved in the control of cell proliferation, apoptosis, invasion, migration, and metastases in various cancers by promoting epithelial-mesenchymal transition, upregulating WNT/beta-catenin, and downregulating AMPK/mTOR pathways [18]. NANOG contributes to carcinogenesis by activating and preserving cancer stem cell properties; it regulates signaling pathways such as STAT3/Snail [20, 21]. OCT4 has a characteristic nuclear staining pattern specific for germ cell neoplasms [22]. Cytoplasmic expression of OCT4 has been described in metastatic pheochromocytomas and in moderately differentiated neuroendocrine tumors [23] but has not been reported before in adrenocortical carcinomas.

ACTH is known to be synthesized by the chromaffin cells of the adrenal medulla and to participate in complex intraglandular autocrine and paracrine loops regulating steroidogenesis in the adrenal cortex [24]. Although exceedingly rare, pheochromocytomas have been known to be a potential source of ectopic ACTH, and only 58 such cases have been reported in the English medical literature between 1977 and 2018 [10, 17]. In most of these patients, the contralateral adrenal gland looks grossly hyperplastic on imaging studies and is most likely the origin of the excessive cortisol secretion; however, contralateral atrophy has also been reported in pheochromocytomas with ectopic production of ACTH. Although many case reports and series do not always make a point of mentioning this, some published cases show similar behavior to that of our patient.

Interestingly, several recent reports of mixed corticomedullary tumors describe the tomographic characteristics of the affected gland but omit describing the state of the contralateral adrenal [7, 8, 17]. However, a direct comparison with other mixed tumors is not possible since the other case reports did not undergo dynamic testing to prove an ectopic ACTH source.

The true reason why the contralateral gland is not enlarged despite the presence of an ectopic source of ACTH cannot be proven at this point. The authors have considered some hypotheses in this regard:

(1) Some of the circulating ACTH may correspond to fragments or inactive ACTH, which has been reported as a common consequence of the faulty mRNA processing and peptide secretory mechanisms of these tumors. These isoforms cannot be detected by our assay.

(2) The glucocorticoid excess may have been present for a longer time, but it may have been insidious or "subclinical" for some weeks or months before the aggressive clinical presentation was detected. Since adrenal glands can change their morphology rapidly (in the course of days to weeks) according to the cholesterol deposits, their metabolic activity and the present stimuli, even a few weeks of hypercortisolism, may cause atrophy in some glands.

(3) The atrophic adrenal gland may be indicative of a persistent and obvious effect of systemic hypercortisolism, while the nonsuppressed ACTH can be related to ACTH dependence, but not necessarily to its trophic effects. We could expect to see less local

effects of the ACTH in the smaller gland if the excessive cortisol signals (atrophy) were stronger than the ACTH signals (hypertrophy).

(4) One atrophic gland is also suggestive of the fact that we were not dealing with a case of bilateral macronodular adrenal hyperplasia.

We should also comment that postoperative ACTH was not performed immediately after surgery, but a few weeks later. Immediate ACTH determination after surgery was not considered to be useful at that point due to the fact that the patient was in critical conditions after surgery and that an appropriate elevation of ACTH in response to stress and a sudden decrease of blood cortisol is expected during the first few days when a normal pituitary gland is present. It is also not possible to distinguish the ectopic ACTH from the pituitary ACTH using our assay. A normal or elevated ACTH was also to be expected after the patient was determined to be hypocortisolic in the postoperative evaluations and treatment with prednisone was started. After the morning serum cortisol came back to normal, prednisone was withdrawn, and then we determined ACTH again, which came back normal or slightly elevated, until the presence of the liver metastasis, when it became suppressed.

Despite having received radiation therapy, but to some extent, expectedly, Cushing's syndrome recurred 16 months after surgery, along with the appearance of new hepatic lesions, likely corresponding to metastases. Although the primary tumor was clearly an ACTH-dependent lesion, such dependency was lost once it became metastatic. It was decided not to biopsy these liver lesions because at this point, the patient was receiving only palliative care. Nevertheless, we concluded based on the patient's hormonal profile that they were hormonally active, secreting cortisol and perhaps androgens in an autonomous, ACTH-independent fashion. Supporting the latter is the fact that the contralateral gland looked somewhat hypoplastic on imaging studies. It is interesting to speculate that the medullary component of this mixed tumor seems to require the adrenal microenvironment to produce a biologically active ACTH that would act in a paracrine/autocrine fashion, stimulating steroidogenesis. We believe that the ectopic ACTH produced by the mixed adrenal tumor acted mostly inside the same adrenal gland in a paracrine manner. The affected gland was enlarged and was the only one producing adrenal steroids, while the other one was suppressed. This suppression could explain the atrophy seen in the contralateral adrenal gland and the transient hypocortisolism seen after adrenalectomy. It also supports the idea that the liver metastases were functioning and ACTH independent. We did not find any other MCAT case reports where ectopic ACTH dependency was completely ruled out by a prolactin-controlled petrous sinus sampling and 3 Tesla, contrasted, and dynamic MRI imaging, but we found some reports where ACTH was abnormally normal (nonsuppressed) or high. These tumors might also have ectopic ACTH production, but they were not tested for it. According to several guidelines, complete hormonal workup is mandatory for all adrenal tumors suspicious for malignancy; screening studies should be followed by appropriate endocrine dynamic tests when necessary. Despite the presence of endocrine dysfunction and the worse outcomes reported for functioning tumors, specialized testing is still underused by many specialists. It has also been shown that a thorough evaluation of atypical cases helps to enlighten the pathophysiology of more common cases, although more cases need to replicate these findings in order to study other hypotheses.

In conclusion, we have described the case of a young woman with a MCAT, consisting of cells with pheochromocytoma and adrenocortical carcinoma features. We have identified by double-labeling immunohistochemistry the presence of a few cells within the tumor that immunostained for both cortical and medullary antigens, which together with the positive immunofluorescence for cancer stem cell biomarkers (OCT4, NANOG, and SOX-2) points towards the involvement of primitive embryonic cells as the origin of this neoplasm.

Abbreviation

ACTH:	Adrenocorticotropic hormone
AMPK:	Activated protein kinase
CgA:	Chromogranin A, biomarker for neuroendocrine cells
CT Scan:	Computed tomography scan
DHEA-s:	Dehydroepiandrosterone sulfate
EAS:	Ectopic ACTH syndrome
FSH:	Follicle-stimulating hormone
HE or H&E:	Hematoxylin eosin
IHC:	Immunohistochemistry
LH:	Luteinizing hormone
MCAT:	Mixed corticomedullary adrenal tumors
MIBG:	Metaiodobenzylguanidine
MRI:	Magnetic resonance imaging
mRNA:	Messenger ribonucleic acid
mTOR:	Mammalian target of rapamycin
NANOG:	Tír Na nÓg, an homeobox transcription factor named after the Irish legend of Oisín
OCT4:	Octamer-binding transcription factor 4
PRA:	Plasmatic renin activity
PS-100:	Protein S 100, biomarker for a nerve sheet origin
RT/PCR:	Real-time polymerase chain reaction
SN:	Synaptophysin
SOX_2:	Transcription factor sex-determining region Y-box 2
STAT3:	Signal transducer and activator of transcription 3
UFC:	Urinary free cortisol
WNT:	Portmanteau of the wingless and int genes, stands for wingless-related integration site
99Tc-HYNIC:	99metastableTechnetium-ethylenodiamine–N-N' diacetic acid-HYNIC-TOC [D-Phe1, Tyr3-Octreotide].

References

[1] J. A. Wienecke, L. D. Thompson, and C. S. Heffess, "Corticomedullary mixed tumor of the adrenal gland," *Annals of Diagnostic Pathology*, vol. 5, no. 5, pp. 304–308, 2001.

[2] A. Y. Chu, V. A. LiVolsi, D. L. Fraker, and P. J. Zhang, "Corticomedullary mixed tumor of the adrenal gland with concurrent adrenal myelolipoma," *Archives of Pathology & Laboratory Medicine*, vol. 127, no. 8, pp. e329–e332, 2003.

[3] K. I. Alexandraki, O. P. Michail, A. Nonni et al., "Corticomedullary mixed adrenal tumor: case report and literature review," *Endocrine Journal*, vol. 56, no. 6, pp. 817–824, 2009.

[4] A. Fassina, R. Cappellesso, F. Schiavi, and M. Fassan, "Concurrent pheochromocytoma and cortical carcinoma of the adrenal gland," *Journal of Surgical Oncology*, vol. 103, no. 1, pp. 103-104, 2011.

[5] A. Turk, H. Asad, J. Trapasso, G. Perilli, and V. LiVolsi, "Mixed corticomedullary carcinoma of the adrenal gland: a case report," *Endocrine Practice*, vol. 18, no. 3, pp. e37–e42, 2012.

[6] G. Donatini, S. Van Slycke, S. Aubert, and B. Carnaille, "Corticomedullary mixed tumor of the adrenal gland-a clinical and pathological chameleon: case report and review of literature," *Updates in Surgery*, vol. 65, no. 2, pp. 161–164, 2013.

[7] G. E. Park, Y. Y. Cho, Y. S. Hong et al., "A functioning adrenal adenoma and pheochromocytoma in the same adrenal gland: two discrete adrenal incidentalomas," *The Korean Journal of Internal Medicine*, vol. 30, no. 1, pp. 114–117, 2015.

[8] M. B. Alsabek, R. Alhmaidi, B. Ghazzawi, G. Hamed, and A. Alseoudi, "Mixed corticomedullary adrenal carcinoma–case report: comparison in features, treatment and prognosis with the other two reported cases," *International Journal of Surgery Case Reports*, vol. 31, pp. 254–261, 2017.

[9] L. Duan, F. Fang, W. Fu et al., "Corticomedullary mixed tumour resembling a small adrenal gland-involvement of cancer stem cells: case report," *BMC Edocrine Disorders*, vol. 17, no. 1, p. 9, 2017.

[10] H. Falhammar, J. Calissendorff, and C. Höybye, "Frequency of Cushing's syndrome due to ACTH-secreting adrenal medullary lesions: a retrospective study over 10 years from a single center," *Endocrine*, vol. 55, no. 1, pp. 296–302, 2017.

[11] L. K. Nieman, B. M. K. Biller, J. W. Findling et al., "The diagnosis of Cushing's syndrome: an endocrine society clinical practice guideline," *The Journal of Clinical Endocrinology & Metabolism*, vol. 93, no. 5, pp. 1526–1540, 2008.

[12] A. Lacroix, R. A. Feelders, C. A. Stratakis, and L. K. Nieman, "Cushing's syndrome," *The Lancet*, vol. 386, no. 9996, pp. 913–927, 2015.

[13] A. K.-Y. Lam, "Update on adrenal tumours in 2017 World Health Organization (WHO) of endocrine tumours," *Endocrine Pathology*, vol. 28, no. 3, pp. 213–227, 2017.

[14] A. M. Isidori, G. A. Kaltsas, C. Pozza et al., "The ectopic adrenocorticotropin syndrome: clinical features, diagnosis, management, and long-term follow-up," *The Journal of Clinical Endocrinology & Metabolism*, vol. 91, no. 2, pp. 371–377, 2006.

[15] I. Ilias, D. J. Torpy, K. Pacak, N. Mullen, R. A. Wesley, and L. K. Nieman, "Cushing's syndrome due to ectopic corticotropin secretion: twenty years' experience at the National Institutes of Health," *The Journal of Clinical Endocrinology & Metabolism*, vol. 90, no. 8, pp. 4955–4962, 2005.

[16] D. A. Mathison and C. A. Waterhouse, "Cushing's syndrome with hypertensive crisis and mixed adrenal cortical adenoma-pheochromocytoma (corticomedullary adenoma)," *The American Journal of Medicine*, vol. 47, no. 4, pp. 635–641, 1969.

[17] J. N. Gabi, M. M. Milhem, Y. E. Tovar, E. S. Karem, A. Y. Gabi, and R. A. Khthir, "Severe cushing syndrome due to an ACTH-producing pheochromocytoma: a case presentation and review of the literature," *Journal of the Endocrine Society*, vol. 2, no. 7, pp. 621–630, 2018.

[18] D. Onichtchouk, "Evolution and functions of Oct4 homologs in non-mammalian vertebrates," *Biochimica et Biophysica Acta (BBA)*, vol. 1859, no. 6, pp. 770–779, 2016.

[19] A. Rizzino and E. L. Wuebben, "Sox2/Oct4: a delicately balanced partnership in pluripotent stem cells and embryogenesis," *Biochimica et Biophysica Acta (BBA)–Gene Regulatory Mechanisms*, vol. 1859, no. 6, pp. 780–791, 2016.

[20] L. Zhao, J. Liu, S. Chen, C. Fang, X. Zhang, and Z. Luo, "Prognostic significance of NANOG expression in solid tumors: a meta-analysis," *Oncology Targets and Therapy*, vol. 11, pp. 5515–5526, 2018.

[21] F. Yang, J. Zhang, and H. Yang, "OCT4, SOX_2, and NAN OG positive expression correlates with poor differentiation, advanced disease stages, and worse overall survival in HER2," *Oncology Targets and Therapy*, vol. 11, pp. 7873–7881, 2018.

[22] L. Cheng, M. T. Sung, Cossu-RoccaP et al., "OCT4: biological function and clinical applications as a marker of germ cell neoplasia," *The Journal of Pathology*, vol. 211, no. 1, pp. 1–9, 2007.

[23] R. E. Alexander, L. Cheng, D. J. Grignon, and M. Idrees, "Cytoplasmic staining of OCT4 is a highly sensitive marker of adrenal medullary-derived tissue," *The American Journal of Surgical Pathology*, vol. 37, no. 5, pp. 727–733, 2013.

[24] H. Lefebvre, M. Thomas, C Duprac, J. Bertherat, and E. Louiset, "Role of ACTH in the interactive/paracrine regulation of adrenal steroid secretion in physiological and pathophysiological conditions," *Frontiers in Endocrinology (Laussanne)*, vol. 7, p. 98, 2016.

9

Development and Resolution of Secondary Adrenal Insufficiency after an Intra-Articular Steroid Injection

Jia Wei Tan[1] **and Sachin K. Majumdar**[2]

[1]Department of Internal Medicine, Bridgeport Hospital, Yale New Haven Health System, Bridgeport, Connecticut, USA
[2]Department of Endocrinology, Bridgeport Hospital, Yale New Haven Health System, Bridgeport, Connecticut, USA

Correspondence should be addressed to Jia Wei Tan; jia.tan094@gmail.com

Academic Editor: Osamu Isozaki

Corticosteroid injections are commonly indicated in inflammatory conditions involving the soft tissues, tendon sheaths, bursae, and joints. Local corticosteroids carry a lower risk of complications than systemic corticosteroid but may be systemically absorbed and subsequently suppress the hypothalamic-pituitary-adrenal (HPA) axis. This can cause secondary adrenal insufficiency (SAI) as well as iatrogenic Cushing's syndrome. We report a 78-year-old female who presented with nonspecific gastrointestinal symptoms after a recent intra-articular steroid injection in her shoulder. She had hyponatremia, low morning cortisol, and failed to respond to high-dose cosyntropin. Further workup revealed the underlying cause to be SAI. Follow-up testing revealed a recovery of HPA responsiveness within 2 weeks of her initial diagnosis. *Conclusion.* Our case highlights how the hypothalamic-pituitary axis (HPA) can be suppressed with intra-articular steroids. The threshold to test corticosteroid users for adrenal insufficiency should be low in clinical practice, especially for those patients with nonspecific symptoms after steroid injections. Once diagnosed, temporary treatment with steroids may be required.

1. Introduction

One of the most common adverse effects of corticosteroid administration is secondary adrenal insufficiency (SAI) from suppression of the hypothalamic-pituitary-adrenal axis (HPA) by negative feedback. Oral and inhaled corticosteroids uses are known to cause SAI, whereas its occurrence with injectable corticosteroids is less common [1]. Local corticosteroids in the forms of inhaled, dermal, and intra-articular were developed to avoid first-pass hepatic metabolism and systemic side effects. However, studies have shown that systemic absorption and complications can occur with the use of local corticosteroids regardless of the treatment route [1]. When adrenal insufficiency is diagnosed, the HPA axis can take weeks to recover, and hence, patients may require glucocorticoid replacement therapy until full recovery of adrenal function [2, 3]. Herein, we report a 78-year-old woman with adrenal insufficiency after an intra-articular corticosteroid injection who subsequently demonstrated HPA recovery within 2 weeks of her initial diagnosis.

2. Case Report

A 78-year-old female presented to the emergency department with nausea, abdominal pain, and fatigue for three to four days. The abdominal pain was diffuse, nonremitting, and sharp in nature. It was not associated with food intake. She denied any fever, vomiting, or altered bowel habits. She received one dose of intra-articular cortisone into her left wrist 1 week prior to admission for the treatment of carpal tunnel syndrome (CTS). She also received one dose of intra-articular steroid injection in her right shoulder 2 months prior to presentation. She reported that her blood glucose levels were elevated after the steroid injection. She denied dizziness, salt craving, hypoglycemic episodes, tanning of skin or mucous membranes, or loss of weight. She has a past medical history of type 2 diabetes mellitus, insomnia, and gastroesophageal reflux disease. Medications include gabapentin, insulin, and mirtazapine.

On admission, her blood pressure was 115/69 mmHg, heart rate 68 beats/min, and she was not orthostatic. Her body mass index (BMI) was 21.03 kg/m^2. She had mild diffuse abdominal tenderness without guarding or rigidity. Blood chemistry revealed a serum sodium of 122 mmol/L (ref: 135–145 mmol/l), 126 mmol/L corrected for glucose, chloride of 87 mmol/L (ref: 98–107 mmol/L), potassium of 5.2 mmol/L (ref: 3.3–5.3 mmol/L), and glucose of 275 mg/dL. Complete blood count showed hemoglobin of 12.9 g/dL (ref 11.7–15.5 g/dL), hematocrit of 35% (ref: 35–45%), and WBC count of 5.8 × 10003/μL (ref: 4.0–11.0 × 1000/μL). Further tests revealed a serum plasma osmolality of 277 mOsm/kg (ref: 275–295 mOsm/kg), urine osmolality of 240 mOsm/kg (ref: 50–1200 mOsm/kg), urine sodium of 55 mmol/L, urine potassium of 9 mmol/L, and serum creatinine of 0.7 mg/dL (ref: 0.40–1.30 mg/dL). Her findings were consistent with euvolemic hypotonic hyponatremia.

A morning cortisol level for this patient was less than 0.5 μg/dL at 6:18 am (ref: Cortisol AM: 6.0–18.4 μg/dL). A high-dose cosyntropin stimulation test was then performed. Table 1 summarizes the findings for initial cortisol and the high-dose (250 mcg) cosyntropin test which revealed subnormal response to cosyntropin and relatively low ACTH. She was diagnosed with secondary adrenal insufficiency (SAI). The rest of the biochemical analysis, including thyroid-stimulating hormone (TSH), calcium, phosphorus, total protein albumin, lipid panel, and globulin, was within the normal range. Additional tests to evaluate adrenal function revealed an ACTH level of 8.7 pg/dl at 4.30 p.m. (ref: 7.2–63.3 pg/mL (a.m. draws), aldosterone <1 ng/dl (ref: supine 8:00–10:00 am 3–16 ng/dL), and plasma renin activity of 1.13 ng/mL/h (ref: 0.25–5.82 ng/mL/h). Her dehydroepiandrosterone sulfate (DHEA-S) was 15.1 μg/dL (ref: 35.0–430.0 μg/dL). Prolactin was 16.2 ng/mL (ref: 4.8–23.3 ng/mL), follicle-stimulating hormone was 56.6 (ref: Post-Menopausal Females: 25.8–134.8 mIU/mL), and luteinizing hormone was 33.1 mIU/mL (ref: Post-Menopausal Females: 7.7–58.5 mIU/mL). Pituitary magnetic resonance imaging (MRI) showed a 3-4-millimeter lesion in the pituitary consistent with a microadenoma. Endocrinology was consulted, and it was deemed unlikely that the microadenoma was causing adrenal suppression. The patient remained hemodynamically stable and her symptoms improved during hospitalization. Her hyponatremia and abdominal pain resolved with supportive management which include fluid restriction (1.5 liters per day) and correction of hyperglycemia. She was discharged from the hospital without steroid replacement.

One week after hospitalization, she was seen in the outpatient clinic of endocrinology and was doing well. However, she was admitted to the hospital the next day for acute gastrointestinal symptoms and was found to have a serum sodium of 118 mmol/L (ref: 136–144 mmol/L). Her random cortisol level drawn at 5:13 AM was 16.4 mcg/dL (ref: Cortisol AM: 6.0–18.4 μg/dL), 8 days after she had initially failed cosyntropin stimulation testing. Because her admitting physicians were aware of her recent diagnosis of adrenal insufficiency, she was placed on empiric hydrocortisone until she could be more completely evaluated. Once her cortisol level returned and she was reassessed clinically, hydrocortisone was discontinued and repeat stimulation testing revealed a normal response to cosyntropin (Table 2). Her symptoms were subsequently found to be primarily gastrointestinal in nature, and she revealed a history of copious water consumption at home. Therefore, her hyponatremia was better explained by nonosmotic antidiuretic hormone release due to nausea and gastrointestinal distress in combination with excess water consumption, and her adrenal insufficiency was considered transient and noncontributory to her second admission. However, concerns remained as to whether she should have been given a brief course of empiric steroids after her first admission.

3. Discussion

We report a 78-year-old woman presenting with hypotonic hyponatremia complicated by transient adrenal insufficiency most likely caused by recent intra-articular steroid injections of the wrist and shoulder. Her serum osmolality and urine sodium were elevated, indicating the effect of antidiuretic hormone (ADH). She appeared euvolemic and had normal orthostatic vital signs, thus narrowing the differential diagnosis to syndrome of inappropriate antidiuresis (SIAD), secondary adrenal insufficiency (SAI), hypothyroidism, and decreased intake of solutes (e.g., beer potomania, tea-and-toast diet). The patient was on mirtazapine, which was continued throughout hospitalization; hence, it is possible that there was a component of mirtazapine-induced SIAD. She appeared well nourished and lacked features of severe hypothyroidism, and her serum albumin and TSH were in normal ranges. Given her history of intra-articular steroid injections, serum cortisol and cosyntropin testing were ordered revealing evidence of SAI. Her serum aldosterone level was low, raising the possibility of primary adrenal insufficiency (PAI). However, her clinical picture is inconsistent with PAI as her blood pressure was mildly elevated, and her serum potassium and acid-base status were normal. She was on losartan which may possibly explain her low aldosterone level. Her ACTH and DHEA-S were low, consistent with SAI.

SAI is the most common form of adrenal insufficiency, and it is commonly seen with exogenous steroid administration and their subsequent withdrawal [5]. Cortisol exhibits negative feedback on the release of corticotropin-releasing hormone (CRH), ACTH, and ADH [6]. Exogenous corticosteroids can result in suppression of the HPA axis that may last after the offending agent is discontinued, and since cortisol levels may remain low, the usual suppressive effect on ADH may also be absent. Therefore, ADH levels can be elevated in adrenal insufficiency resulting in diminished free water excretion and predisposition to hyponatremia, particularly when water is consumed in excess, as occurred with our patient. Cortisol secretion is diurnal, and a low morning cortisol level is indicative of adrenal insufficiency. However, levels at other times lack

Table 1: Initial admission cosyntropin stimulation test.

	ACTH level [7.2–63.3 pg/mL (a.m. draws)]	AM cortisol (6.0–18.4 μg/dL)	After 30 minutes (μg/dL)	After 60 minutes (μg/dL)	The next day AM ACTH (7.2–63.3 pg/mL)
Baseline	8.7	<0.5			1.6
Cosyntropin stimulation			5.3	7.7	

Table 2: Second admission (8 days after initial cosyntropin testing) cosyntropin stimulation test.

	ACTH level* [7.2–63.3 pg/mL (a.m. draws)]	AM cortisol* (6.0–18.4 μg/dL)	After 30 minutes** (μg/dL)	After 90 minutes** (μg/dL)
Baseline	14.4	16.4		
Cosyntropin stimulation			8.1	14.5

*8 days after initial cosyntropin stimulation test. **11 days after initial cosyntropin test, blood drawn late so second result is at 90 minutes. Our laboratory uses the Roche Diagnostics Elecsys® cortisol II assay which results in cortisol values approximately 30% lower than prior assays. Previously a value of >18 mcg/dL was considered normal, but with the assay in use a value of >13.5 mcg/dL was adopted as a normal response [4].

diagnostic utility and might be difficult to interpret on their own. An ACTH level would differentiate between primary and secondary adrenal insufficiency [7]. A low-normal ACTH points towards SAI and warrants an MRI of the hypothalamic-pituitary area to rule out hypothalamic or pituitary lesions such as craniopharyngioma, metastasis, and pituitary adenoma [8]. DHEA-S, which is an ACTH-responsive hormone, has a long half-life (about 20 h) and less diurnal variation than cortisol [9] and can serve as an adjunct measure in the diagnosis of adrenal insufficiency. A middle to upper range of normal reference value of DHEA-S indicates that the underlying pathology is less likely due to SAI [7].

Interestingly, she revealed evidence of HPA recovery on a subsequent admission one week later. This highlights how the transient suppression of the HPA axis by exogenous steroids can complicate the diagnosis and management of steroid-associated adrenal insufficiency since the degree of morbidity caused and the time course of full HPA recovery are unclear. The distinction between transient HPA suppression and adrenal insufficiency is challenging and may confound the evaluation of patients when they present with features such as hyponatremia, hypotension, and hypoglycemia since they can indicate adrenal insufficiency as well as alternative diagnoses.

In our case, we found that patient underwent a local corticosteroid injection for CTS. There is no published literature on the association of adrenal insufficiency with a local steroid injection for CTS to date. A randomized clinical trial with a 5-yearfollow-up reported improvement in quality of life among CTS patients who received local corticosteroid injection and did not observe adverse effects of local steroid injection [10]. Therefore, we postulate that the culprit was the intra-articular corticosteroid injection that the patient received two months prior to admission but cannot exclude an effect of the recent one for CTS either.

The incidence of adrenal insufficiency is higher with intra-articular corticosteroid injections than with oral corticosteroids [52.2% (95% CI, 40.5–63.6) vs 48.7% (95% CI, 36.9–60.6)]. SAI has been reported after local corticosteroid injections into various locations including the greater trochanter, epidural space, knee, and ankle [11]. After an intra-articular triamcinolone injection, a significant decrease in serum cortisol and urine cortisol excretion was seen [12]. Postinjection, the serum cortisol was nadired in 24 hours and normalised in 7 to 14 days [12]. Duclos et al. found that 90% of the patients had adrenal insufficiency 2 days post-intra/periarticular glucocorticoid injection, and serum cortisol remained suppressed 7 and 14 days postinjection [11]. They have also found that the degree of adrenal suppression was directly proportional to the steroid dose injected. Habib et al. found that 25% of patients who received an intra-articular corticosteroid injection for the knee joint [80 mg of methylprednisolone acetate (MPA)] had adrenal suppression for at least 2 to 4 weeks postinjection, and the adrenal function recovered in all patients by week 8 [13]. Interestingly, none of the adrenal insufficiency patients were symptomatic. The group subsequently conducted a study using 6 mg of betamethasone acetate/betamethasone sodium phosphate and found that only 0.05% of the patients who received intra-articular corticosteroid injections had SAI 3 weeks postinjection [14]. Eighty mg of MPA is approximately equivalent to 15 mg of betamethasone, suggesting that the systemic absorption of steroids and subsequent risk of SAI are likely dose-dependent.

Although HPA suppression typically lasts for weeks, the duration could be prolonged to 9 months [1]. This could be due to atrophy of the zona fasciculata and reticularis with chronic ACTH deficiency resulting in a decrease production of cortisol [15]. Given some uncertainty exists about the duration of suppression, education regarding symptoms and management of adrenal insufficiency should be given to patients who are vulnerable to adrenal crises in times of stress or illness while the HPA is suppressed.

There are no specific guidelines concerning the monitoring and evaluation of the HPA axis for recovery in the setting of SAI related to intra-articular glucocorticoid injections. Most cases are dealt with on an individual basis depending on the patient's treatment plan and most likely go undiagnosed and unnoticed. If SAI is suspected, a cosyntropin stimulation test can be performed to evaluate HPA axis recovery. Situations, where it would be reasonable to perform testing, would be in the setting of symptoms concerning for adrenal insufficiency within three months of a corticosteroid injection, in the setting of anticipated stressors such as planned surgery, or acute stressors such as illness or hospitalization, and if there is a concern for suppression prior to repeated intra-articular steroid injections. The insulin tolerance test (ITT) is another dynamic test that assesses HPA integrity. This test is contraindicated in cardiac dysrhythmias patients and requires close supervision [16]. In our case, ITT was deemed unsafe to perform on this elderly lady with multiple comorbidities who were acutely ill, especially since we had access to the cosyntropin stimulation test which is simpler and less invasive than the ITT.

The high-dose (250 μg of corticotrophin) ACTH stimulation test is supra-physiological and may miss mild forms of adrenal insufficiency, and the low-dose (1 μg of corticotrophin) ACTH stimulation testing gives results that are comparable or even more sensitive than that of high-dose testing [17, 18]. Ospina et al. found that both high- and low-dose stimulation tests had similar diagnostic accuracy in SAI. For the high-dose stimulation test, the sensitivity is 0.64 (95% CI 0.52–0.73), and the specificity is 0.93 (95% CI 0.89–0.96). For the low-dose stimulation test, the sensitivity is 0.83 (95% CI 0.75–0.89), and the specificity is 0.86 (95% CI 0.78–0.91) [19]. However, low-dose testing has not been validated in patients with acute illnesses, hypoalbuminemia, or acute hypothalamic-pituitary disorders. Furthermore, there are no commercially available preparations for the low-dose cosyntropin. There is a possibility of misdiagnosis and inconsistency in dosing due to errors in preparation since 250 mcg needs to be diluted to 1 mcg by the pharmacy on demand. Therefore, the low-dose ACTH testing is not recommended as first-line testing for adrenal insufficiency.

In conclusion, we describe a patient with transient SAI in the setting of recent corticosteroid injections who had a quick recovery of her HPA axis; however, her course was complicated by uncertainty as to how much adrenal impairment contributed to her presentation. This case illustrates the dilemma of managing patients with low cortisol levels in the weeks to months following corticosteroid injections and highlights the need for more detailed studies and clinical guidelines.

Abbreviations

HPA: Hypothalamic-pituitary-adrenal axis
SAI: Secondary adrenal insufficiency
PAI: Primary adrenal insufficiency.

Authors' Contributions

Dr. Tan wrote the manuscript, and Dr. Majumdar guided the clinical case management, review, and editing of the manuscript.

References

[1] L. H. A. Broersen, A. M. Pereira, J. O. L. Jørgensen, and O. M. Dekkers, "Adrenal insufficiency in corticosteroids use: systematic review and meta-analysis," *Journal of Clinical Endocrinology and Metabolism*, vol. 100, no. 6, pp. 2171–2180, 2015.

[2] J. H. Baek, S. K. Kim, J. H. Jung, J. R. Hahm, and J. Jung, "Recovery of adrenal function in patients with glucocorticoids induced secondary adrenal insufficiency," *Endocrinol Metab (Seoul)*, vol. 31, no. 1, pp. 153–160, 2016.

[3] S. Dinsen, B. Baslund, M. Klose et al., "Why glucocorticoid withdrawal may sometimes be as dangerous as the treatment itself," *European Journal of Internal Medicine*, vol. 24, no. 8, pp. 714–720, 2013.

[4] V. Raverot, C. Richet, Y. Morel, G. Raverot, and F. Borson-Chazot, "Establishment of revised diagnostic cut-offs for adrenal laboratory investigation using the new roche diagnostics elecsys® cortisol ii assay," *Annales d'endocrinologie*, 2016.

[5] E. Charmandari, N. C. Nicolaides, and G. P. Chrousos, "Adrenal insufficiency," *The Lancet*, vol. 383, no. 9935, pp. 2152–2167, 2014.

[6] J. K. Gjerstad, S. L. Lightman, and F. Spiga, "Role of glucocorticoid negative feedback in the regulation of HPA axis pulsatility," *Stress: The International Journal on the Biology of Stress*, vol. 21, no. 5, pp. 403–416, 2018.

[7] L. M. Gruber and I. Bancos, "Secondary adrenal insufficiency: recent updates and new directions for diagnosis and management," *Endocrine Practice*, vol. 28, no. 1, pp. 110–117, 2022.

[8] I. Bancos, S. Hahner, J. Tomlinson, and W. Arlt, "Diagnosis and management of adrenal insufficiency," *Lancet Diabetes & Endocrinology*, vol. 3, no. 3, pp. 216–226, 2015.

[9] W. Leowattana, "DHEAS as a new diagnostic tool," *Clinica Chimica Acta*, vol. 341, no. 1-2, pp. 1–15, 2004.

[10] M. Hofer, J. Ranstam, and I. Atroshi, "Extended follow-up of local steroid injection for carpal tunnel syndrome: a randomized clinical trial," *JAMA Network Open*, vol. 4, no. 10, Article ID e2130753, 2021.

[11] M. Duclos, M. Guinot, M. Colsy et al., "High risk of adrenal insufficiency after a single articular steroid injection in athletes," *Medicine & Science in Sports & Exercise*, vol. 39, no. 7, pp. 1036–1043, 2007.

[12] T. Weitoft and L. Rönnblom, "Glucocorticoid resorption and influence on the hypothalamic-pituitary-adrenal axis after intra-articular treatment of the knee in resting and mobile patients," *Annals of the Rheumatic Diseases*, vol. 65, no. 7, pp. 955–957, 2005.

[13] G. Habib, A. Jabbour, S. Artul, and G. Hakim, "Intra-articular methylprednisolone acetate injection at the knee joint and the hypothalamic-pituitary-adrenal axis: a randomized controlled study," *Clinical Rheumatology*, vol. 33, no. 1, pp. 99–103, 2014.

[14] G. Habib, S. Artul, M. Chernin, G. Hakim, and A. Jabbour, "The effect of intra-articular injection of betamethasone acetate/betamethasone sodium phosphate at the knee joint on the hypothalamic-pituitary-adrenal Axis," *Journal of Investigative Medicine*, vol. 61, no. 7, pp. 1104–1107, 2013.

[15] D. G. Gardner and D. M. Shoback, *Greenspan's Basic and Clinical Endocrinology*, McGraw-Hill Education, New York, NY, USA, 2017.

[16] A. B. Grossman, "The diagnosis and management of central hypoadrenalism," *Journal of Clinical Endocrinology and Metabolism*, vol. 95, no. 11, pp. 4855–4863, 2010.

[17] K. Tordjman, A. Jaffe, Y. Trostanetsky, Y. Greenman, R. Limor, and N. Stern, "Low-dose (1 μg) adrenocorticotrophin (ACTH) stimulation as a screening test for impaired hypothalamo-pituitary-adrenal axis function: sensitivity, specificity and accuracy in comparison with the high-dose (250 μg) test," *Clinical Endocrinology*, vol. 52, no. 5, pp. 633–640, 2000.

[18] S. R. Rose, R. H. Lustig, S. Burstein, P. Pitukcheewanont, D. C. Broome, and G. A. Burghen, "Diagnosis of ACTH deficiency," *Hormone Research in Paediatrics*, vol. 52, no. 2, pp. 73–79, 1999.

[19] N. S. Ospina, A. Al Nofal, I. Bancos et al., "ACTH stimulation tests for the diagnosis of adrenal insufficiency: systematic review and meta-analysis," *Journal of Clinical Endocrinology and Metabolism*, vol. 101, no. 2, pp. 427–434, 2016.

10

Therapeutic Challenges for Elderly Patients with Primary Hyperparathyroidism

Kenneth Sluis, Hyon Kim, Yuling He, Beatrice Wong, and Xiangbing Wang

Division of Endocrinology, Metabolism, and Nutrition, Department of Medicine, Rutgers University-Robert Wood Johnson Medical School, New Jersey, NJ 08903, USA

Correspondence should be addressed to Xiangbing Wang; wangx9@rwjms.rutgers.edu

Academic Editor: Mihail A. Boyanov

Primary hyperparathyroidism (PHPT) predominantly affects older adults, and parathyroidectomy can achieve definitive cure in symptomatic PHPT and asymptomatic meeting surgical criteria. As the population continues to age, the treatment of PHPT in octogenarians and nonagenarians presents a clinical conundrum. This case series presents the management of eight patients 85 years of age and older diagnosed with PHPT. A retrospective chart review of patients diagnosed with primary hyperparathyroidism were identified in a single institution. Those patients 85 years of age and older who were followed up for over one year were included in this case series. The literature on treatment options for this age group was also reviewed. Eight cases of PHPT patients aged 88 ± 2.5 years old with a follow-up average of 5.6 ± 4.4 years were reported in our case series. Six PHPT patients were medically managed and two PHPT patients underwent parathyroid resection. Most of the medically managed PHPT patients except for one had long-term stability of disease for over five years. The treatment of PHPT diagnosed in patients over 85 years of age presents a clinical challenge for which there is no clear consensus guideline. Our case series supports that medical therapy is a feasible option for PHPT patients over 85 years old.

1. Introduction

Primary Hyperparathyroidism (PHPT) is a common disease that increases in prevalence with advancing age. Prevalence peaks in women around 70–79 years of age (492 per 100,000) and in men over 80 years old (264 per 100,000) [1]. Most patients with PHPT initially present with asymptomatic hypercalcemia. Those that are symptomatic present with axial and extremity fractures, nephrolithiasis, and psychiatric disturbance [2]. Surgical resection of the involved glands is the standard of care for young or symptomatic patients with PHPT. Medical management is used as a bridge to surgery or in patients who refuse or cannot safely undergo surgery. Strategies include hydration with expectant management, stopping offending agents such as calcium supplementation and medications (thiazides, lithium) and using diuretics, bisphosphonates, selective estrogen receptor modulators, and cinacalcet [2]. Expectant management involves serial monitoring for worsening of symptoms without specific therapeutic intervention [3, 4].

Most of the literature on the treatment of PHPT is not age-specific. About 1.5% of patients over the age of 70 have PHPT [5]. As our population continues to age and as average life expectancy increases, the proportion of elderly patients with PHPT will also grow. Though the standard of care to manage PHPT is surgery to achieve cure, the role of surgery is less clear in the very elderly. The objective of our study is to report eight cases of PHPT patients over 85 years of age who were managed using medical or surgical treatment to elucidate differences in prognosis and outcomes.

2. Cases Presentation

We conducted a retrospective chart review of PHPT patients evaluated at Robert Wood Johnson University Hospital from January 2000 to September 2016. Our institution's IRB provided approval for our investigations. There were 556 patients diagnosed with PHPT during this time. The diagnostic criteria of PHPT included: (1) intact PTH > 65 pg/mL (normal range:

Table 1: Eight cases of PHPT in patients over age 85.

Case #	Clinical description
Case 1	An 86-year-old woman with a history of osteopenia, hyperlipidemia, and GERD was diagnosed with PHPT with a calcium level of 13 mg/dl, iPTH level of 66 pg/ml, 25OHD 34 ng/ml and creatinine 1.07 mg/dl. She underwent surgery and had successful removal of a right upper parathyroid gland. She achieved surgical cure with normalized calcium and iPTH levels. Her last calcium was 9.7 mg/dl, iPTH 12.4 pg/ml and 25OHD 54 ng/ml at her 2 year follow up visit.
Case 2	A 91-year-old woman with a history of hyperparathyroidism with parathyroidectomy of 3.5 glands 5 years ago, hypothyroidism, osteoporosis, and goiter presented with a calcium level of 11.6 and iPTH level of 500. She was diagnosed with relapse of PHPT, and was managed with cinacalcet, furosemide, and risendronate. Serum calcium was controlled for about 8 years, but creatinine started to rise. Ten years after the recurrence of PHPT, cinacalcet had to be lowered and her bisphosphonate had to be discontinued after a further increase in creatinine. She suffered a left hip fracture and a possible aspiration event during the subsequent hospitalization. She passed away from sepsis after 10 years' medical treatment of recurrence of PHPT.
Case 3	An 85-year-old woman with a history of a resected follicular Hurthle cell neoplasm presented with a calcium level of 11.5 mg/dl and iPTH of 279 pg/ml. She was diagnosed with PHPT and treated with cessation of hydrochlorothiazide, initiation of furosemide, and cinacalcet for 5 years. Cinacalcet dosage had to be increased after a year, but then subsequently discontinued due to worsening renal function (Cr 2.98–3.3 mg/dl). Five years after diagnosis her PTH level increased (483–511 pg/ml) but calcium was 10–11 mg/dL. She was hospitalized for cellulitis 6 years later and was discharged to hospice care for end-stage renal disease. She passed away at the age of 91.
Case 4	A 91-year-old man with a history of type 2 diabetes, hyperlipidemia, dementia, atrial fibrillation, and congestive heart failure was hospitalized for sepsis. He was found to have a calcium level of 11.1 mg/dl, iPTH 59 pg/ml, 24-hour calcium 203 mg, and 25OHD 26 ng/ml. He was diagnosed with PHPT. He was treated with calcitonin, oral hydration and furosemide. He was discharged to his long-term care facility. His calcium level remained normal up to 10.9 mg/dL with Cr 1.8 mg/dl at 1-year follow up.
Case 5	A 96-year-old woman with a history vitamin D deficiency, osteoporosis, and hypothyroidism was found to have a calcium level of 11.2 mg/dl, iPTH 165 pg/ml, and 24-hour urine calcium of 204 mg. A parathyroid scan showed a possible left lower pole adenoma. She refused surgery and was treated with zoledronic acid infusion for her osteoporosis. Calcium decreased to 10.2 mg/dL three years after diagnosis she was given a second zoledronic acid infusion. She was followed for 4 years and did well with serum calcium maintained from 10.2 to 10.7 md/dL and iPTH 147 pg/ml.
Case 6	An 86-year-old woman with a history of osteoporosis, hypertension and dementia was found to have a calcium level of 11.1 mg/dl, iPTH 100 pg/ml, and 25OHD 32 ng/mL. She did not tolerate bisphosphonate therapy and was treated with oral hydration, cessation of thiazide diuretic, and encouragement of physically activity. Two years after diagnosis, calcium levels were maintained in the high-normal range (10.2–10.5 mg/dl). Her dementia worsened and she suffered a left hip fracture 8 years after diagnosis. She passed away on hospice from a gangrenous wound after 8 years of expectant medical management of PHPT at age of 96.
Case 7	An 86-year-old woman with osteopenia treated with bisphosphonates and a selective estrogen receptor modulator, hypothyroidism, vitamin D deficiency and DVT was found to have a calcium level of 11.8 mg/dl, iPTH 128 pg/ml, 24-hour urine 142 mg, and 25OHD 31 ng/mL Sestamibi scan did not locate an adenoma. Expectant management with increased oral hydration, decreased milk intake, cessation of thiazides, and encouragement to increase activity was begun. Her calcium rose as high as 12.9 mg/dL but then settled to 11.2 mg/dL on subsequent measurement. She was followed without incident for 3 years.
Case 8	An 89-year-old woman with a history of hypothyroidism was found with a calcium level of 11.5 mg/dl, iPTH 95 pg/ml and 25OHD 24.6 ng/mL. She was asymptomatic and was managed expectantly with oral hydration and increased physical activity. Calcium was maintained from 10.2to 10.9 mg/dL and PTH 77–107 pg/ml. She was hospitalized for hypertensive urgency but otherwise had no sequelae for 6 years.

Note: PHPT = Primary hyperparathyroidism, iPTH = Intact parathyroid hormone, 25OHD = 25 hydroxyvitamin D.

10–65 pg/mL) or inappropriately normal levels in the presence of elevated serum calcium, (2) serum calcium > 10.6 mg/dL (normal range: 8.5–10.4 mg/dL), and (3) 24-hour urinary calcium > 100 mg/day (normal range: 100–250 mg/day). Eight PHPT patients aged 85 years and older with follow-up duration longer than one year were included for this study. Patient demographics, baseline characteristics, clinical presentation and overall clinical follow-up were examined.

Eight patients diagnosed with PHPT at the age of 85 years or older were included. The average age at diagnosis was 88 ± 2.5 years old. The average follow-up duration was 5.6 ± 4.4 years. The average calcium was 11.3 ± 0.78 mg/dL, iPTH was 166 ± 154 pg/mL and 24-hour urine calcium was 183 ± 35.5 mg at the time of diagnosis. All eight patients met guidelines [2, 5] for surgery by the serum calcium levels >1 mg/dl upper limit of normal, creatinine clearance <60 cc/min or *T*-score <2.5 (Table 1). Six PHPT patients were medically managed for one to eight years and two PHPT patients underwent parathyroid resection. The surgical group had a pre-operative serum calcium of 12.3 mg/dL while the medically managed group had an average of 10.9 mg/dL. For two patients treated surgically, one patient was cured with normal calcium and PTH levels but was only followed up for two years. One patient had recurrence of PHPT five years after surgery and required medical management with cinacalcet, loop diuretic, and bisphosphonate for ten years. Six patients were managed medically for an average of 5.2 years with minimal complications. Only one of the six patients experienced PHPT-related mortality. This patient had severe dementia, was on medical treatment for eight years, and passed away on hospice after a hip fracture. Of the other medically managed patients, three patients were managed with pharmaceutical therapy, one with bisphosphonate and two with cinacalcet. Two other patients were treated with nonpharmaceutical expectant management, which included oral hydration, discontinuation of HCTZ and maintaining physical activity. They had favorable outcomes after three to six years.

Patient vignettes are demonstrated in Table 1.

3. Discussion

The Endocrine Society consensus guidelines recommend parathyroidectomy for both symptomatic and asymptomatic PHPT. Surgery is readily offered for biochemical cure in younger, symptomatic or asymptomatic patients with PHPT meeting surgical criteria [2]. The benefits of parathyroidectomy include advantages in survival, increased bone density, reduced fatigue, and other subjective measures [6, 7].

Much of the current literature advocates for more aggressive surgical therapy for the elderly. However, the benefit of surgery at achieving cure for octogenarians and nonagenarians is less straightforward than for the young. There is increased risk for complications, prolonged operation time and increased length of stay in hospitals for patients over the age of 80 years [7, 8]. As our understanding of PHPT has evolved, different phenotypes of the disease have been recognized, the symptoms of which can be confounded by the aging process in this population [9]. Studies have shown that medically managed patients with PHPT could have stable disease for over ten years [9, 10]. Our expanded case series supports medical management as a reasonable option in the very elderly, especially those with comorbidities.

Literature in favor of medical management of the very old shows promise despite its smaller scope. Khan et al. [4] and Marcocci et al. [11] reviewed the rationale and evidence behind medical management and expectant monitoring. They found that medical management can be effective, and that patients' quality of life can be similar to those treated surgically. Jacobs et al. [3] described four patients with PHPT aged 79 to 87 years treated with medical management as a bridge to surgery or as sole therapy in poor surgical candidates or those refusing surgery. They employed saline hydration, pamidronate and cinacalcet. Medical therapy was a successful bridge to surgical cure with parathyroidectomy for two patients after two weeks to two months of treatment. Medical therapy was not tolerated for another and pursued indefinitely for the final patient. Wong reported two PHPT patients over the age of 90 treated with oral rehydration, bisphosphonate or cinacalcet. They experienced no PHPT related complications or fractures in a follow-up duration of seven months to four years [12].

The limitations of our study include small sample size and short duration of follow-up. One patient had baseline dementia, and 3 nonagenarian patients passed away after 6–10 years follow up, we did not have the data and therefore cannot compare quality of life, cognitive and muscle function before and after intervention.

In summary, our data suggest that medical therapy is a reasonable option for PHPT patients over 85 years old. As life expectancy increases and more patients are diagnosed with PHPT later in life, further consensus guidelines may need to specifically address treatment recommendations for patients over the age of 85 years. Studies with larger patient populations and randomized controlled trials are needed to support our findings.

References

[1] M. W. Yeh, P. H. Ituarte, H. C. Zhou et al., "Incidence and prevalence of primary hyperparathyroidism in a racially mixed population," *The Journal of Clinical Endocrinology & Metabolism*, vol. 98, no. 3, pp. 1122–1129, 2013.

[2] J. P. Bilezikian, M. L. Brandi, R. Eastell et al., "Guidelines for the management of asymptomatic primary hyperparathyroidism: summary statement from the fourth international workshop," *The Journal of Clinical Endocrinology & Metabolism*, vol. 99, no. 10, pp. 3561–3569, 2014.

[3] L. Jacobs, M. M. Samson, H. J. Verhaar, and H. L. Koek, "Therapeutic challenges in elderly patients with symptomatic hypercalcemia caused by primary hyperparathyroidism," *The Netherlands Journal of Medicine*, vol. 70, no. 1, pp. 35–38, 2012.

[4] A. Khan, A. Grey, and D. Shoback, "Medical management of asymptomatic primary hyperparathyroidism: proceedings of the third international workshop," *Journal of Clinical Endocrinology & Metabolism*, vol. 94, no. 2, pp. 373–381, 2009.

[5] H. Chen, S. Parkerson, and R. Udelsman, "Parathyroidectomy in the elderly: do the benefits outweigh the risks?" *World Journal of Surgery*, vol. 22, no. 6, pp. 531–536, 1998.

[6] J. Bollerslev, S. Jansson, C. L. Mollerup et al., "Medical observation, compared with parathyroidectomy, for asymptomatic primary hyperparathyroidism: a prospective, randomized trial," *The Journal of Clinical Endocrinology & Metabolism*, vol. 92, no. 5, pp. 1687–1692, 2007.

[7] G. B. Talpos, H. G. Bone3rd, M. Kleerekoper et al., "Randomized trial of parathyroidectomy in mild asymptomatic primary hyperparathyroidism: patient description and effects on the SF-36 health survey," *Surgery*, vol. 128, no. 6, pp. 1013–1021, 2000.

[8] D. C. Thomas, S. A. Roman, and J. A. Sosa, "Parathyroidectomy in the elderly: analysis of 7313 patients," *Journal of Surgical Research*, vol. 170, no. 2, pp. 240–246, 2011.

[9] J. P. Bilezikian, "Primary hyperparathyroidism," *The Journal of Clinical Endocrinology & Metabolism*, vol. 103, no. 11, pp. 3993–4004, 2018.

[10] M. R. Rubin, J. P. Bilezikian, D. J. McMahon et al., "The natural history of primary hyperparathyroidism with or without parathyroid surgery after 15 years," *The Journal of Clinical Endocrinology & Metabolism*, vol. 93, no. 9, pp. 3462–3470, 2008.

[11] C. Marcocci, J. Bollerslev, A. A. Khan, and D. M. Shoback, "Medical management of primary hyperparathyroidism: proceedings of the fourth international workshop on the management of asymptomatic primary hyperparathyroidism," *The Journal of Clinical Endocrinology & Metabolism*, vol. 99, no. 10, pp. 3607–3618, 2014.

[12] B. Wong and X. Wang, "Treatment of nonagenarians with primary hyperparathyroidism," *Journal of the American Geriatrics Society*, vol. 64, no. 10, pp. e112–e113, 2016.

11

Laparoscopic Bilateral Adrenalectomy in a Young Female Patient with Recurrent Cushing's Disease

W. G. P. Kanchana,[1] P. A. D. M. Kumarathunga,[2] Gajawathana Shakthilingham,[2] Charles Antonypillai,[2] Sonali Gunatilake,[2] D. D. Karunasagara,[1] T. Jayasingharachchi,[3] V. Pinto,[3] and K. B. Galketiya[1]

[1]*Department of Surgery, Teaching Hospital Peradeniya, Kandy, Sri Lanka*
[2]*Diabetes and Endocrine Clinic, National Hospital Kandy, Kandy, Sri Lanka*
[3]*Department of Anaesthesiology, Teaching Hospital Peradeniya, Kandy, Sri Lanka*

Correspondence should be addressed to W. G. P. Kanchana; pulasthi@live.com

Academic Editor: Mihail A. Boyanov

Introduction. Synchronous bilateral adrenalectomy is undertaken less often due to numerous perioperative challenges and rare circumstances of patients needing this procedure. Bilateral adrenalectomy is an important second-line option for patients with persistent or recurrent hypercortisolism following transsphenoidal surgery for Cushing's disease. Here, we present a challenging case of synchronous laparoscopic bilateral adrenalectomy for a young female patient with recurrent Cushing's disease and fertility wishes. *Case Presentation.* A 21-year-old recently married patient who was diagnosed with Cushing's disease with a pituitary microadenoma had undergone two attempts of transsphenoidal excision of the pituitary tumour. Follow-up evaluation showed an unresectable residual tumour with invasion of the intracavernous part of the left internal carotid artery. As the patient had the hypothalamic-pituitary-ovarian axis intact with strong fertility wishes, she was offered bilateral adrenalectomy instead of radiotherapy. She was prepared for the surgery with close perioperative support from the endocrinology and anaesthesia teams. Intravenous hydrocortisone infusion was started at the induction of anaesthesia. Transperitoneal approach was used with the patient positioned in left and right lateral positions for right and left glands, respectively. A meticulous surgical technique was used for the identification of adrenal veins to clip them before division followed by handling of the glands. The patient had minimal haemodynamic disturbances during surgery. Intraoperative blood loss was less than 100 ml, and operative time was 220 minutes. She had a gradual recovery following postoperative respiratory distress due to basal atelectasis and consolidation. Cortisol levels were less than 20 nmol/L postoperatively, suggesting successful surgical intervention. Two months after surgery, she continued on maintenance therapy of oral hydrocortisone and fludrocortisone and was encouraged to go ahead with pregnancy. *Conclusion.* Although bilateral adrenalectomy is considered a high-risk procedure, these risks can be mitigated and performed safely while maintaining close multidisciplinary perioperative support.

1. Introduction

Synchronous bilateral adrenalectomy is undertaken less often due to numerous perioperative challenges and rare circumstances of patients needing this procedure [1]. Bilateral adrenalectomy is an important second-line option for patients with persistent or recurrent hypercortisolism following transsphenoidal surgery for Cushing's disease [2]. Other indications for bilateral adrenalectomy include ectopic ACTH-dependent Cushing's syndrome, adrenocortical hyperplasia, bilateral adrenal adenomas, and bilateral pheochromocytomas [3]. A majority of bilateral adrenalectomies are being done on Cushing's disease patients as seen in several case series [1, 3, 4].

Cushing's disease causes ACTH- (adrenocorticotropic hormone-) dependent rise in cortisol levels due to pituitary macro- or microadenoma. First-line therapy is transsphenoidal excision of the pituitary tumour. Persistent or recurrent Cushing's disease after transsphenoidal excision is often treated medically or by radiotherapy when the residual pituitary tumour is unresectable. Patients with failed medical therapy and fertility wishes which preclude radiotherapy are selected for bilateral adrenalectomy which aims to halt cortisol production and its effects [5].

Here, we present a challenging case of synchronous laparoscopic bilateral adrenalectomy for a young female patient with recurrent Cushing's disease and fertility wishes.

2. Case Presentation

A 21-year-old recently married female patient was evaluated for weight gain, oligomenorrhoea, and hirsutism which progressed over a duration of 2 years. She had a typical Cushingoid appearance and elevated blood pressure on examination. Her visual field assessment was normal. Overnight dexamethasone suppression test (ODST) and low-dose dexamethasone suppression test (LDST) failed to suppress the HPA (hypothalamic-pituitary-adrenal) axis confirming the diagnosis of Cushing's syndrome (CS). Subsequent evaluation revealed elevated ACTH levels and a 9.6 mm × 6.7 mm nonenhancing lesion in the pituitary fossa (pituitary microadenoma) leading to a diagnosis of Cushing's disease (CD).

She underwent transsphenoidal excision of the pituitary microadenoma in May 2018, which resulted in remission. Histology was suggestive of a pituitary lesion with strong cytoplasmic positivity to ACTH. Follow-up revealed recovery of HPA axis within 6 months to preoperative values. Re-evaluation at 1 year revealed nonsupressed ODST and LDST with MRI evidence of recurrent tumour in the pituitary fossa with left-side cavernous sinus invasion confirming recurrent Cushing's disease (Figure 1).

She underwent repeated transsphenoidal excision of the pituitary tumour in August 2019. Histology was consistent with a pituitary adenoma with strong cytoplasmic staining for ACTH. No malignant features were seen in the histology, and the Ki-67 index was 8 to 10%. The immediate postoperative evaluation revealed persistently high ACTH and cortisol levels suggestive of persistent Cushing's disease. MRI showed residual tumour measuring 9 × 10 × 12 mm in size after 4 months from surgery with invasion of the intracavernous part of the left internal carotid artery.

At this point, with an unresectable residual pituitary tumour and medical management failing to control hypercortisolism, she was left with either radiotherapy or bilateral adrenalectomy for control of hypercortisolism. Since she had the hypothalamic-pituitary-ovarian axis intact with strong fertility wishes, she was offered bilateral adrenalectomy. Her preoperative ultrasound scan showed prominent bilateral adrenal glands.

She was prepared for surgery with close perioperative support from the endocrinology and anaesthesia teams. Particular attention was given to pulmonary prehabilitation, blood pressure, and blood sugar control. Intravenous hydrocortisone was initiated at the induction of anaesthesia and continued as an infusion.

She was initially operated on the left lateral position for the right adrenal gland. We employed the Veress needle technique with 5-port entry. The liver was retracted to expose the hepatorenal pouch. Blunt and sharp dissection continued to expose the inferior vena cava (IVC) and the upper pole of the right kidney. The right adrenal gland was identified. Dissection continued in the right side of the IVC and behind the IVC, separating the right adrenal gland from the IVC. The adrenal vein was identified above the level of the renal vein and clipped before division. The right adrenal gland was dissected off from the upper pole of the kidney and perinephric fat using ultrasonic shears and by bipolar diathermy. The specimen was delivered in a bag. Port sites were closed with a drain at the hepatorenal pouch.

The patient was placed in the right lateral position for the left side procedure. The large pendulous abdomen of the patient resulted in all right-side ports being well away from the left surgical site. Thus, none of the ports used for the right side could be utilized for left side surgery (Figure 2). Veress needle technique with 5-port entry was employed. Splenic flexure was brought down by division of gastrocolic omentum and splenocolic attachments. Descending colon mobilized medially to expose the left kidney. The hilum and upper pole of the left kidney was exposed. The left renal vein, tail of the pancreas, and splenic hilum was exposed and identified using blunt and sharp dissection. The left adrenal vein originating from the left renal vein was identified and clipped before division. The left adrenal gland with surrounding perinephric fat was dissected with ultrasonic shears and bipolar diathermy. The specimen was retried in a bag. Port sites were closed with a drain at the left paracolic gutter. Figure 2 shows the large pendulous abdomen with closed port sites. The patient had minimal haemodynamic disturbances during surgery. Intraoperative blood loss was less than 100 ml, and operative time was 220 minutes.

The patient had a smooth recovery initially and was sent to ward from the intensive care unit (ICU). She developed respiratory distress and low oxygenation on the 2nd postoperative day. Pulmonary embolism was excluded with a CT pulmonary angiogram. CT showed basal atelectasis and consolidation which was treated with CPAP (continuous positive airway pressure) mask, high-flow oxygen therapy, and antibiotics. Intravenous hydrocortisone infusion was continued to support the stress response to possible chest infection. She had a gradual recovery since then and was discharged on the 10th postoperative day on oral hydrocortisone and fludrocortisone therapy.

Cortisol levels were performed on day 14 from surgery after withholding oral steroid therapy for 12 hours. Cortisol levels were less than 20 nmol/L suggestive of successful surgical intervention. Histology report showed bilateral hyperplastic adrenal glands. Two months after surgery, she continued on maintenance therapy of oral hydrocortisone and fludrocortisone and was encouraged to go ahead with pregnancy with close follow-up for the development of Nelson's syndrome.

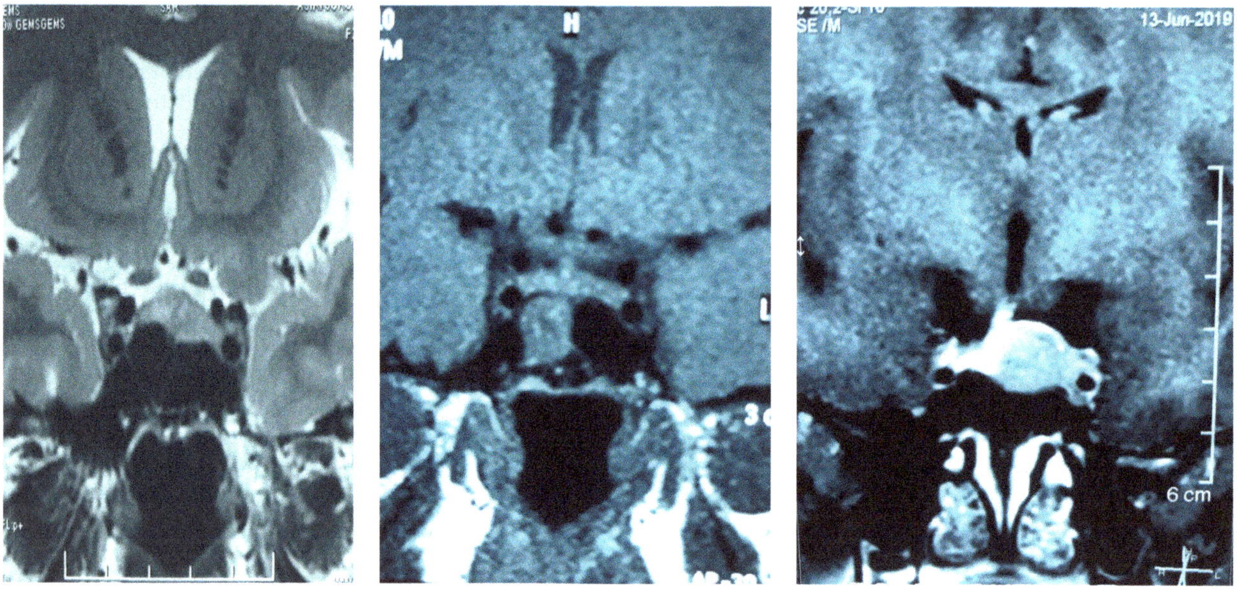

(a) (b) (c)

Figure 1: (a) 9.6 mm × 6.7 mm nonenhancing lesion in the pituitary fossa, (b) postsurgical changes with no evidence of adenoma, and (c) a 1.3 × 1.2 × 1.1 cm recurrent lesion in the left pituitary with left cavernous sinus invasion.

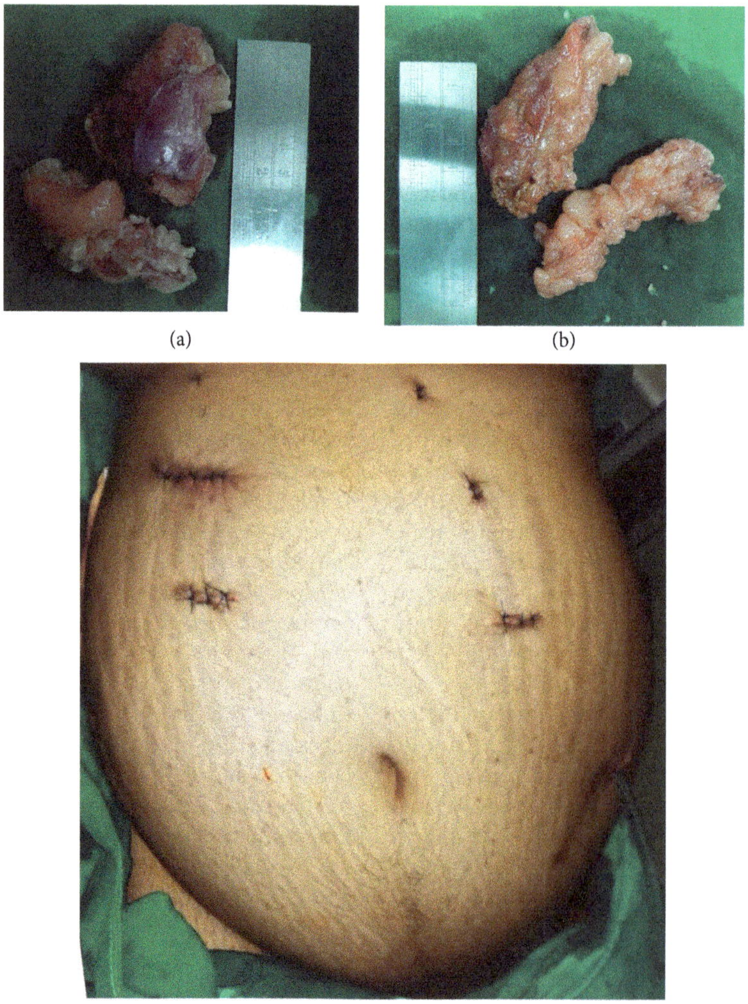

(c)

Figure 2: (a) Right adrenal gland with perinephric fat. (b) Left adrenal gland with perinephric fat. (c) Port placement and surgical wounds.

3. Discussion

Since the first laparoscopic adrenalectomy was performed in 1992 by Gagner et al., laparoscopic adrenalectomy gained increasing popularity and is considered the gold standard in modern day surgical practice as the relatively small size of the adrenal gland does not justify a large surgical wound [6]. Laparoscopic approach is advantageous in Cushingoid patients as the open approach could lead to difficult access and large surgical wounds which in turn could lead to poor pulmonary function, chest infections, and wound infections following surgery [1, 7]. Apart from wound-related complications, open bilateral adrenalectomy has shown to be associated with higher rates of intraoperative and postoperative bleeding and higher morbidity (40% vs. 13%), and mortality (5.6% vs. 2.4%) rates when compared to the laparoscopic approach [1]. The patient presented did not require narcotic analgesics from day one and was very comfortable on the following day after surgery. However, she became tachypnoeic by postoperative day two and required readmission to ICU.

Bilateral adrenalectomy presents numerous perioperative and intraoperative challenges. Preoperative control of comorbidities is of great importance as uncontrolled diabetes or hypertension could further complicate perioperative care. Preoperative medical therapy may be indicated in patients with high mean cortisol burden. Intraoperative complications including bleeding, need for conversion to open surgery, and haemodynamic disturbances due to excessive handling of the gland can be avoided when meticulous and thorough surgical techniques are used [3, 6]. Our patient was stable throughout the procedure.

Commonly employed technique in adrenal surgery is the laparoscopic transperitoneal approach [8]. This allows visualization of other intraabdominal viscera, thus achieveing better spatial orientation and control when compared with the retroperitoneoscopic approach. The retroperitoneoscopic approach could be helpful in avoiding adhesions in patients with past abdominal surgeries as well as bilateral cases. Even though studies evaluating unilateral adrenal surgery using these two techniques have demonstrated no additional benefits for the retroperitoneoscopic approach, some authors have suggested benefits in bilateral surgeries as the prone position can allow access to both surgical sites avoiding the need for repositioning of the patient [1, 8]. We used the transperitoneal approach which is the standard technique in our unit.

Adrenal crisis remains the most feared complication after bilateral adrenalectomy and requires intravenous hydrocortisone therapy until the patient can tolerate oral hydrocortisone therapy. Some authors have reported infectious and thromboembolic complication rates as high as 40% and 13%, respectively [1]. Thus, mechanical and pharmacological thromboprophylaxis is warranted until the patient is fully mobilized. Our patient developed postoperative respiratory distress for which timely investigations and interventions were instituted, leading to satisfactory patient recovery.

Patients undergoing bilateral adrenalectomies need to be assessed for the development of Nelson's syndrome as the loss of feedback inhibition on the pituitary gland can lead to flare up of the tumour. Thus, assessment of ACTH levels and pituitary fossa MRI is necessary in the follow-up [5].

4. Conclusion

Although bilateral adrenalectomy is considered a high-risk procedure, these risks can be mitigated and performed safely while maintaining close multidisciplinary perioperative support.

Additional Points

Patient Perspective. "I was worried about going for radiotherapy to treat the residual tumour as doctors explained to me that I could have problems in conceiving. This was especially sensitive issue to me as I was married for 3 years and awaiting completion of my treatments to have children. Doctors explained that removing both adrenal glands is a procedure that should not be taken lightly as it might have complications. But having discussed with my husband, I took the decision to go ahead with this surgery with the hope of having children one day. At the end I am doing well following surgery and I am happy that I took this decision."

Consent

Informed consent was taken from the patient regarding the publication of the case report.

References

[1] D. Maccora, G. Walls, G. Sadler, and R. Mihai, "Bilateral adrenalectomy: a review of 10 years' experience," *The Annals of The Royal College of Surgeons of England*, vol. 99, no. 2, pp. 119–122, 2017.

[2] A. Wong, J. A. Eloy, and J. K. Liu, "The role of bilateral adrenalectomy in the treatment of refractory Cushing's disease," *Neurosurgical Focus*, vol. 38, no. 2, p. E9, 2015.

[3] D. Malley, R. Boris, S. Kaul et al., "Synchronous bilateral adrenalectomy for adrenocorticotropic-dependent Cushing's syndrome," *JSLS: Journal of the Society of Laparoendoscopic Surgeons*, vol. 12, no. 2, pp. 198–201, 2008.

[4] M. C. Takata, E. Kebebew, O. H. Clark, and Q.-Y. Duh, "Laparoscopic bilateral adrenalectomy: results for 30 consecutive cases," *Surgical Endoscopy*, vol. 22, no. 1, pp. 202–207, 2008.

[5] H. Nishioka and S. Yamada, "Cushing's disease," *Journal of Clinical Medicine*, vol. 8, no. 11, 2019.

[6] N. Tsuru and K. Suzuki, "Laparoscopic adrenalectomy," *Journal of Minimal Access Surgery*, vol. 1, no. 4, pp. 165–172, 2005.

[7] Y. N. Pierpont, T. P. Dinh, R. E. Salas et al., "Obesity and surgical wound healing: a current review," *ISRN Obesity*, vol. 2014, Article ID 638936, 13 pages, 2014.

[8] M. J. Mellon, A. Sethi, and C. P. Sundaram, "Laparoscopic adrenalectomy: surgical techniques," *Indian Journal of Urology IJU: The Urological Society of India*, vol. 24, no. 4, pp. 583–589, 2008.

12

The Incidence of Erosive Esophagitis as a Complication of Pediatric Diabetic Ketoacidosis

Sungeeta Agrawal,[1] Serife Uysal,[2] Meghan Fredette,[3] Lisa Swartz Topor,[3] Shara R. Bialo,[3] Michael Herzlinger,[4] Jason Shapiro,[4] Linda K. Snelling,[5] Charlotte M. Boney,[6] and Jose Bernardo Quintos[3]

[1]*Division of Pediatric Endocrinology, Tufts Children's Hospital, Boston, MA, USA*
[2]*Division of Pediatric Endocrinology, Texas Children's Hospital, Houston, TX, USA*
[3]*Division of Pediatric Endocrinology and Diabetes, Rhode Island Hospital, Providence, RI, USA*
[4]*Division of Pediatric Gastroenterology, Rhode Island Hospital, Providence, RI, USA*
[5]*Division of Critical Care, Rhode Island Hospital, Providence, RI, USA*
[6]*Department of Pediatrics, Baystate Children's Hospital, Springfield, MA, USA*

Correspondence should be addressed to Jose Bernardo Quintos; jbquintos@brown.edu

Academic Editor: J. Paul Frindik

Introduction. Gastrointestinal (GI) symptoms commonly occur during diabetic ketoacidosis (DKA) and typically resolve with treatment. However, GI complications can persist after DKA resolves. The incidence of upper GI bleeding during DKA in adults has been described, with erosive esophagitis one of the most common lesions. The incidence of GI bleeding or erosive esophagitis in children with DKA has not been previously reported. We performed a retrospective chart review of DKA admissions in children 0 to <18 years with type 1 diabetes mellitus (T1DM) at a pediatric hospital between January 2009 and July 2016. Among 395 episodes of DKA over 7.5 years, erosive esophagitis occurred during two DKA admissions (0.5%) and there were no episodes of GI bleeding. *Case presentations.* Both episodes of erosive esophagitis occurred in adolescent males with known T1DM who presented with severe DKA. Both developed odynophagia after resolution of DKA and were readmitted for DKA recurrence. Upper endoscopy for both patients showed erosive esophagitis. Biopsies were negative for infection, though candida was found during one patient's endoscopy. Both had resolution of their esophagitis symptoms with medication management; neither has had recurrence. *Conclusion.* Erosive esophagitis, a rare complication of pediatric DKA, can manifest with odynophagia or substernal chest pain. This complication can lead to DKA recurrence, likely due to increased insulin resistance from inflammation and pain and from reduced oral intake and insulin administration. Patients with odynophagia associated with DKA should be monitored closely to allow timely evaluation and treatment of esophagitis.

1. Introduction

The incidence of type 1 diabetes mellitus (T1DM) is rising, and diabetic ketoacidosis (DKA) occurs in approximately 30% of children with new onset T1DM [1]. Common gastrointestinal (GI) symptoms of DKA include abdominal pain, nausea, and vomiting, and these symptoms often resolve with treatment [2]. GI complications that persist after resolution of DKA can also occur, such as pancreatitis and GI bleeding [3]. The incidence of upper GI bleeding in adults with DKA is around 9%, and erosive esophagitis is one of the most common lesions found during endoscopy [4, 5]. The incidence of GI bleeding or acute esophagitis in youth with DKA has not been reported.

The mechanisms of DKA-associated GI bleeding are unknown. Acute hyperglycemia can lead to delayed gastric emptying, resulting in reflux and mucosal damage [6]. Clinical parameters associated with increased risk of GI bleeding during DKA include longer duration of diabetes and diabetes complication such as gastroparesis [5]. Use of proton pump inhibitors and H2 receptor antagonists, suggestive of antecedent symptoms of peptic acid disease, has also been associated with increased risk of GI bleeding during DKA [5]. Laboratory values associated with increased risk of upper GI bleeding during DKA include elevated BUN, creatinine, and glucose [4, 5].

Given the lack of data about GI bleeding and esophagitis during DKA in the pediatric population, we sought to determine the incidence of these GI complications associated with DKA in pediatric patients.

2. Case Presentation

2.1. Methods. We performed a retrospective cohort study of children 0 to <18 years admitted to Hasbro Children's Hospital for pediatric DKA, between January 1, 2009, and July 31st, 2016, as previously described [7]. DKA was defined in accordance with the International Society of Pediatric and Adolescent Diabetes (ISPAD) consensus guidelines: pH ≤ 7.3 or bicarbonate ≤15 mEq/L (15 mmol/L), with blood glucose ≥200 mg/dl (11.1 mmol/L), and ketosis or ketonuria [8]. Treatment was also in accordance with ISPAD and pediatric guidelines [8, 9]. Information collected included vital signs, anthropometrics, laboratory data, past medical history, physical exam, and complications. Charts for patients with erosive esophagitis were reviewed in detail. REDCap (Research Electronic Data Capture) electronic data capture tools, hosted by Lifespan Corporation, were used to collect and manage study data [10].

2.2. Results. We identified 395 episodes of DKA over 7.5 years, with average age 12.7 years (range 0.6–17.9 years). As described previously, 214 of the 395 DKA episodes occurred in males (54%), and 176 episodes occurred in those with new onset diabetes mellitus (NODM) (45%) [7].

2.3. Cases. Erosive esophagitis occurred in two male patients (0.5%) with known T1DM who presented with severe DKA (Table 1). Neither patient had other complications of diabetes, including microalbuminuria, retinopathy, or neuropathy. Patient A presented with DKA in the setting of inadequate sick day management during illness, and he developed substernal chest pain during hospitalization. He was prescribed ranitidine and carafate and was discharged home. He was readmitted two days later with recurrent DKA and odynophagia. Patient B presented with severe DKA in the setting of a GI illness. Two days after discharge, he was readmitted for management of pancreatitis without DKA. He had abdominal pain at that time, with no episodes of emesis. Pancreatitis resolved, and he developed odynophagia over the next two weeks and was readmitted with recurrent DKA. Upper endoscopy for both patients showed erosive esophagitis. Figure 1 shows biopsy results for patient B. Biopsies were negative for infection, though brushings from patient B were positive for candida and he was treated with fluconazole. Patient A was empirically treated with fluconazole prior to his endoscopy, and his brushings were negative for candida. Neither had oral candidiasis. Both patients were discharged home on proton pump inhibitors and had resolution of their symptoms; neither has had recurrence during 4 years of follow-up.

3. Discussion

Erosive esophagitis is a rare complication of pediatric DKA and occurred in 0.5% of DKA admissions at a pediatric hospital. In both cases, the erosive esophagitis was associated with DKA recurrence. To our knowledge, this is the first study to report the incidence of erosive esophagitis in pediatric DKA.

Abnormal gastric motility may contribute to the development of erosive esophagitis during DKA. Gastroparesis is a known long-term complication of diabetes that occurs due to autonomic neuropathy and is associated with increased risk of GI bleeding during DKA [5]. Gastroparesis affects up to 50% of patients with diabetes in moderate control (both T1 and T2DM) [11]. The T1D Exchange Registry found that 4.8% of adult patients with a diabetes duration of at least 2 years were clinically diagnosed with gastroparesis [11, 12]. The incidence of gastroparesis among children with T1DM has not been reported, and neither of our patients had a diagnosis of gastroparesis. However, acute hyperglycemia can also result in delayed gastric emptying, even without the underlying diagnosis of gastroparesis [6].

Esophageal candidiasis may also contribute to risk of erosive esophagitis during DKA. One of our patients had findings of candida on endoscopy, while the other patient was treated empirically with fluconazole. In adults, diabetes mellitus is a known risk factor for esophageal candidiasis [13, 14] and has been reported in a child with poorly controlled T1DM [15]. Further studies are needed to study the role of candidal infection in esophagitis in DKA.

Both of our patients experienced erosive esophagitis in the setting of DKA recurrence. The esophagitis was likely a contributing factor to the DKA recurrence, due to increased insulin resistance from pain and inflammation [16–18], and reduced insulin administration due to decreased food intake. Therefore, while erosive esophagitis is a rare event, consequences are significant. In patients with DKA and odynophagia, we recommend clinicians consider early GI evaluation, work-up, and management. Prompt treatment can reduce pain, improve oral intake, improve insulin sensitivity, and reduce risk of DKA recurrence.

Interestingly, we did not find any episodes of GI bleeding during DKA, a complication which has been reported in adults with DM. It is possible that erosive esophagitis is a less severe presentation and that treatment prevented subsequent GI hemorrhage or that the manifestation of this type of GI complication differs in pediatric patients compared to adults. In adults with diabetes, those with peptic disease treated with acid suppression are more likely to develop a GI bleed in the setting of DM that those not requiring acid suppression, suggesting that individuals at higher risk for GI bleed may have had antecedent symptoms that led to initiation of acid suppressive therapy [5]. Thus, it is possible that patients with acid reflux symptoms prior to DKA

TABLE 1: Clinical characteristics of patients presenting with esophagitis as a complication of severe diabetes ketoacidosis.

	Patient A	Patient B
Chronologic age (yrs)	16	13
Sex	Male	Male
Diabetes duration (yrs)	7.3	3.5
HbA1c prior to admission (%, (mmol/mol))	12 (108)	7.1 (54)
Average HbA1c over the past year (%, (mmol/mol))	10.2 (88)	7.5 (58)
pH	6.9	6.9
Serum glucose (mg/dl)	217	952
HCO3 (meq/L)	<5	3
Sodium (meq/L)	138	137
Potassium (meq/L)	3	5.8
BUN (mg/dl)	13	54
Creatinine (mg/dl)	0.76	1.9
Upper GI endoscopy	Moderate to severe esophagitis in entire esophagus	Severe esophagitis in entire esophagus

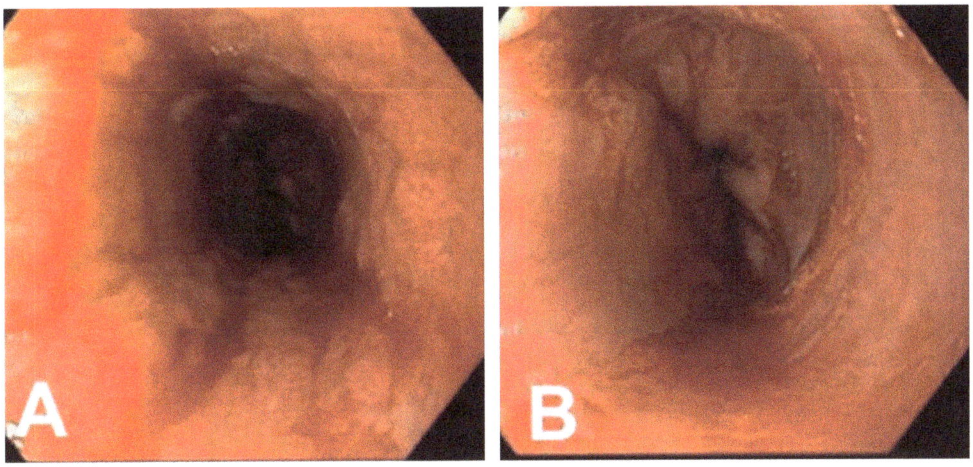

FIGURE 1: (a) Severe mucosal abnormality with erythema, friability (with spontaneous bleeding), and hemorrhagic appearance in the middle and distal esophagus. (b) Mucosal friability and sloughing in the distal esophagus (both images from Patient B).

presentation such as heartburn, dysphagia, or odynophagia may be at higher risk for GI bleeding/erosive esophagitis. As erosive esophagitis is a rare event in pediatric DKA, larger studies including multiple diabetes centers are needed to better characterize this complication of DKA.

4. Conclusion

While erosive esophagitis is a rare complication of pediatric diabetic ketoacidosis, it is associated with increased morbidity, including DKA recurrence. Patients with odynophagia or substernal chest pain during or after DKA should be evaluated for erosive esophagitis and monitored closely for recurrent ketosis and acidosis.

Abbreviations

T1DM: Type 1 diabetes mellitus
DKA: Diabetic ketoacidosis
GI: Gastrointestinal
ISPAD: International society of pediatric and adolescent diabetes
REDCap: Research electronic data capture
NODM: New onset diabetes mellitus.

References

[1] D. Dabelea, A. Rewers, J. M. Stafford et al., "Trends in the prevalence of ketoacidosis at diabetes diagnosis: the SEARCH for diabetes in youth study," *Pediatrics*, vol. 133, no. 4, pp. e938–e945, 2014.

[2] E. J. Barrett and R. S. Sherwin, "Gastrointestinal manifestations of diabetic ketoacidosis," *Yale Journal of Biology and Medicine*, vol. 56, no. 3, pp. 175–178, 1983.

[3] S. R. Bialo, S. Agrawal, C. M. Boney, and J. B. Quintos, "Rare complications of pediatric diabetic ketoacidosis," *World Journal of Diabetes*, vol. 6, no. 1, pp. 167–174, 2015.

[4] K. R. Badipatla, P. Jadhav, S. Vaddigiri et al., "Predictors of acute gastrointestinal bleeding in diabetic ketoacidosis: a retrospective observational study in minority population," *Gastroenterology Report*, vol. 5, no. 4, pp. 293–297, 2017.

[5] D. O. Faigel and D. C. Metz, "Prevalence, etiology, and prognostic significance of upper gastrointestinal hemorrhage in diabetic ketoacidosis," *Digestive Diseases and Sciences*, vol. 41, no. 1, pp. 1–8, 1996.

[6] G. S. Hebbard, M. Samsom, W. M. Sun, J. Dent, and M. Horowitz, "Hyperglycemia affects proximal gastric motor and sensory function during small intestinal triglyceride infusion," *American Journal of Physiology-Gastrointestinal and Liver Physiology*, vol. 271, no. 5, pp. G814–G819, 1996.

[7] S. Agrawal, R. Kremsdorf, S. Uysal, M. E. Fredette, and L. S. Topor, "Nephrolithiasis: a complication of pediatric diabetic ketoacidosis," *Pediatric Diabetes*, vol. 19, no. 2, pp. 329–332, 2018.
[8] J. I. Wolfsdorf, J. Allgrove, M. E. Craig et al., "Diabetic ketoacidosis and hyperglycemic hyperosmolar state," *Pediatric Diabetes*, vol. 15, no. S20, pp. 154–179, 2014.
[9] A. L. Rosenbloom, "The management of diabetic ketoacidosis in children," *Diabetes Therapy*, vol. 1, no. 2, pp. 103–120, 2010.
[10] P. A. Harris, R. Taylor, R. Thielke, J. Payne, N. Gonzalez, and J. G. Conde, "Research electronic data capture (REDCap)-A metadata-driven methodology and workflow process for providing translational research informatics support," *Journal of Biomedical Informatics*, vol. 42, no. 2, pp. 377–381, 2009.
[11] A. E. Bharucha, Y. C. Kudva, and D. O. Prichard, "Diabetic gastroparesis," *Endocrine Reviews*, vol. 40, no. 5, pp. 1318–1352, 2019.
[12] G. Aleppo, P. Calhoun, N. C. Foster, D. M. Maahs, V. N. Shah, and K. M. Miller, "Reported gastroparesis in adults with type 1 diabetes (T1D) from the T1D Exchange clinic registry," *Journal of Diabetes and Its Complications*, vol. 31, no. 12, pp. 1669–1673, 2017.
[13] N. S. SaleemIajz and O. Lodhi, "Esophageal candidiasis in a patient with uncontrolled diabetes mellitus and recurrent abdominal pain, symptomatic or incidental? A case report and brief literature review," *Journal of Medical Cases*, vol. 6, no. 11, pp. 523–526, 2015.
[14] G. A. Bartolomew, B. Rodu, and D. S. Bell, "Oral candidiasis in patients with diabetes mellitus: a thorough analysis," *Diabetes Care*, vol. 10, no. 5, pp. 607–612, 1987.
[15] A. Saeed, A. Assiri, Z. Zaidi, and A. Alsheikh, "Fungal esophagitis in a child with insulin dependent diabetes mellitus," *Journal of the College of Physicians and Surgeons—Pakistan: JCPSP*, vol. 26, no. 8, pp. 712-713, 2016.
[16] S. E. Shoelson, J. Lee, and A. B. Goldfine, "Inflammation and insulin resistance," *Journal of Clinical Investigation*, vol. 116, no. 7, pp. 1793–1801, 2006.
[17] L. Chen, R. Chen, H. Wang, and F. Liang, "Mechanisms linking inflammation to insulin resistance," *International Journal of Endocrinology*, vol. 2015, Article ID 508409, 9 pages, 2015.
[18] H. Zand, N. Morshedzadeh, and F. Naghashian, "Signaling pathways linking inflammation to insulin resistance," *Diabetes & Metabolic Syndrome: Clinical Research & Reviews*, vol. 11, no. S1, pp. S307–S309, 2017.

13

Metastatic Papillary Thyroid Carcinoma in a Paediatric Patient

Nthabiseng Ellen Mothata[1], **Takalani Gidion Morulana**[2], **Nyaweleni Tshifularo**[2], **Phumudzo Bridgett Nemutaduni**[3], **Nozipho Elizabeth Nyakale**[3], **and Moshawa Calvin Khaba**[1]

[1]*Department of Anatomical Pathology, Dr George Mukhari Academic Laboratory, National Health Laboratory Services, Sefako Makgatho Health Sciences University, Ga-Rankuwa, South Africa*
[2]*Department of Paediatric Surgery, Dr George Mukhari Academic Hospital, Sefako Makgatho Health Sciences University, Ga-Rankuwa, South Africa*
[3]*Department of Nuclear Medicine, Dr George Mukhari Academic Hospital, Sefako Makgatho Health Sciences University, Ga-Rankuwa, South Africa*

Correspondence should be addressed to Moshawa Calvin Khaba; ckhaba@yahoo.co.uk

Academic Editor: Mihail A. Boyanov

Papillary thyroid carcinoma is the most common endocrine cancer in the paediatric population. Although the disease is diagnosed at a later stage, the prognosis is favourable. When these patients present with lymph nodal and/or pulmonary metastases, they may be initially confused for infectious diseases such as tuberculosis. Therefore, thorough clinical assessment including radiology and microbiological and histopathological assessment is important for early and correct diagnosis. We report an 11-year-old female patient who presented with cervical lymphadenopathy and the histopathological assessment confirmed metastatic papillary thyroid carcinoma. Subsequent radiological investigation revealed further metastasis to the lung. This manuscript highlights the difficulties that might be encountered in the initial management of paediatric PTC which present atypically.

1. Introduction

Paediatric thyroid carcinomas are rare endocrine cancers, majority of which are comprised of papillary thyroid carcinoma (PTC) followed by follicular carcinoma [1]. They are associated with radiation exposure, thyroid disease such as Hashimoto's thyroiditis, and inherited condition such as familial adenomatous polyposis. They are more common in older children and adolescence with a female-to-male ratio of 5 : 1 [2, 3]. Approximately less than 3% of the patients have thyroid nodules which should raise a high index of suspicion for malignancy [1, 4]. A definite diagnosis is usually delayed due to the subtle presentation of the primary malignancy, and therefore, they may present late with metastatic disease [1]. The gold standard of diagnosis is histopathology. Surgery and radioactive iodine are the treatment of choice in these patients and are dependent on the risk groups [5]. Although they present with metastatic disease, the prognosis still remains good [2]. We present a paediatric patient who presented atypically with metastatic PTC to the cervical lymph nodes and lungs.

2. Case Presentation

An 11-year-old African female patient presented to paediatric surgery department with a 4 months' history of lump on the left side of the neck. She gave a history of a painless and slow-growing lump on the left side of the neck that was treated with antibiotics by several general practitioners with no improvement. She did not have any comorbidities; however, her mother has a thyroidectomy for nodular goiter. She appeared chronically ill without pallor, jaundice, or proptosis. Her vital signs were within normal limits. She had a lateral neck mass that measured $50\,mm \times 40\,mm$ which was mobile, nontender, and hard with attachment to the skin. Other systemic examinations were unremarkable. Blood investigation was within normal limits including thyroid function tests. A neck ultrasound showed an enlarged left cervical lymph node with a normal blood flow in the right and left thyroid lobes. There was a macrolobulated lesion (TIRADS 5) with increased flow and mass effect to the internal jugular vein (Figure 1(a)). A lymph node biopsy was done and confirmed a metastatic papillary thyroid carcinoma. A subsequent staging computed tomography (CT) scan showed a distinct focal peripheral mass lesion on the inferior pole of the left thyroid lobe with calcifications, mass effect on the left internal jugular vein (Figure 1(b)), and bilateral upper lung lobe nodules. An uneventful total thyroidectomy with a modified neck dissection was done and sent for histopathological assessment.

Gross pathology showed a thyroid tumour that measured 55 × 35 × 10 mm and matted lymph nodes. The tumour was unencapsulated, hemorrhagic, and firm without necrosis.

Microscopic examination confirmed papillary variant of PTC evidenced by tumour arranged in papillae, nests, and follicles (Figures 2(a) and 2(b)). These structures were lined by follicular cells with nuclei exhibiting grooves, clearing, pseudoinclusions, overlapping, and crowding. In addition, five lymph nodes that were sampled showed metastatic disease.

An iodine-123 single photon emission computed tomography (SPECT) scan done postsurgery, under high thyrotropin stimulation (>30 mU/L), showed increased nonuniform uptake in level II, III, and IV cervical lymph nodes, mild residual uptake in the thyroid bed, and increased uptake in the lungs bilaterally (Figure 3(a)). These features confirmed metastatic disease to the lymph nodes and lungs.

A left lateral lymph node clearance was done which further confirmed metastatic papillary thyroid carcinoma. Four weeks postsurgery, the patient received 100 mCi of I-131 therapy. This was under TSH stimulation with the withdrawal of eltroxin for 4 weeks and given I^{131} under maximally stimulated TSH. Prophylactic dose of prednisone was given in conjunction with this therapy to minimize inflammatory response that may result from the radiation.

The posttherapeutic iodine-131 images (Figure 3(b)) done prior to discharge were congruent in pattern to the staging iodine-123 scan images. Thyroid function tests were low (thyroxine: 10.4 pmol/L, tri-iodo thyronine: 5.6 pmol/L, and thyroid-stimulating hormone: 0.54 mIU/L). The patient was discharged on eltroxin daily.

At the 6th month follow-up visit, she tolerated the RAI well with improved nutritional status. She was euthyroid with TSH: 4.13 mIU/L, T4: 9.4 pmol/L, T3: 6.0 pmol/L, and thyroglobulin: >300 μg/L. She was put on lifetime thyroid hormone replacement therapy.

3. Discussion

Papillary thyroid carcinoma is the leading cause of paediatric endocrine cancers with an incidence of 6% of all cancers [1]. In typical cases of PTC, patients present as multifocal involving both lobes and 50% of children present with cervical lymph node metastasis and lung metastasis. The initial evaluation of thyroid nodule or neck mass is serum TSH and T4 which in most cases is normal at presentation, followed by neck ultrasound. This is followed by a confirmatory fine-needle aspiration (FNA) [6]. Our patient presented with atypical feature, an asymptomatic neck mass on the left side of the neck; therefore, a normal workup for thyroid disease was not followed. She did not have risk factors for thyroid malignancy; hence, a clinical diagnosis of thyroid malignancy was not entertained. Whilst Hashimoto's thyroiditis (HT) is the commonest risk factor associated with paediatric PTC [7], the patient did not report any history of autoimmune disease. Furthermore, histopathological assessment of thyroid did not reveal background HT. While thyroid function tests would not have helped as they are usually normal, FNA of the mass should still be done. This helps to exclude nonmalignant and malignant disease. Clinician should always have a high index of suspicion for malignancy in children who presents with asymptomatic neck mass.

The histomorphological features of PTC in children are the same as in adults. Although it may present with varied growth patterns including papillary, follicular, and solid, amongst others, the diagnosis is based on typical nuclear features. These features include Orphan Annie eye nuclei which are optically clear. They also exhibit pseudoinclusion and grooves [8]. The diagnosis on the index patient was done based on these features.

The management of PTC involves extensive planning from staging preoperatively and deciding on approach that will benefit both the patient and family. Given the very high rate of metastatic disease in this population, preoperative neck ultrasound to identify suspicious lymph nodes and chest X-ray and/or chest CT should be considered in these patients as it will guide on the type of surgical treatment to be followed.

The latest American Thyroid Association (ATA) children's guidelines, published in 2015, recommend radioactive iodine therapy (RAI) after total thyroidectomy for intermediate- and high-risk groups who have extensive central neck lymph node involvement or locally invasive or extensive lateral neck cervical lymph nodes. The aim of RAI is to increase the response rate to surgical management. It has been reported that when radioactive iodine therapy is used in conjunction with thyroid-stimulating hormone (TSH) suppression, the rate for complete response is 47.32% and for partial response is 38.39%. Postsurgical RAI therapy is indicated in paediatric PTC due to its increased risk of bilateral (30%) or multifocal involvement (65%) [6, 8].

Lymph node dissection is recommended to reduce the risk of recurrence and increase the efficacy of RAI therapy in patients with extrathyroidal invasion or locoregional metastasis [8–10].

The index patient was in the high-risk group, and hence, a total thyroidectomy with radical neck dissection and radioactive therapy was the preferred choice of treatment.

The follow-up guidelines include serum thyroglobulin on levothyroxine every 3–6 months for 2–3 years then

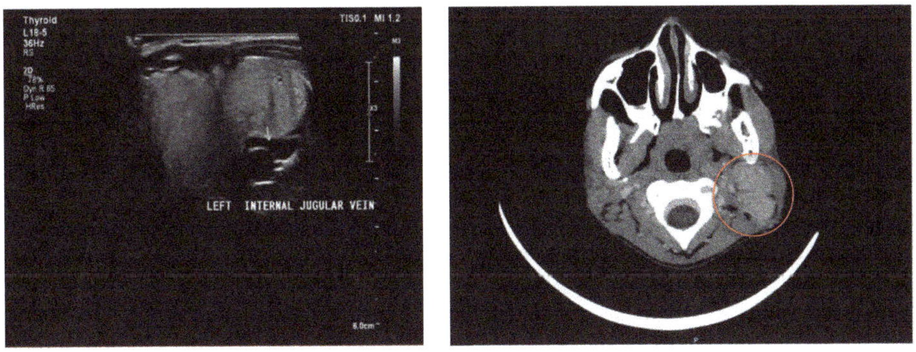

(a) (b)

FIGURE 1: (a) Neck ultrasound shows enlarged left cervical lymph node compressing on the left internal jugular vein; (b) CT scan shows mattered left cervical lymphadenopathy (○).

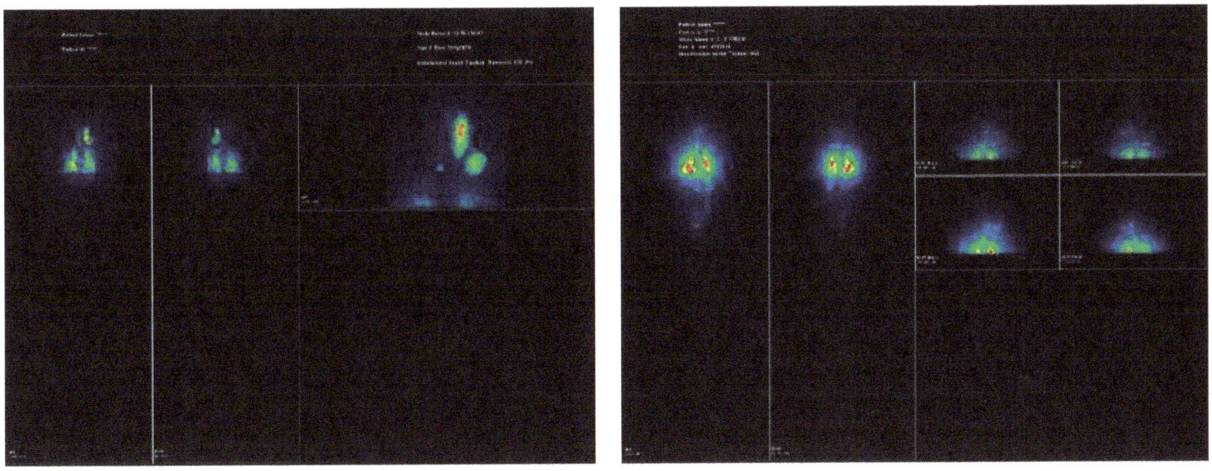

(a) (b)

FIGURE 2: (a) I^{123} and (b) I^{131} show increased nonuniform uptake in level II, III, and IV cervical lymph nodes, mild residual uptake in the thyroid bed, and increased uptake in the lungs bilaterally.

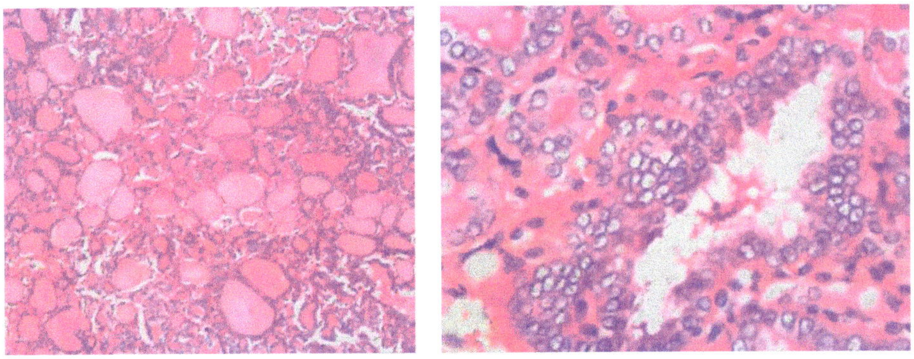

(a) (b)

FIGURE 3: (a) Thyroid tumour with papillary and follicular pattern; (b) typical nuclear features of PTC: nuclear overlapping, clearing, and occasional grooves.

annually and thyroid ultrasound including cervical lymph nodes for 6–12 months for intermediate- and high-risk groups and annually for low-risk patients. In case the thyroglobulin level is elevated, and the thyroid ultrasound is negative, then a CT scan of the chest and neck is recommended. In children, more than 98% of cases have a good survival rate at 10 years while few patients develop progressive or refractory disease not amenable to surgical intervention or resistant to radioactive therapy.

The prognosis for PTC is excellent with low mortality rate. The survival rate for different risk groups is as follows: 99% for low-risk groups, 83% for intermediate-risk groups, and 43% for high-risk groups [11].

The survivors of childhood ductal thyroid carcinoma need a follow-up for life since recurrence has been reported at 40 years after initial therapy [8].

In conclusion, fine-needle aspiration may provide early diagnosis in children with neck mass and avoid delayed management. A high index of suspicion for PTC should be maintained, regardless of risk factors. This allows for early targeted treatment with reduction in morbidity and mortality in this population. Surgical treatment with or without lymph node dissection and radiotherapy remains the cornerstone of management in paediatric PTC.

Ethical Approval

Sefako Makgatho University Research Ethics Committee (SMUREC) approved the publication of this case report.

Consent

Written, informed consent was obtained from the parent of the patient for publication of this case report. A copy of the consent form is available for review.

Acknowledgments

The authors all express their gratitude to the patient's parents who gave consent for this case to be presented in this paper.

References

[1] V. A. Paulson, E. R. Rudzinski, and D. S. Hawkins, "Thyroid cancer in the pediatric population," *Genes (Basel)*, vol. 10, no. 9, p. 723, 2019.

[2] K. A. Lee, M. T. A. Sharabiani, D. Tumino et al., "Differentiated thyroid cancer in children: a UK multicentre review and review of the literature," *Clinical Oncology*, vol. 31, no. 6, pp. 385–390, 2019.

[3] J. Chen, N. Huang, Q. Ji, Y. Wang, Y. Zhu, and D. Li, "Multifocal papillary thyroid cancer in children and adolescents: 12-year experience in a single center," *Gland Surgery*, vol. 8, no. 5, pp. 507–515, 2019.

[4] A. I. Stefan, A. Piciu, A. Mester, D. Apostu, M. Badan, and C. I. Badulescu, "Pediatric thyroid cancer in Europe: an overdiagnosed condition? a literature review," *Diagnostics*, vol. 10, no. 2, p. 112, 2020.

[5] P. K. Prasad, P. Mahajan, D. S. Hawkins, S. Mostoufi-Moab, and R. Venkatramani, "Management of pediatric differentiated thyroid cancer: an overview for the pediatric oncologist," *Pediatric Blood and Cancer*, vol. 67, no. 6, p. e28141, 2020.

[6] J. D. Prescott and M. A. Zeiger, "The RET oncogene in papillary thyroid carcinoma," *Cancer*, vol. 121, no. 13, pp. 2137–2146, 2015.

[7] M. L. Sur, R. Gaga, C. Lazăr, C. Lazea, C. Aldea, and D. Sur, "Papillary thyroid carcinoma in children with Hashimoto's thyroiditis-a review of the literature between 2000 and 2020," *Journal of Pediatric Endocrinology and Metabolism*, vol. 33, no. 12, pp. 1511–1517, 2020.

[8] G. L. Francis, S. G. Waguespack, A. J. Bauer et al., "Management guidelines for children with thyroid nodules and differentiated thyroid cancer," *Thyroid*, vol. 25, no. 7, pp. 716–759, 2015.

[9] H. D. Baumgarten, A. J. Bauer, A. Isaza, S. Mostoufi-Moab, K. Kazahaya, and N. S. Adzick, "Surgical management of pediatric thyroid disease: complication rates after thyroidectomy at the children's hospital of philadelphia high-volume pediatric thyroid center," *Journal of Pediatric Surgery*, vol. 54, no. 10, pp. 1969–1975, 2019.

[10] L. Massimo, D. Zarri, and D. Caprino, "Psychosocial aspects of survivors of childhood cancer or leukemia," *Minerva pediatrica*, vol. 57, no. 6, pp. 389–397, 2005.

[11] I. D. Hay, T. Gonzalez-Losada, M. S. Reinalda, J. A. Honetschlager, M. L. Richards, and G. B. Thompson, "Long-term outcome in 215 children and adolescents with papillary thyroid cancer treated during 1940 through 2008," *World Journal of Surgery*, vol. 34, no. 6, pp. 1192–1202, 2010.

14

An Infant with Asymptomatic Vitamin D Intoxication: A Prolonged and Sustainable Recovery

Ibrahim Al Alwan,[1,2,3] **Nouf Al Issa**,[2] **Yousef Al Anazi**,[2,4] **Khalid Al Noaim**,[2,5] **M. Zulf Mughal**,[6,7] **and Amir Babiker**[1,2,3]

[1]*College of Medicine, King Saud Bin Abdulaziz University for Health Sciences, Riyadh, Saudi Arabia*
[2]*Endocrine Division, Department of Pediatrics, King Abdullah Specialized Children Hospital, Riyadh, Saudi Arabia*
[3]*King Abdullah International Medical Research Centre, Ministry of the National Guard Health Affairs, Riyadh, Saudi Arabia*
[4]*Department of Pediatrics, College of Medicine, Majmaah University, Majmaah, Saudi Arabia*
[5]*Department of Pediatrics, College of Medicine, King Faisal University, Al-Ahsa, Saudi Arabia*
[6]*Department of Paediatric Endocrinology, Royal Manchester Children's Hospital, Manchester University NHS Foundation Trust, Manchester, UK*
[7]*Faculty of Biology, Medicine and Health, University of Manchester, Manchester, UK*

Correspondence should be addressed to Ibrahim Al Alwan; alwani@ksau-hs.edu.sa

Academic Editor: Toshihiro Kita

Vitamin D intoxication (VDI) usually develops due to inappropriate use of vitamin D in high doses by the families of infants with complaints suggestive of vitamin D deficiency such as delayed teething, knock knees, or delayed walking. We present here an experience of treating an infant with asymptomatic VDI that had a prolonged course of recovery and a sustainable level of vitamin D over a follow-up period of 2.5 years. In our patient, vitamin D started to drop steadily after a month of stopping vitamin D supplements but not to a normal level. It reached an acceptable level only after six months. This case emphasizes the importance of educating parents about the empirical use of vitamin D over the counter, assessing the baseline level of serum vitamin D level prior to initiation of treatment and highlights the value of verifying additional dietary sources of vitamin D or oral supplements in patient's history.

1. Background

Vitamin D exists in three inactive forms, that is, cholecalciferol, ergocalciferol, and 7-dehydrocholesterol. Cholecalciferol is found in animal-sourced foods, whereas ergocalciferol mainly comes from plant sources and fortified foods. During sun exposure, 7-dehydrocholesterol is produced endogenously in the skin; then, the above three inactive forms are converted to 25-hydroxyvitamin D (25(OH)D) in the liver. A final hydroxylation to 1,25-dihydroxyvitamin D (1,25-(OH)2D) occurs in the kidney to the active form of vitamin D [1]. The active form binds to the vitamin D receptor (VDR) to increase intestinal calcium and phosphate absorption [2, 3].

Serum 25-hydroxyvitamin D reflects an individual's vitamin status. Vitamin D level >50 nmol/L is considered as vitamin D sufficiency, while, levels between 30 to 50 nmol/l are considered as vitamin D insufficiency and <30 nmol/l is vitamin D deficiency. Physiologically, the body maintains serum 25(OH)D concentration within a narrow range of 75–220 nmol/L across vitamin D supplies through a homeostatic process [4]. That includes critical points of metabolism that controls the level of 25(OH)D through catabolism of 25(OH)D by the liver with execration of the excess into the bile and in tissues throughout the body by the side-chain cleavage pathway into the inactive form of 24,25(OH)D [5].

A routine use of vitamin D supplements guided by physician prescription is rationalized in children with a high risk of vitamin D deficiency, such as breastfed babies, lack of exposure to sunlight, having a darker complexion, obesity, difficulty in absorbing fat in the diet, or gastric bypass surgery as well as in osteoporosis or other metabolic bone diseases [6]. However, the easy accessibility of vitamin D to patients over the counter and the empirical prescription by doctors, given its importance in general wellbeing as above, are risk factors for overdose and intoxication [7, 8]. More recently, there has been increased interest in the assessment of vitamin D level during pregnancy and the effect of vitamin D deficiency on fetus and baby [9]. However, VDI is as important as vitamin D deficiency as there is no consensus on when to start vitamin D supplementation, the optimum dose, and duration of treatment as well as the optimum level vitamin D during pregnancy [10].

VDI usually develops due to inappropriate use of vitamin D in high doses by the families of infants with complaints suggestive of vitamin D deficiency such as a delay in teething or knock knees in lower limbs and delayed walking. Other causes of VDI include empirical prescription of vitamin D supplements by health care providers before a precise diagnosis of vitamin D deficiency [11]. Estimated tolerable upper limits of vitamin D by the American Academy of Pediatrics per age are 1000 IU/day for 0-1-year-old, 2500 IU/day for 1–3 years old, 3000 IU/day for 4–8 years old, and 4000 IU/day for nine years old and above [12]. Patients with VDI usually present with symptoms of hypercalcemia such as polyuria and polydipsia with a decrease in appetite, weight loss, and gastrointestinal manifestation as nausea, vomiting, and constipation; they might also present with dehydration and seizure in severe cases [9, 10]. In VDI, high concentrations of either free 1,25(OH)2D, or 25-hydroxyvitamin D leads to hypercalcemia by intestinal calcium absorption and bone resorption [13]. Hypercalcemia increases the load in the kidney due to calcium excretion in the distal tubules, causing hypercalciuria. Persistently elevated serum calcium concentration impairs the concentrating ability of the kidneys and causes polyuria and dehydration. It can also result in nephrocalcinosis [9].

Vitamin D intoxication (VDI) is rare but probably not unusual, with a recent increase in its reporting [11]. Overdose and intoxication can occur because of prescribing, manufacturing, or formulation errors [14]. Patients and physicians should be more aware of the potential dangers of vitamin D overdose. According to the American Academy of Pediatrics, serum 25-hydroxyvitamin D (25(OH)D) level above 250 nmol/L (100 ng/ml) is considered as hypervitaminosis D. In contrast, serum 25(OH)D level above 375 nmol/L (150 ng/ml) is associated with vitamin D intoxication (VDI) [15].

We present here an experience of treating an infant with asymptomatic VDI that had a prolonged course of resolution and sustainable level of vitamin D over a lengthy period of follow-up of 2.5 years, compared with previously reported cases.

2. Case Presentation

An eleven-months-old girl, a full-term baby that was an outcome of cesarean section with a birth weight of 2.67 kg, had grade 1 hydronephrosis in antenatal care. She was discharged with her mother in good condition. Mother was healthy with a serum 25(OH)D level of 30.3 nmol/l in the second trimester, indicating insufficient vitamin D. She was only on ferrous sulfate but not on vitamin D supplements.

During the child's routine visit at the age of 11 months to the well-baby clinic for vaccination, she grew well and was asymptomatic with a height of 72.5 cm (25–50th centile) and a 9.2 kg (50th centile) weight. Her vital signs were acceptable. She was alert and well-hydrated, vitally stable afebrile on examination with acceptable growth parameters for her age. The other examination was unremarkable, and there was no alopecia.

The primary physician requested routine laboratory tests due to the mother's concerns of delayed teething and hair loss. It showed a serum 25(OH)D level of 555 nmol/L (reference range >250 nmol/L toxicity) with normal adjusted calcium and phosphate level 2.49 nmol/l, 1.77 mmol/l, respectively; she was on a supplementary formula with a multivitamin that contains 400 IU of vitamin D once daily for one month prescribed over the counter. Moreover, the mother applied an ampule of vitamin D (Steril Devit-3 I.M/oral ampule) that contains 300,000 IU on the baby's gum one month before that visit as recommended by one of her relatives. The child remained asymptomatic during follow-up, and her serum 25(OH)D level normalized to 105.3 nmol/L after 6 months of discontinuing vitamin D supplements (Figure 1). In addition, the patient had normal other chronological investigations of the bone profile including serum calcium levels (Table 1). The level of 25(OH)D remained normal after 2.5 years of discontinuing treatment despite no additional sources of vitamin D supplements or extra exposure to sunlight (Figure 1). Repeated renal ultrasound showed persistent bilateral grade 1 hydronephrosis with no nephrocalcinosis.

3. Discussion

Our patient exceeded the tolerable upper limits of vitamin D level for her age. However, she remained asymptomatic and maintained a normal level of 25(OH)D for 2.5 years post ingestion of a supraphysiologic dose of vitamin D.

Systematic studies on vitamin D intoxication (VDI) have been conducted in a variety of different animal species. These studies showed that the plasma 25(OH)D concentrations associated with toxicity were always over 375 nmol/L [16]. For ethical reasons, no systematic experimental studies have examined VDI in humans. However, numerous anecdotal reports over the years have described accidental VDI. Jones, in a review of pharmacokinetics of vitamin D toxicity, found that all reported cases with overt symptoms of VDI had a concentration of 25(OH)D well above the normal range at 710–1587 nmol/L, with several patients exhibiting values consistently around 750 nmol/L [16]. Supporting a previous conclusion by Vieth et al., Jones established that hypercalcemia only results when 25(OH)D3 concentrations have always been above 375–500 nmol/L [7, 16]. In a recent review, the Pediatric Endocrine Society assessed the risk of VDI in infants and children, and reports on VDI in infants and young children were presented with severe hypercalcemia and serum 25(OH)D level in a range of 250–670 ng/

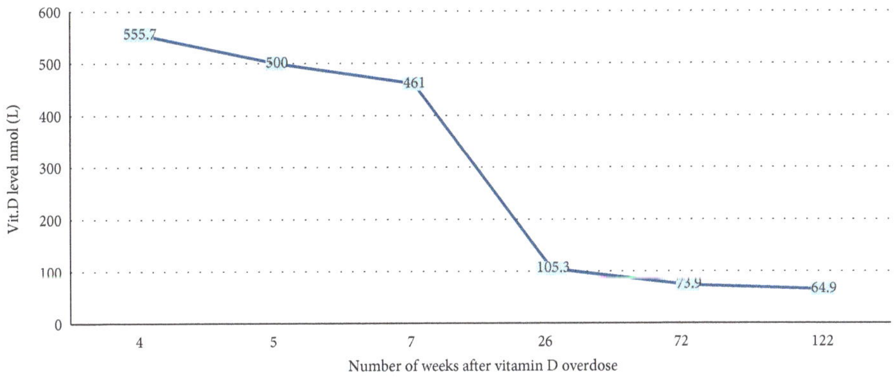

Figure 1: Vitamin D levels over 2.5 years of follow-up.

Table 1: Biochemical values in our patients over 2 years follow-up.

Investigation	Reference value	21/03/2019 at 11 months of age	25/03/2019 at 11 months of age	3/4/2019 at 12 months of age	18/09/2019 at 17 months of age	16/08/2020 at 28 months of age	4/08/2021 at 38 months of age
Total 25-OH vit D	nmol/L	555.7	500	461	105.3	73.9	64.9
Adj Ca	2.20–2.70 mmol/L	2.49	2.47	2.33	2.46	2.42	2.28
Albumin	38–54 g/L	44	41	44	44	45	46
Ca	2.20–2.70 mmol/L	2.57	2.49	2.41	2.54	2.52	2.54
Phosphorus	1.10–1.95 mmol/L	1.74	1.81	1.62	1.88	1.82	1.61
Alkaline phosphatase	156–369 U/L	284	214	221	270	262	246

mL (625–1675 nmol/L). There is significant variability in the amount of vitamin D administered and the resulting serum 25(OH)D concentrations among these cases. Rather than a specific level of 25(OH)D, the diagnosis of VDI was based on elevated serum 25(OH)D concentrations associated with hypercalcemia or hypercalciuria, whereas serum 1,25(OH)2D levels were normal and PTH was suppressed.

Despite the randomized clinical trials with evidence that symptomatic toxicity has only been reported with serum levels of 25(OH)D at levels >500 nmol/L. To allow a large safety margin, the global consensus on nutritional rickets defined Vitamin D toxicity as hypercalcemia and serum 25(OH)D >250 nmol/L with hypercalciuria and suppressed PTH [6].

Our patient was asymptomatic with an accidental finding of a high vitamin D level exceeding 500 nmol/L a month after ingesting a single dose of oral vitamin D3 in a routine visit, with normal adjusted calcium and phosphorus levels as well as normal PTH levels. She had no prior vitamin D level reported results.

Reviewing previous literature of infants with VDI (Supplement A), we postulate that variations in the duration and frequency of the overdose could lead to variability in associated symptoms due to variable hormonal responses that control vitamin D metabolism. In previous reports, infants with symptomatic vitamin D intoxication had received daily large doses (50,000–200,000 IU of vitamin D3) over a longer duration (1–4 months) [13, 17–24]. On the other hand, those with an asymptomatic course of illness had received relatively much smaller doses (10,000–12,000 IU of vitamin D3) over a shorter duration (less than a month) before presentation [23, 24]. Moreover, it might also be important to evaluate patients with VDI, especially when asymptomatic, for polymorphism of vitamin D binding protein (DBP) and gene mutations of CYP24A1, which code for 24-hydroxylase enzyme that change vitamin D into an inactive form. Unfortunately, these tests were not performed on our patient.

Our patient, a ten-month-old child, ingested a single mega dose of vitamin D that was accidentally recognized after a month of that event. The duration of receiving toxic amounts of vitamin D supplements (a stagnant dose) and the resultant serum calcium level seem to affect symptomatology. Probably, a single nonrepeated large dose in our patient did not "soak up" DBP compared to the stagnant dose over a more extended period described in previous reports that made our patient asymptomatic. In addition, as in previous reports, the cut point of vitamin D level beyond which one would expect symptoms was 750 nmol/l, and our patient vitamin D level was less than that level [16]. Despite that a vitamin D level of 375 nmol/l was described as the critical level for VDI in previous reports, the cut points of Ca levels associated with symptoms using Spearman's correlation in that Turkish reports was found to be above 3.5 mmol/l [11, 25]. Since we do not have previous laboratory results of calcium level in our patient, she probably had have mild (2.5–2.9 mmol/l) to moderate (3.0–3.5 mmol/l) serum calcium levels before her initial presentation a month after the ingestion of vitamin D overdose. Absence or mild soaked-up effect of DBP, a vitamin D level less than 750 nmol/l, and a possible mild to moderate hypercalcemia prior to presentation could all contribute to our patient' asymptomatic course of illness.

The half-life of vitamin D3 is approximately 15 days; however, VDI might take several months to resolve even after stopping the medication because it is a lipophilic vitamin and is stored in fat [9]. In our patient, vitamin D started to drop steadily after a month of stopping vitamin D supplements but not to a normal level until after six months from the initial presentation. Last but not least, all previous reports have focused on the effect of VDI to the point of time when the patients recovered, i.e., when vitamin D level is normalized. In our patient, a follow-up of 2.5 years after recovery, i.e., a normal vitamin D level after six months of follow-up, revealed a steady level of vitamin D (around 65 nmol/l) without additional sources of vitamin D, including extra exposure to sunlight.

4. Conclusion

Physicians have to assess baseline blood levels of vitamin D in children before starting vitamin D supplements to avoid using higher doses that can lead to asymptomatic, yet, potentially harmful course of VDI with a prolonged recovery and sustainable high levels even without extra supplements of vitamin D in the diet as in our patient.

Consent

Our patient's mother has signed consent for this material to be published.

Authors' Contributions

All authors conceived and designed the study, acquired the data, analysed and interpreted the data, approved the final version to be published, and agreed to be accountable for the article and to ensure that all questions regarding the accuracy or integrity of the article are investigated and resolved. IA, NA, YA, and AB drafted the article. ZM, IA, and AB revised it critically for important intellectual content.

Acknowledgments

The authors would like to thank the patient and the family for their kind agreement for this data to be published.

Supplementary Materials

Figure 1: vitamin D levels per number of weeks over 2.5 years of follow-up. Table 1: biochemical values related to vitamin D metabolism in our patients over 2 years follow-up. Supplement A: clinical, biochemical, and management characteristics of previous infants reported with vitamin D intoxication highlighting the course of illness in symptomatic and asymptomatic patients. (*Supplementary Materials*)

References

[1] S. Kimball, G. E.-H. Fuleihan, and R. Vieth, "Vitamin D: a growing perspective," *Critical Reviews in Clinical Laboratory Sciences*, vol. 45, no. 4, pp. 339–414, 2008.

[2] R. Bouillon, S. V. Cromphaut, and G. Carmeliet, "Intestinal calcium absorption: molecular vitamin D mediated mechanisms," *Journal of Cellular Biochemistry*, vol. 88, no. 2, pp. 332–339, 2003.

[3] T. D. Bell, M. B. Demay, and S.-A. M. Burnett-Bowie, "The biology and pathology of vitamin D control in bone," *Journal of Cellular Biochemistry*, vol. 111, no. 1, pp. 7–13, 2010.

[4] C. F. Munns, N. Shaw, M. Kiely et al., "Global consensus recommendations on prevention and management of nutritional rickets," *Journal of Clinical Endocrinology & Metabolism*, vol. 101, no. 2, pp. 394–415, 2016.

[5] R. Vieth, "Vitamin D supplementation, 25-hydroxyvitamin D concentrations, and safety," *American Journal of Clinical Nutrition*, vol. 69, no. 5, pp. 842–856, 1999.

[6] R. Nair and A. Maseeh, "Vitamin D: the "sunshine" vitamin," *Journal of Pharmacology and Pharmacotherapeutics*, vol. 3, no. 2, pp. 118–126, 2012.

[7] M. G. Vogiatzi, E. Jacobson-Dickman, and M. D. DeBoer, "Vitamin D supplementation and risk of toxicity in Pediatrics: a review of current literature," *Journal of Clinical Endocrinology & Metabolism*, vol. 99, no. 4, pp. 1132–1141, 2014.

[8] A. Anık, G. Çatlı, A. Abacı, C. Dizdarer, and E. Böber, "Acute vitamin D intoxication possibly due to faulty production of a multivitamin preparation," *Journal of Clinical Research in Pediatric Endocrinology*, vol. 5, no. 2, pp. 136–139, 2013.

[9] I. A. Alwan, M. A. Badi, M. Badri et al., "Higher serum alkaline phosphatase activity in infants born to vitamin D-deficient mothers," *Archives of Osteoporosis*, vol. 14, no. 1, p. 102, 2019.

[10] G. K Küçükali, M. Keskin, Ş. S Erdeve, and S. Çetinkaya, "Perinatal outcomes of high-dose vitamin D administration in the last trimester," *Turkish Journal of Obstetric and Gynecology*, vol. 18, no. 2, pp. 159–162, 2021.

[11] B. Ozkan, S. Hatun, and A. Bereket, "Vitamin D intoxication," *Turkish Journal of Pediatrics*, vol. 54, no. 2, pp. 93–98, 2012.

[12] A. C. Ross, J. E. Manson, S. A. Abrams et al., "The 2011 report on dietary reference intakes for calcium and vitamin D from the Institute of Medicine: what clinicians need to know," *Journal of Clinical Endocrinology & Metabolism*, vol. 96, no. 1, pp. 53–58, 2011.

[13] N. Waheed, H. A. Cheema, A. Saeed et al., "Vitamin D intoxication in 7-month-old infant with recommended daily intake of vitamin D," *Journal of Ayub Medical College, Abbottabad*, vol. 30, no. 4 Suppl 1, pp. S673–S675, 2018.

[14] K. Galior, S. Grebe, and R. Singh, "Development of vitamin D toxicity from overcorrection of vitamin D deficiency: a review of case reports," *Nutrients*, vol. 10, no. 8, p. 953, 2018.

[15] M. Misra, D. Pacaud, A. Petryk, P. F. Collett-Solberg, M. Kappy, and Drug and Therapeutics Committee of the Lawson Wilkins Pediatric Endocrine Society, "Vitamin D deficiency in children and its management: review of current knowledge and recommendations," *Pediatrics*, vol. 122, no. 2, pp. 398–417, 2008.
[16] G. Jones, "Pharmacokinetics of vitamin D toxicity," *The American Journal of Clinical Nutrition*, vol. 88, no. 2, pp. 582S–586S, 2008.
[17] K. Mühlendahl and J. Nawracala, "Vitamin D intoxication," *European Journal of Pediatrics*, vol. 158, p. 266, 1999.
[18] V. Talarico, M. Barreca, R. Galiano, M. C. Galati, and G. Raiola, "Vitamin D and risk for vitamin A intoxication in an 18-month-old boy," *Case Reports in Pediatrics*, vol. 2016, Article ID 1395718, 3 pages, 2016.
[19] L. Cantrell and E. Hogen, "Vitamin D overdosage in an infant from nonprescription vitamin D drops," *American Journal of Health-System Pharmacy*, vol. 72, no. 15, pp. 1262-1263, 2015.
[20] H. Ketha, H. Wadams, A. Lteif, and R. J. Singh, "Iatrogenic vitamin D toxicity in an infant--a case report and review of literature," *Journal of Steroid Biochemistry and Molecular Biology*, vol. 148, pp. 14–18, 2015.
[21] N. A. Bilbao, "Vitamin D toxicity in young breastfed infants: report of 2 cases," *Global Pediatric Health*, vol. 4, Article ID 2333794X1773169, 2017.
[22] C. Kara, F. Gunindi, A. Ustyol, and M. Aydin, "Vitamin D intoxication due to an erroneously manufactured dietary supplement in seven children," *Pediatrics*, vol. 133, no. 1, pp. e240–e244, 2014.
[23] N. Radlović, Z. Leković, D. Ristić et al., "Case report of acute vitamin D intoxication in an infant," *Srpski Arhiv Za Celokupno Lekarstvo*, vol. 142, no. 11–12, pp. 736–739, 2014.
[24] K. Rajakumar, E. C. Reis, and M. F. Holick, "Dosing error with over-the-counter vitamin D supplement: a risk for vitamin D toxicity in infants," *Clinical Pediatrics*, vol. 52, no. 1, pp. 82–85, 2013.
[25] K. Demir, H. Döneray, C. Kara et al., "Comparison of treatment regimens in management of severe hypercalcemia due to vitamin D intoxication in children," *Journal of Clinical Research in Pediatric Endocrinology*, vol. 11, no. 2, pp. 140–148, 2019.

15

Challenging Diagnosis of Addison's Disease Presenting with Adrenal Crisis

Ni Wayan Wina Dharmesti,[1] Made Ratna Saraswati,[2] Ketut Suastika,[2] Wira Gotera,[2] and I Made Pande Dwipayana[2]

[1]*Resident: Internal Medicine Department, Faculty of Medicine Udayana University, Sanglah Hospital, Denpasar, Bali, Indonesia*
[2]*Endocrine and Metabolism Division, Internal Medicine Department, Faculty of Medicine Udayana University, Sanglah Hospital, Denpasar, Bali, Indonesia*

Correspondence should be addressed to Made Ratna Saraswati; ratnasaraswati@unud.ac.id

Academic Editor: Toshihiro Kita

Primary adrenal insufficiency, also known as Addison's disease, is a rare but potentially fatal condition resulting from the failure of the adrenal cortex to produce glucocorticoid and/or mineralocorticoid hormones. Unfortunately, the clinical manifestation of primary adrenal insufficiency is not specific and often progresses insidiously, resulting in late diagnosis, or in severe cases, life-threatening circulatory collapse. Adrenal insufficiency should be considered in patients with unexplained vascular collapse. We report the case of a woman who presented to the emergency ward with unexplainable shock that was later diagnosed as adrenal crisis due to Addison's disease. The presence of hyperpigmentation in patients with rapid progression of adrenal insufficiency suggests the diagnosis of Addison's disease presenting with adrenal crisis.

1. Introduction

Addison's disease is characterized by the failure of the adrenal cortex to produce sufficient glucocorticoids and/or mineralocorticoids (primary adrenocortical insufficiency) to meet metabolic needs because of the destruction or primary dysfunction of the adrenal glands. Decreased secretion of glucocorticoid and/or mineralocorticoid hormones in primary adrenal insufficiency leads to decreased negative feedback to the pituitary gland, which in turn results in increased secretion of adrenocorticotropin hormone (ACTH), which differentiates it from secondary adrenocortical insufficiency (deficiency of ACTH secretion) [1–3]. Addison's disease is a rare disorder with a prevalence of 35–140 cases per million people and an incidence of 4 per million people per year in Caucasian populations [4, 5]. Autoimmunity (autoimmune adrenalitis) accounts for 90% of primary adrenal insufficiency cases reported in western countries [1, 2, 6]. Autoimmune adrenalitis may present as a part of the autoimmune polyglandular syndrome (APS) or as an isolated illness [4, 7]. There is a slight female predominance in the case of autoimmune adrenalitis, with a 2 : 1 female to male ratio [1]. Other conditions that may cause primary adrenocortical insufficiency in addition to autoimmunity include infections, genetic disorders, malignancy, medication, and critical illness.

Primary adrenal insufficiency is a potentially life-threatening condition that demonstrates the vital role of glucocorticoid and mineralocorticoid hormones in maintaining the homeostasis of energy, electrolytes, and body fluids [2]. However, clinical symptoms and signs are usually nonspecific, thereby posing a challenge to diagnosis and, consequently, to providing appropriate treatment. Acute adrenal crisis represents acute adrenocortical insufficiency, with prominent features of hypotension and shock that may rapidly lead to death if patients are left untreated [2]. With the aim of increasing awareness and knowledge of Addison's disease, we report the case of a 27-year-old woman who presented to the emergency ward with shock, which was later found to be caused by primary adrenal insufficiency.

2. Case Presentation

A 27-year-old woman was referred to the emergency ward of Sanglah Hospital with a diagnosis of shock caused by suspected hypovolemia or septic shock, acute gastroenteritis with dehydration, suspected autoimmune disease, and suspected pneumonia. The patient had fever for 7 days before admission, accompanied by a productive cough with yellowish phlegm, but no shortness of breath. She had nausea, vomiting, and diarrhea before the onset of fever. Diarrhea was defined as watery stool (without blood) at least three times per day. The patient also reported loss of appetite and loss of body weight (approximately 10 kg within 2 months). The patient had an irregular menstrual cycle since the age of 17 years, and the last menstruation was 18 months ago. She reached menarche at the age of 13 years with a normal growth of breasts and pubic hair. A history of chronic cough, diabetes, or cancer was ruled out. A family history of the same conditions was also excluded. The patient was not taking any regular medication, except for menstruation pills prescribed by her obstetrician several times. The patient was hospitalized for 3 days in another private hospital before admission to Sanglah Hospital and was treated with fluid resuscitation with 1000 ml of crystalloid, intravenous cefoperazone, intravenous paracetamol, intravenous ondansetron, and norepinephrine drip 0.1 mcg/kg BW/h. The patient was unmarried and worked as an employee in a private company.

The patient appeared very ill and somnolent upon her first presentation to the emergency ward. Her blood pressure was 90/70 mmHg (on continuous infusion of norepinephrine), heart rate was 108 beats per minute, respiration rate was 22 breaths per minute, and axillary temperature was 37°C. Physical examination revealed a whitish plaque on the tongue, hyperpigmentation of the gingival mucosa, and bilateral skin hyperpigmentation of the interphalangeal joints of fingers and toes as well as knees; her extremities felt cold and moist with a capillary refill time of 2–3 s. No abnormal breath sounds were detected on lung auscultation, and abdominal examination findings were normal (Figure 1).

Laboratory results from a previous hospital showed a high leukocyte count ($20.4 \times 10^3\,\mu$L) with lymphocytosis, normal hemoglobin and platelet levels, increased serum creatinine level (1.2 mg/dL), and slightly decreased sodium (134 mmol/L), potassium, and blood glucose level both within normal limit. Serial complete blood count examination showed a decrease in leukocyte count ($10.6 \times 10^3\,\mu$L) before the patient was referred to our hospital. We repeated the examination in the emergency ward and found no abnormalities in complete blood count and levels of serum creatinine, random blood glucose, or liver enzymes. Blood gas analysis showed respiratory alkalosis with a pH of 7.47, pCO_2 of 22.2 mmHg, slightly decreased sodium level (132 mmol/L), and a normal potassium level (4.87 mmol/L). Urine examination and chest radiography were performed to determine possible sources of infection, and both showed normal results. Feces examination could not be performed because the patient did not pass stool while at our hospital. A pregnancy test was performed using a urine sample, and the result was negative.

Our initial assessment was acute diarrhea with possible bacterial or viral causes, severe community-acquired pneumonia with sepsis and septic shock, and secondary amenorrhea. An immunocompromised state was also suspected in our case with a differential diagnosis of systemic lupus erythematosus and human immunodeficiency virus (HIV) infection. Fluid resuscitation was continued in the emergency ward by administering 1000 ml of crystalloid and 0.9% NaCl at 30 drops/min. Antibiotic treatment was also continued with intravenous cefoperazone (1 g every 12 h), intravenous levofloxacin (750 mg every 24 h), oral fluconazole (150 mg every 24 h) to treat oral candidiasis, and continuous infusion of norepinephrine (0.1 mcg/kg BW/h). To determine the cause of amenorrhea, the Obstetric-Gynecologic Department was consulted. However, no abnormality or signs of pregnancy were noted on gynecologic examination. The test results for hepatitis B virus and HIV infection were nonreactive.

The patient's symptoms of nausea, vomiting, weakness, and fever did not improve with the initial treatment. Moreover, despite fluid resuscitation, blood pressure needed to be maintained by administering a continuous infusion of norepinephrine. There was an improvement in the appearance of the whitish plaque on the tongue after 4 days of fluconazole and a hyperpigmentation plaque appeared on the tongue, as shown in Figure 1(a). Following the observation of generalized hyperpigmentation on the skin and mucosa, Addison's disease was suspected, which warranted the evaluation of morning cortisol level. The ACTH level could not be examined because this test is not available in Indonesia. On the following day, morning cortisol hormone level test revealed a very low level (0.84 μg/dL; normal range: 4.3–22.4 μg/dL). The patient was diagnosed as having Addison's disease on day 6 of hospitalization in our hospital, followed immediately by administering intravenous infusion of hydrocortisone (100 mg over 30 min, every 24 h). Abdominal ultrasound was performed to further evaluate the possible underlying conditions, and we found no enlarged lymph nodes, no intra-abdominal masses, and no adrenal gland calcifications. Antibiotic and norepinephrine drip was discontinued 2 days after starting intravenous hydrocortisone, as the patient showed marked clinical improvement, and we found no pathogenic microorganisms in blood and sputum cultures. Repeated examination of sodium and potassium levels, while administering intravenous hydrocortisone, showed that the values were within normal limits. Therefore, we switched to oral hydrocortisone after 7 days of intravenous preparation. The oral dose was started with 20 mg of hydrocortisone in the morning and 10 mg in the afternoon, after which the patient was discharged from hospital. The oral dose was maintained for one month, during which the patient reported disappearance of weakness and return of appetite. The patient also gained her weight and evaluation of electrolytes level was

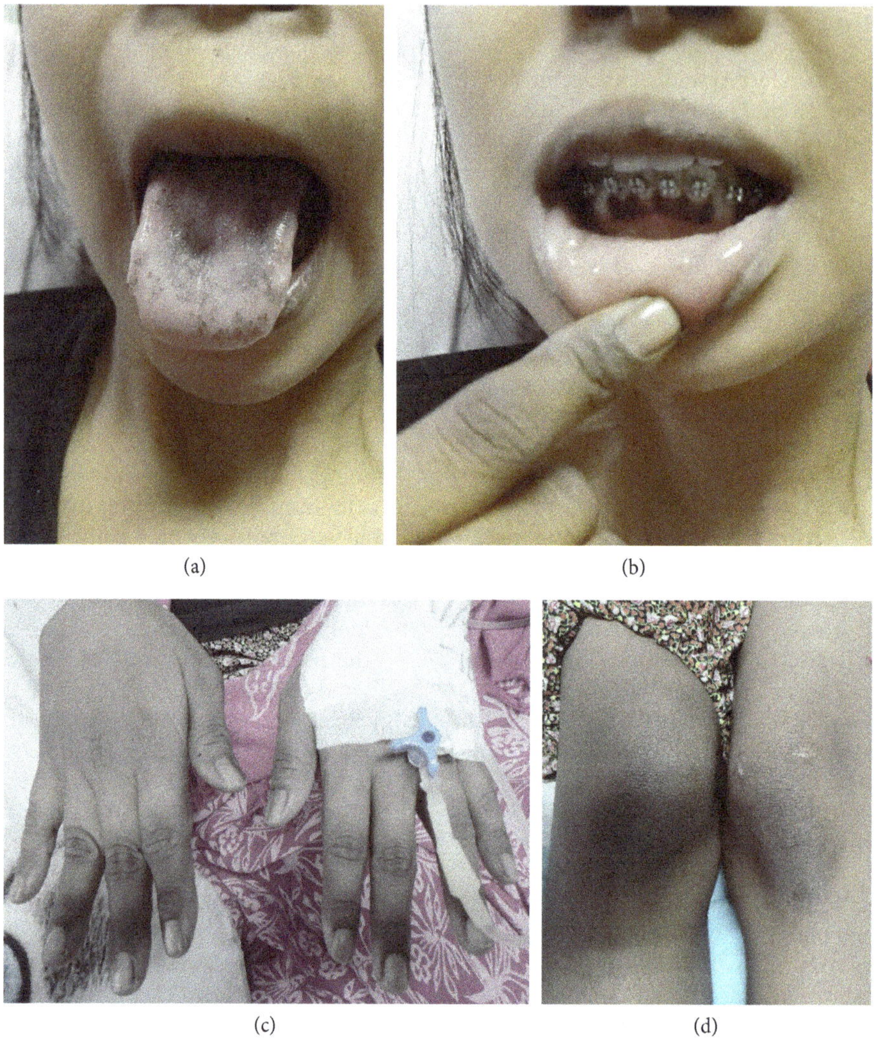

Figure 1: Hyperpigmentation on skin and mucosa: (a) tongue, (b) gum, (c) hands, and (d) knee.

normal. Therefore, we slowly decreased the dose in the second month to 20 mg hydrocortisone taken once daily in the morning.

3. Discussion

Primary adrenal insufficiency poses a diagnostic challenge due to its rare incidence and its nonspecific clinical manifestations, which often develop slowly over a long period of time that may cause delay in diagnosis or patients presenting with acute life-threatening condition [3, 8]. Clinical pictures of primary adrenal insufficiency correlate closely with the degree of adrenal gland destruction and is classified as chronic primary adrenal insufficiency and acute adrenal crisis [1]. Patients with chronic primary adrenal insufficiency may show signs and symptoms of hyperpigmentation, weakness and fatigue, loss of body weight, loss of appetite, gastrointestinal disturbances, hypotension, salt craving, and postural symptoms. Hyperpigmentation of the skin and mucosal membrane is an early and classical manifestation of Addison's disease that results from increased ACTH levels; consequently, it does not appear in secondary adrenal insufficiency. Hypotension is present in 90% of the cases and is accompanied by orthostatic symptoms, which in severe chronic cases or acute illness can develop into shock. Amenorrhea is common in Addison's disease due to weight loss, chronic illness, or primary ovarian failure due to polyglandular autoimmune syndrome [1]. Our patient was admitted with nonspecific symptoms of fever, weakness, lethargy, nausea and vomiting, and refractory shock despite the continuous infusion of norepinephrine. Before admitted to the hospital, the patient was complaining of nonspecific symptoms such as loss of appetite, weight loss, and irregular menstruation. The presence of skin and mucosal hyperpigmentation was noticed while the patient was admitted in our hospital and this was the suggestive sign of primary adrenal insufficiency in our patient. However, the diagnosis of primary adrenal insufficiency in our case was suspected after six days of hospitalization after the hyperpigmentation on oral mucosa was clearly seen as the oral thrush was improved.

Acute adrenal crisis, or simply adrenal crisis, is marked by life-threatening, rapid clinical deterioration in patients with adrenal insufficiency and hypotension (systolic blood pressure < 100 mmHg) [9–13]. Adrenal crisis is associated with several risk factors such as chronic adrenal insufficiency, infection, trauma, or surgery [10, 14, 15]. It might appear as the first manifestation of adrenal insufficiency in around 8 per 100 patients with adrenal insufficiency per year, but it is often diagnosed late due to its nonspecific symptoms [16]. Other clinical symptoms that may appear are fever, dehydration, nausea and vomiting, anorexia, weakness, hypoglycemia, and loss of consciousness [1]. Since hypovolemic shock is a common presentation, adrenal insufficiency should be considered in patients with unexplained vascular collapse. The presence of hyperpigmentation of the skin and mucosa in patients with unexplained vascular collapse suggests the diagnosis of primary adrenal insufficiency [1]. Rapid clinical deterioration and refractory shock that did not respond to norepinephrine infusion likely signaled an adrenal crisis in our patient. The adrenal crisis in our case might have been precipitated by lung infection, although no pathogen was found in sputum or blood cultures probably because the culture specimen was taken after several days of antibiotic administration.

The diagnosis of primary adrenal insufficiency is based on a low level of morning (basal) cortisol hormone (either serum or plasma), which is confirmed by low levels of stimulated cortisol by performing corticotropin stimulation test. Primary adrenal insufficiency is also suspected when the basal cortisol level is less than 140 nmol/L (5 μg/dL) and the concentration of plasma ACTH is increased by 2-fold from the upper limit of normal [2]. Corticotropin stimulation test, also known as cosyntropin test or ACTH test, is considered the gold standard for the diagnosis of primary adrenal insufficiency [17] and should be performed to confirm diagnosis in patients with clinical signs and symptoms of primary adrenal insufficiency, unless the results of basal cortisol levels are indicative of adrenal insufficiency [18]. Accordingly, it is recommended that therapy is started in patients with severe symptoms of adrenal insufficiency or adrenal crisis, without waiting for the result of a confirmatory test [2, 12, 16]. Presently, there is no laboratory marker available to confirm adrenal crisis, and diagnosis is based on the clinical presentation of the patient [9]. The diagnosis of Addison's disease in our case was based on a very low level of morning cortisol (0.84 μg/dL) and the appearance of hyperpigmentation on the skin and mucosa, which is the classical clinical finding of primary adrenal insufficiency resulting from elevated levels of ACTH. Confirmatory examination with corticotropin stimulation test could not be performed because of limitations in laboratory facilities and this was not lead to any delay to start administering glucocorticoid treatment in our patient. The immediate administration of intravenous hydrocortisone was followed by significant clinical improvement, which also supports the diagnosis of primary adrenal insufficiency in our patient.

Other laboratory or radiological examinations have a limited role in confirming the diagnosis of adrenal insufficiency but have a greater role in evaluating its etiology. Determining the etiology or underlying conditions of adrenal insufficiency is the next step after confirming primary adrenal insufficiency based on hormonal levels [2]. The most common cause is autoimmune adrenalitis, either as isolated autoimmune adrenalitis or as a part of a group of autoimmune disorders known as autoimmune polyglandular syndrome, which is clinically classified into type 1 (APS-1) and type 2 (APS-2). Autoimmune adrenalitis in the case of APS-1 is associated with other immune disorders, such as hypoparathyroid, chronic mucocutaneous candidiasis, and other less common disorders (Hashimoto's thyroiditis, vitiligo, and premature ovarian failure), while in the case of APS-2, autoimmune adrenalitis is associated with hypothyroidism, type 1 diabetes mellitus, premature ovarian failure, and pernicious anemia. All of these disorders should be fully evaluated before confirming the diagnosis of isolated autoimmune adrenalitis. However, infection remains a common underlying cause in developing countries. Other possible etiologies that should be evaluated are medication use and malignancy [1, 5]. While ketoconazole, an antifungal agent, is known to possibly induce adrenal insufficiency, little is known about the effect of administering fluconazole [19]. Several case reports have demonstrated the evidence of a temporal reversible relationship between adrenal insufficiency (cosyntropin test) and the administration of high-dose intravenous fluconazole in critically ill patients [19]. Our patient received 150 mg of oral fluconazole every 24 h for the treatment of oral candidiasis, which was improved after 4 days of fluconazole doses. Administration of fluconazole in our case was unlikely an additional factor that exacerbated adrenal insufficiency, as significant clinical improvement was not observed after discontinuing fluconazole but by administering hydrocortisone.

Investigation of possible etiology in our case helped to exclude HIV infection, tuberculosis (based on chest X-ray examination), malignant tumors, or use of medication, although other autoimmune diseases associated with APS were not fully evaluated (hypoparathyroidism, autoimmune thyroid disease, and primary ovarian failure). Based on available practice guidelines, the evaluation of possible etiology or underlying conditions was still regarded as best practice (unrated evidence) [2]. Possible underlying conditions can be evaluated through serial examinations following the initiation of glucocorticoid therapy, based on symptoms that may appear later. Evaluation of other autoimmune diseases in our case were more focused on APS-2, since patients with APS-1 commonly have chronic mucocutaneous candidiasis since childhood, and APS-2 has a higher prevalence than APS-1 and more often progresses to adrenal crisis [5, 20]. Further evaluation of the possibility of primary ovarian failure in our case was planned by checking the level of follicle stimulating hormone, luteinizing hormone, and prolactin on the next outpatient visit; however, these hormone levels had not been evaluated before reporting this case.

Glucocorticoid therapy is recommended in all patients with primary adrenal insufficiency [2]. The suggested regimen is 15–25 mg of hydrocortisone or 20–35 mg of cortisone acetate in two or three divided oral doses per day. An alternative regimen is prednisolone (3–5 mg/day) administered orally in one or two doses. Dexamethasone should not be used in the case of primary adrenal insufficiency because of the risk of cushingoid effect, due to difficulties in titrating dexamethasone doses [2]. Adjusting the dose of hydrocortisone to body surface area (5.5 mg/m^2) or body weight (0.12 mg/kg) may result in more physiological cortisol levels in primary adrenal insufficiency patients than fixed dose regimens [2]. Patients who present with critical illness or adrenal crisis should be administered parenteral hydrocortisone at an initial dose of 100 mg along with fluid resuscitation with isotonic saline. The dose of parenteral hydrocortisone is continued with 200 mg of hydrocortisone administered as continuous infusion over 24 h. On the next day, hydrocortisone is administered intravenously (100 mg every 24 h). Switching to oral preparation is based on the clinical improvement of the patient. Monitoring of therapy and adjustment of oral dose are also based on clinical presentations, not done by repeating hormonal evaluation [2]. The patient in our case had refractory shock that could not be stabilized by continuous infusion of norepinephrine, which led to the diagnosis of adrenal crisis. Therefore, we decided to administer intravenous hydrocortisone (100 mg every 24 h) and 30 min of continuous infusion of 100 ml normal saline for 7 days until hemodynamic and clinical symptoms were improved. Supportive therapy with fluid resuscitation was also administered to the patient. Following clinical symptom improvement, intravenous hydrocortisone was switched to an oral preparation, 20 mg in the morning and 10 mg in the afternoon, to resemble physiological cortisol secretion. Due to patient's good clinical response with oral hydrocortisone, the dose was reduced to single dose of 20 mg hydrocortisone in the morning. Cortisol in twice-daily dose gives satisfactory response in most patients; however, some patients may require only a single morning dose to maintain well-being and normal energy levels [1]. Outcome study of glucocorticoid therapy in the patient with adrenal insufficiency also found that less-frequent dosing may be associated with better compliance [21].

In conclusion, adrenal crisis should be considered in patients presenting with unexplainable vascular collapse. Presence of skin and/or mucosal hyperpigmentation would suggest primary adrenocortical insufficiency as underlying condition. Examination of basal cortisol level and ACTH test are recommended to diagnose Addison's disease. However, treatment with glucocorticoid should be started in patients with severe symptoms of adrenal insufficiency or adrenal crisis, without waiting for the result of a confirmatory test.

Consent

Written informed consent was obtained from the patient for publication of this case report and the accompanying images.

References

[1] T. B. Carroll, D. C. Aron, J. W. Findling, and J. B. Tyrell, D. G. Gardner and D. Shoback, *Glucocorticoids and Adrenal Androgens in Greenspan Basic and Clinical Endocrinology*pp. 303–312, McGraw-Hill, New York, NY, USA, 9th edition, 2011.

[2] S. R. Bornstein, B. Allolio, W. Arlt et al., "Diagnosis and treatment of primary adrenal insufficiency: an endocrine society clinical practice guideline," *The Journal of Clinical Endocrinology & Metabolism*, vol. 101, no. 2, pp. 364–389, 2016.

[3] S. R. Bornstein, "Predisposing factors for adrenal insufficiency," *New England Journal of Medicine*, vol. 360, no. 22, pp. 2328–2339, 2009.

[4] A. Michels and N. Michels, "Addison disease: early detection and treatment principles," *American Family Physician*, vol. 89, no. 7, pp. 563–568, 2014.

[5] I. Wallace, S. Cunningham, and J. Lindsay, "The diagnosis and investigation of adrenal insufficiency in adults," *Annals of Clinical Biochemistry: International Journal of Laboratory Medicine*, vol. 46, no. 5, pp. 351–367, 2009.

[6] M. M. Erichsen, K. Løvås, K. J. Fougner et al., "Normal overall mortality rate in Addison's disease, but young patients are at risk of premature death," *European Journal of Endocrinology*, vol. 160, no. 2, pp. 233–237, 2009.

[7] W. Arlt, J. L. Jameson, *Disorders of Adrenal Cortex in Harrison's Endocrinology*pp. 118–124, McGraw-Hill, New York, NY, USA, 3rd edition, 2013.

[8] B. Bleicken, M. Ventz, M. Quinkler, and S. Hahner, "Delayed diagnosis of adrenal insufficiency is common: a cross-sectional study in 216 patients," *The American Journal of the Medical Sciences*, vol. 339, no. 6, pp. 525–531, 2010.

[9] M. Iwasaku, M. Shinzawa, S. Tanaka, K. Kimachi, and K. Kawakami, "Clinical characteristics of adrenal crisis in adult population with and without predisposing chronic adrenal insufficiency: a retrospective cohort study," *BMC Endocrine Disorders*, vol. 17, no. 1, p. 58, 2017.

[10] L. C. C. J. Smans, E. S. Van der Valk, A. R. M. M. Hermus, and P. M. J. Zelissen, "Incidence of adrenal crisis in patients with adrenal insufficiency," *Clinical Endocrinology*, vol. 84, no. 1, pp. 17–22, 2016.

[11] B. Allolio, "Extensive expertise in endocrinology. Adrenal crisis," *European Journal of Endocrinology*, vol. 172, no. 3, pp. R115–R124, 2015.

[12] T. H. K. Puar, N. M. M. L. Stikkelbroeck, L. C. C. J. Smans, P. M. J. Zelissen, and A. R. M. M. Hermus, "Adrenal crisis: still a deadly event in the 21st century," *The American Journal of Medicine*, vol. 129, no. 3, pp. e1–339, 2016.

[13] R. L. Rushworth, D. J. Torpy, and H. Falhammar, "Adrenal crises: perspectives and research directions," *Endocrine*, vol. 55, no. 2, pp. 336–345, 2017.

[14] S. Hahner, C. Spinnler, M. Fassnacht et al., "High incidence of adrenal crisis in educated patients with chronic adrenal insufficiency: a prospective study," *The Journal of Clinical Endocrinology & Metabolism*, vol. 100, no. 2, pp. 407–416, 2015.

[15] S. Hahner, M. Loeffler, B. Bleicken et al., "Epidemiology of adrenal crisis in chronic adrenal insufficiency: the need for new prevention strategies," *European Journal of Endocrinology*, vol. 162, no. 3, pp. 597–602, 2010.

[16] R. Dineen, C. J. Thompson, and M. Sherlock, "Adrenal crisis: prevention and management in adult patients," *Therapeutic Advances in Endocrinology and Metabolism*, vol. 10, Article ID 2042018819848218, 2019.

[17] I. L. Schmidt, H. Lahner, K. Mann, and S. Petersenn, "Diagnosis of adrenal insufficiency: evaluation of the corticotropin-releasing hormone test and basal serum cortisol in comparison to the insulin tolerance test in patients with hypothalamic-pituitary-adrenal disease," *The Journal of*

Clinical Endocrinology & Metabolism, vol. 88, no. 9, pp. 4193–4198, 2003.

[18] R. Kazlauskaite, A. T. Evans, C. V. Villabona et al., "Corticotropin tests for hypothalamic-pituitary- adrenal insufficiency: a metaanalysis," *The Journal of Clinical Endocrinology & Metabolism*, vol. 93, no. 11, pp. 4245–4253, 2008.

[19] S. G. Albert, M. J. DeLeon, and A. B. Silverberg, "Possible association between high-dose fluconazole and adrenal insufficiency in critically ill patients," *Critical Care Medicine*, vol. 29, no. 3, pp. 668–670, 2001.

[20] G. Meyer, K. Badenhoop, and R. Linder, "Addison's disease with polyglandular autoimmunity carries a more than 2·5-fold risk for adrenal crises: German Health insurance data 2010-2013," *Clinical Endocrinology*, vol. 85, no. 3, pp. 347–353, 2016.

[21] M. Forss, G. Batcheller, S. Skrtic, and G. Johannsson, "Current practice of glucocorticoid replacement therapy and patient-perceived health outcomes in adrenal insufficiency - a worldwide patient survey," *BMC Endocrine Disorders*, vol. 12, no. 1, p. 8, 2012.

16

Functional Adrenal Collision Tumor in a Patient with Cushing's Syndrome

Cathy Zhou[1] **Ghaneh Fananapazir**[1] **and Michael J. Campbell**[2]

[1]*Department of Radiology, University of California, Davis Medical Center, Sacramento, CA, USA*
[2]*Department of Surgery, University of California, Davis Medical Center, Sacramento, CA, USA*

Correspondence should be addressed to Michael J. Campbell; mjcampb@ucdavis.edu

Academic Editor: J. Paul Frindik

Adrenal collision tumors are rare and produce unique diagnostic challenges for clinicians. We report the case of a 45-year-old woman with obesity and diabetes mellitus and an incidentally-discovered adrenal mass containing macroscopic fat, thought to be a myelolipoma. A functional workup confirmed adrenocorticotropic hormone- (ACTH-) independent Cushing's syndrome. The patient underwent a successful laparoscopic adrenalectomy with pathology showing an adrenal collision tumor consisting of an adrenocortical adenoma and a myelolipoma. Postoperatively, the clinical symptoms, body mass index, and hemoglobin A1C all improved. Clinicians should consider a functional workup in patients with radiographically diagnosed myelolipomas as some may prove to be hormonally active collision tumors.

1. Introduction

"Adrenal collision tumor" is the radiographic term used to describe the appearance of a single radiographic mass consisting of two histologically distinct adrenal neoplasms. Adrenal collision tumors involving a myelolipoma are particularly challenging because radiologists are trained to label adrenal lesions with any amount of macroscopic fat as myelolipomas [1]. Clinicians are trained that radiographically diagnosed myelolipomas do not need further imaging or a biochemical evaluation for autonomous hormone production like other adrenal tumors. We report a case of a 45-year-old woman with Cushing's syndrome secondary to an adrenal tumor diagnosed as a myelolipoma on abdominal imaging. Ultimately, the patient was found to have an adrenal collision tumor composed of a functioning adrenocortical adenoma and a myelolipoma. Only five similar cases have been previously described and are reviewed in this report [2–6].

1.1. Case Presentation. In November 2012, a 45-year-old Caucasian woman presented to her primary care physician with lower abdominal pain. At the time of presentation, her medical history was notable for obesity (weight = 183.2 kg and body mass index (BMI) 61.6 mg/m^2), type 2 diabetes mellitus (hemoglobin A1C (HbA1C) = 7.5%), hypertension, and recurrent episodes of cellulitis. A contrast-enhanced CT scan of the abdomen and pelvis in the portal venous phase was obtained that showed no source for her abdominal pain but did note an incidental 5.5 × 4.0 cm left adrenal tumor containing macroscopic fat and reported as a myelolipoma (Figure 1(a)). This tumor had grown from a CT scan in April 2007, where it measured 4.4 × 3.3 cm (Figure 1(b)). The right adrenal appeared normal on both scans.

In September 2014, the patient was referred to an endocrinologist for worsening diabetes mellitus. At this visit, her weight was 184.7 kg with a BMI of 61.9 mg/m^2 and HbA1C of 9.2%. Because of clinical concern for hypercortisolism, a functional workup was initiated. A 1 mg dexamethasone suppression test revealed a postsuppression cortisol of 9.3 μg/d (reference range <1.8 μg/dL). Serum aldosterone was 4.7 ng/dL with a renin activity of 0.3 ng/ml/hr. Plasma free metanephrines were less than the upper limit of normal, and a morning adrenocorticotropic hormone (ACTH) was 16 ng/L (reference range 6–50 ng/L). The patient was lost to follow-up before completing further testing.

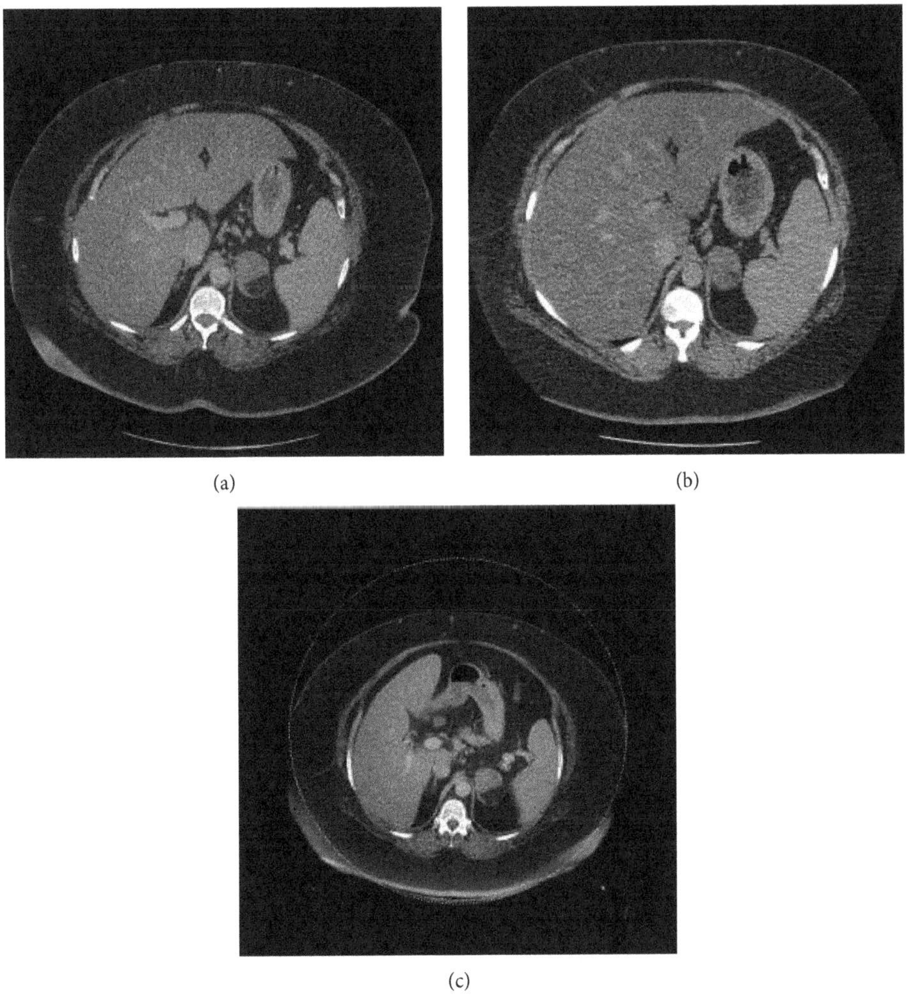

FIGURE 1: A CT for abdominal pain in November 2012 revealed a presumed adrenal myelolipoma with a focus of macroscopic fat (a). In comparing to a prior exam from April 2007 (b), this mass had grown in size, and subsequent imaging from April 2016 (c) continued to demonstrate growth.

In June 2015, she reestablished care with her endocrinologist. Physical exam was notable for obesity, but without other clinical signs of Cushing's syndrome, including moon facies, buffalo hump, or striae. A dual-energy X-ray absorptiometry (DEXA) scan showed normal bone health. The 24-hour urine cortisol level was 54.1 μg/day (reference range <45 μg/day). Repeat 24-hour urine cortisol was again elevated at 47.5 μg/day. ACTH was 8 ng/L (reference range 6–50 ng/L) and dehydroepiandrosterone sulfate (DHEAS) was suppressed at <15 μg/dL (reference range 32–240 μg/dL). Repeat 1-mg dexamethasone suppression test was elevated at 13.5 μg/dL (reference range <1.8 μg/dL). BMI was 62.4 kg/m^2 (weight 186.1 kg), and HgA1C was 9.0%. Given continued symptomatology and positive lab values, the patient was then referred to endocrine surgery with suspicion for Cushing's syndrome from her left adrenal myelolipoma but failed to make her appointments.

In March 2016, the patient was seen by endocrine surgery for consideration of a laparoscopic left adrenalectomy for Cushing's syndrome. A repeat CT showed the tumor had increased in size to 5.8 cm and was still partially composed of macroscopic fat and consistent with a myelolipoma (Figure 1). BMI was 65.1 kg/m^2 (weight = 188.7 kg) and HbA1C was 10.0%. She underwent an uncomplicated laparoscopic adrenalectomy in October 2017. The case was performed via a standard transabdominal approach. The patient had a generous amount of intraabdominal fat which was mobilized with the colon and spleen from the left adrenal gland. She required an increased pneumoperitoneum pressure to facilitate exposure (17 cm of water). The remainder of her case and postoperative course were unremarkable. On surgical pathology, she was noted to have a 6.7 cm adrenal collision tumor comprised of a 4 cm adrenocortical adenoma and a 2.7 cm myelolipoma (Figure 2). Postoperatively, the patient was placed on corticosteroid replacement, which was tapered over the course of a year and a half without significant symptoms of adrenal insufficiency. 24 hour urine cortisol following discontinuation of steroids normalized to 7.6 μg/24 hours. Her weight decreased to 149.4 kg with a BMI of 51.6 and HbA1c of 7.3% (Figure 3).

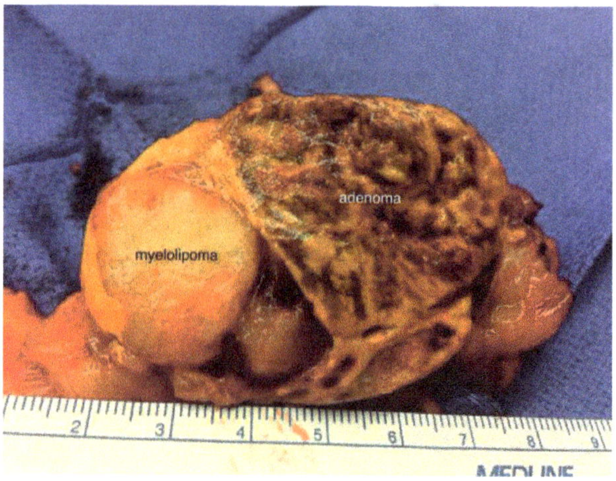

FIGURE 2: The surgical specimen demonstrates the characteristic macroscopic fat component of the myelolipoma with an adjacent well-circumscribed solid golden yellow adenoma.

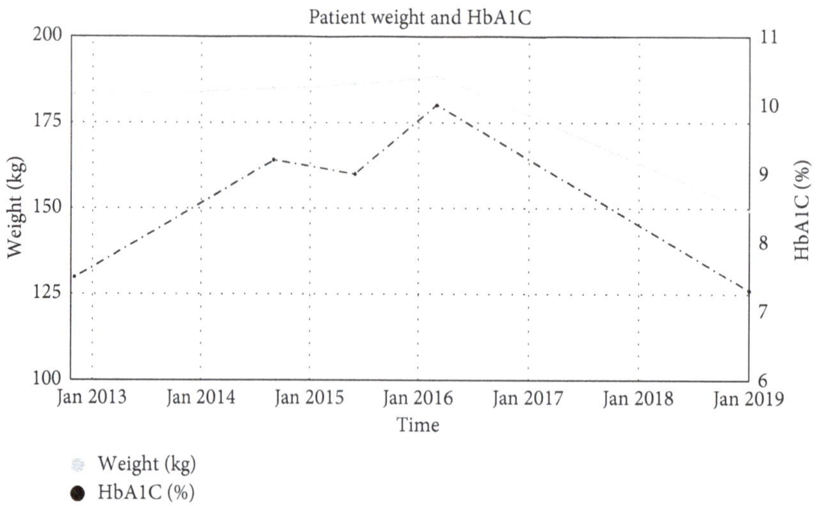

FIGURE 3: Patient weight and hemoglobin A1C graphed over time.

2. Discussion

We present the case of a 45-year-old woman with a radiographically diagnosed myelolipoma and ACTH independent Cushing's syndrome that underwent laparoscopic left adrenalectomy with surgical pathology showing a collision tumor with a 4 cm adrenocortical adenoma and 2.7 cm myelolipoma. Following surgery, her weight and diabetes improved and 24 hour urine cortisol normalized.

Incidentally discovered adrenal tumors, adrenal incidentalomas (AIs), are common, occurring in 3–7% of abdominal imaging performed for other reasons [1]. The majority of AIs are benign adrenocortical adenomas [7]. It is generally accepted that most AIs should undergo evaluation for the autonomous secretion of cortisol, catecholamines, and aldosterone (in hypertensive or hypokalemic patients) [1]. About 10–12% of AIs are cortisol secreting [7].

The presence of macroscopic fat on CT in an AI is considered virtually diagnostic of myelolipoma [8]. Adrenal myelolipomas are uncommon tumors that are composed of mature adipose and myeloid tissue and thought to be benign tumors which are not capable of autonomous hormone production [9]. It is generally accepted that myelolipomas do not warrant an evaluation for autonomous hormone production. The diagnosis of myelolipoma is made radiographically by the presence of an adrenal tumor containing macroscopic fat [10], but our group has previously reported that the accuracy of this diagnosis may depend on the amount of macroscopic fat seen in the tumor [11]. While adrenal myelolipomas are hormonally inactive, there is an increased association of myelolipomas and multiple endocrine disorders, including Cushing's syndrome. Although the exact etiology is unknown, one theory suggests a hormonally induced transformation of adrenal tissue into myeloid and lipomatous cells [12, 13].

Alternatively, others have suggested adrenal tissue necrosis may lead to myelolipomatous change [9, 10]. Both theories may account for the incidence of myelolipomas coupled with adrenal hyperplasia and Cushing's syndrome, as it has been reported [12, 14, 15].

Table 1: Case reports of adrenal myelolipoma and functioning adrenal adenoma.

Case authors	Age	Gender	ACTH	Cortisol	Side	Tumor size (cm)	Symptoms
Vyberg et al. [16]	31	F	↓	↑	L	2.5	Weight gain, hair loss, ecchymoses
Selye et al. [13]	58	F	↓	↑	R	$7 \times 4 \times 4$	Diabetes mellitus
Jenkins et al. [15]	67	F	↓	↑	L	$3.5 \times 3 \times 2$	Diabetes mellitus
Su et al. [9]	29	F	↓	—	R	$3.3 \times 2.2 \times 1.7$	Transient hypertension
Guresci et al. [14]	1.5	F	—	↑	L	$7 \times 6 \times 4.5$	Hypertension, weight gain, excessive body hair growth

Long-term hypercortisolism is associated with diabetes mellitus, hypertension, hyperlipidemia, and osteoporosis. Laparoscopic adrenalectomy has been shown to improve outcomes over nonsurgical therapy [16] and is the recommended treatment for patients with unilateral cortisol-secreting adrenal tumors [17]. Long-term autonomous secretion of cortisol from an adrenal tumor leads to suppression of the contralateral adrenal gland. Therefore, patients undergoing adrenalectomy for unilateral hypercortisolism require postoperative glucocorticoid replacement until the recovery of their remaining adrenal gland. There can be a delayed recovery taking up to 24 months [18].

Only five other case reports have chronicled a combination of an adrenal myelolipoma and functioning adrenal adenoma in a patient with Cushing's syndrome [2–6] (Table 1). An additional case of an adrenal myelolipoma and a functioning adrenal adenoma in a patient with Conn's syndrome have also been described [17]. As with our patient, Lu et al. previously reported that the majority of myelolipoma-adrenocortical adenoma collision tumors were found in female patients, involved the left adrenal gland, and if functional, demonstrated hormonal profiles compatible with Cushing's syndrome [17].

3. Conclusion

Adrenal lesions with macroscopic fat on imaging are typically labelled as myelolipomas and may not undergo a functional evaluation. This case report demonstrates that clinicians should consider a functional evaluation of select patients with radiographically diagnosed myelolipomas as they may prove to be functional collision tumors.

References

[1] W. W. Mayo-Smith, J. H. Song, G. L. Boland et al., "Management of incidental adrenal masses: a white paper of the acr incidental findings committee," *Journal of the American College of Radiology*, vol. 14, no. 8, pp. 1038–1044, 2017.

[2] T. Matsuda, H. Abe, M. Takase et al., "Case of combined adrenal cortical adenoma and myelolipoma," *Pathology International*, vol. 54, no. 9, pp. 725–729, 2004.

[3] R. Armand, A. R. Cappola, R. B. Horenstein, C. B. Drachenberg, H. Sasano, and J. C. Papadimitriou, "Adrenal cortical adenoma with excess black pigment deposition, combined with myelolipoma and clinical Cushing's syndrome," *International Journal of Surgical Pathology*, vol. 12, no. 1, pp. 57–61, 2004.

[4] I. A. Cardinalli, A. G. de Oliveira-Filho, M. J. Mastellaro, R. C. Ribeiro, and S. S. Aguiar, "A unique case of synchronous functional adrenocortical adenoma and myelolipoma within the ectopic adrenal cortex in a child with Beckwith-Wiedemann syndrome," *Pathology-Research and Practice*, vol. 208, no. 3, pp. 189–194, 2012.

[5] H. Hisamatsu, H. Sakai, S. Tsuda, K. Shigematsu, and H. Kanetake, "Combined adrenal adenoma and myelolipoma in a patient with Cushing's syndrome: case report and review of the literature," *International Journal of Urology*, vol. 11, no. 6, pp. 416–418, 2004.

[6] M. Vyberg and L. Sestoft, "Combined adrenal myelolipoma and adenoma associated with Cushing's syndrome," *American Journal of Clinical Pathology*, vol. 86, no. 4, pp. 541–545, 1986.

[7] M. Fassnacht, W. Arlt, I. Bancos et al., "Management of adrenal incidentalomas: European society of endocrinology clinical practice guideline in collaboration with the European network for the study of adrenal tumors," *European Journal of Endocrinology*, vol. 175, no. 2, pp. G1–G34, 2016.

[8] N. Khater and R. Khauli, "Myelolipomas and other fatty tumours of the adrenals," *Arab Journal of Urology*, vol. 9, no. 4, pp. 259–265, 2011.

[9] H. C. Su, X. Huang, W. L. Zhou et al., "Pathologic analysis, diagnosis and treatment of adrenal myelolipoma," *Canadian Urological Association Journal*, vol. 8, no. 9-10, pp. E637–E640, 2014.

[10] E. M. Schaeffer and L. R. Kavoussi, "Adrenal myelolipoma," *Journal of Urology*, vol. 173, no. 5, p. 1760, 2005.

[11] M. J. Campbell, M. Obasi, B. Wu, M. T. Corwin, and G. Fananapazir, "The radiographically diagnosed adrenal myelolipoma: what do we really know?" *Endocrine*, vol. 58, no. 2, pp. 289–294, 2017.

[12] A. Ishay, A. Ishay, M. Dharan, M. Dharan, R. Luboshitzky, and R. Luboshitzky, "Combined adrenal myelolipoma and medullary hyperplasia," *Hormone Research*, vol. 62, no. 1, pp. 23–26, 2004.

[13] H. Selye and H. Stone, "Hormonally induced transformation of adrenal into myeloid tissue," *The American Journal of Pathology*, vol. 26, no. 2, pp. 211–233, 1950.

[14] S. Guresci, C. Kara, D. T. Ertugrul, and A. Unsal, "Combined adrenal medullary hyperplasia and myelolipoma: a mimicker of pheochromocytoma," *Turkish Journal of Endocrinology and Metabolism*, vol. 13, pp. 84–86, 2009.

[15] P. J. Jenkins, S. L. Chew, D. G. Lowe, R. H. Reznek, and J. A. H. Wass, "Adrenocorticotrophin-independent unilateral macronodular adrenal hyperplasia occurring with myelolipoma: an unusual cause of Cushing's syndrome," *Clinical Endocrinology*, vol. 41, no. 6, pp. 827–830, 1994.

[16] A. Toniato, I. Merante-Boschin, G. Opocher, M. R. Pelizzo, F. Schiavi, and E. Ballotta, "Surgical versus conservative management for subclinical cushing syndrome in adrenal incidentalomas: a prospective randomized study," *Annals of Surgery*, vol. 249, no. 3, pp. 388–391, 2009.

[17] H. S. Lu, M. F. Gan, H. S. Chen, and S. Q. Huang, "Adrenal myelolipoma within myxoid cortical adenoma associated with Conn's syndrome," *Journal of Zhejiang University Science B*, vol. 9, no. 6, pp. 500–505, 2008.

[18] M. Välimäki, R. Pelkonen, L. Porkka, A. Sivula, and A. Kahri, "Long-term results of adrenal surgery in patients with Cushing's syndrome due to adrenocortical adenoma," *Clinical Endocrinology*, vol. 20, no. 2, pp. 229–236, 1984.

17

Syndrome of Inappropriate Antidiuretic Hormone Secretion (SIADH) and Subsequent Central Diabetes Insipidus: A Rare Presentation of Pituitary Apoplexy

S. B. Smedegaard,[1] J. O. Jørgensen,[2] and N. Rittig[1,2,3]

[1]*Department of Internal Medicine, Horsens Regional Hospital, Sundvej 30, 8700 Horsens, Denmark*
[2]*Department of Diabetes and Hormone Diseases (DoH), Aarhus University Hospital, Palle Juul-Jensens Blvd 99, 8200 Aarhus N, Denmark*
[3]*Steno Diabetes Center Aarhus, Aarhus University Hospital, Palle Juul-Jensens Blvd 99, 8200 Aarhus N, Denmark*

Correspondence should be addressed to N. Rittig; nikolaj.rittig@clin.au.dk

Academic Editor: Hidetoshi Ikeda

Pituitary apoplexy (PA) is a rare endocrine emergency that occasionally presents with sodium disturbances. Here we present a rare case with a previously healthy 41-year-old female who presented with acute onset headache and nausea without visual impairment or overt pituitary dysfunction. Plasma sodium concentrations declined abruptly during the first two days of admission to a nadir of 111 mmol/l. Urine and blood chemistry were consistent with syndrome of inappropriate antidiuretic hormone secretion (SIADH). Magnetic resonance imaging revealed recent bleeding into a pituitary cystic process. Hyponatremia was successfully corrected with fluid restriction and both visual function and anterior pituitary function remained intact. Subsequently, the patient developed central diabetes insipidus (CDI), which responded well to desmopressin substitution. To our knowledge, this is the first case of PA presenting predominantly with posterior pituitary dysfunction that transitioned from SIADH to permanent CDI.

1. Introduction

Pituitary apoplexy (PA) is a rare clinical emergency induced by sudden haemorrhage or infarction into the pituitary gland, which predominantly occurs into an existing pituitary adenoma [1]. Abrupt onset of severe headache is the main symptom, but neurological symptoms, nausea, visual impairment, ocular palsy, and endocrine disturbances frequently occur [1–3]. Severe hyponatremia due to the syndrome of inappropriate antidiuretic hormone secretion (SIADH) is occasionally reported in PA [4–7] and also occurs in ≈ 6% of patients undergoing pituitary surgery [8].

In general, SIADH is caused by inappropriate excretion of vasopressin from the pituitary gland, ectopic vasopressin production, or increased ADH sensitivity [9]. The condition was first detected by William Schwartz and Frederic Bartter in 1967, who also established the clinical criteria for SIADH, which includes serum sodium < 135 mmol/l, serum osmolality < 275 mmol/kg, urine sodium > 40 mmol/l, urine osmolality > 100 mmol/kg, absence of clinical signs of volume depletion, absence of known conditions causing hyponatremia, and successful correction of sodium levels with fluid restriction [10]. Various conditions can cause SIADH including granulomatous diseases, malignant tumours, central nervous disease, and drug intake [9]. Rare causes of SIADH such as PA may be overlooked, not least since the two conditions share symptoms and signs including nausea and hyponatremia.

Central diabetes insipidus (CDI) is another rare condition, which is characterized by polyuria (> 3 L per day), excessive thirst, polydipsia, and elevated serum sodium levels [11]. It is known that CDI complicates PA with a prevalence of less than 5% and that the condition most often is temporary and resolves within the following weeks [1, 3]. To our knowledge,

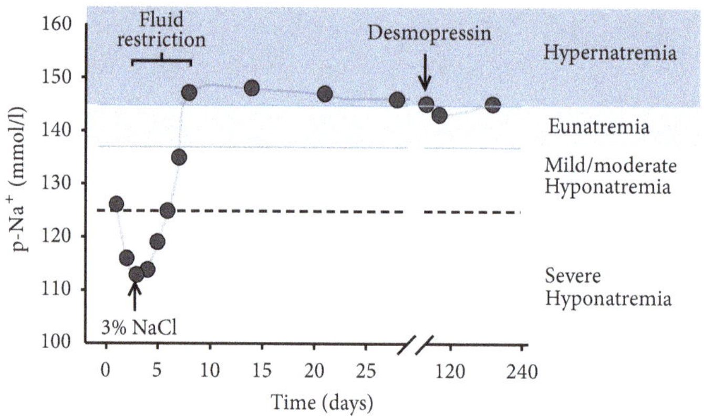

FIGURE 1: Plasma concentrations of sodium. Horizontal axis depicts time course from hospital admission (day 0) until 180 days' follow-up. Vertical axis depicts plasma sodium concentrations (p-Na$^+$). Hyponatremia was treated with intravenous hyperosmolar sodium infusion (3% NaCl at day 2) and fluid restriction (day 2 to day 5). The subsequent development of central diabetes insipidus (CDI) was treated with low dose desmopressin (initiated around day 60).

a case of PA dominated by SIADH and subsequent CDI in the absence of overt anterior pituitary deficits has not previously been reported.

2. Case Presentation

A previously healthy 41-year-old Caucasian woman was admitted to the Emergency Department at the Regional Hospital of Horsens with a three-day history of severe headache, nausea, and dizziness. The physical examination was unremarkable with no evidence of impaired vision. Regular medication only included oral contraceptives (75 microgram desogestrel). Initial blood screen tests revealed moderate hyponatremia (126 mmol/l) and borderline low levels of iodothyronines (T_3 and T_4) and thyroid-stimulating hormone (TSH, Table 1). An acute cerebral computed tomography (CT) did not show haemorrhage or infarction, and no mass lesion in the sellar region. Lumbar puncture showed no signs of infection or bleeding. Additional blood tests showed normal anterior pituitary function (Table 1) except moderate hyperprolactinemia. During the first two days of admission, plasma sodium concentrations dropped to a nadir level of 111 mmol/l (Figure 1). On the third day, a magnetic resonance imaging [MRI] of the brain showed recent bleeding into a cystic process (10x10x8 mm) in the sellar region in close proximity to the optic chiasm with displacement of the pituitary gland to the right (Figure 2). Urine and blood examination at day two (Table 1) were consistent with SIADH according to standard criteria [10]. The patient was treated with fluid restriction (day two to day five) and an intravenous bolus of hypertonic saline 3% (day two only), which induced a gradual increase in plasma sodium concentrations (Figure 1). During the following weeks, the patient developed polyuria, polydipsia, and persistent hypernatremia. She was diagnosed with central diabetes insipidus (CDI) and successfully treated with desmopressin (dose 0.1 mg daily).

A MRI follow-up after three and ten months showed no change in the size of the cystic adenoma and automated perimetry showed a normal visual field. Anterior pituitary function remained intact, whereas the patient's CDI is considered permanent.

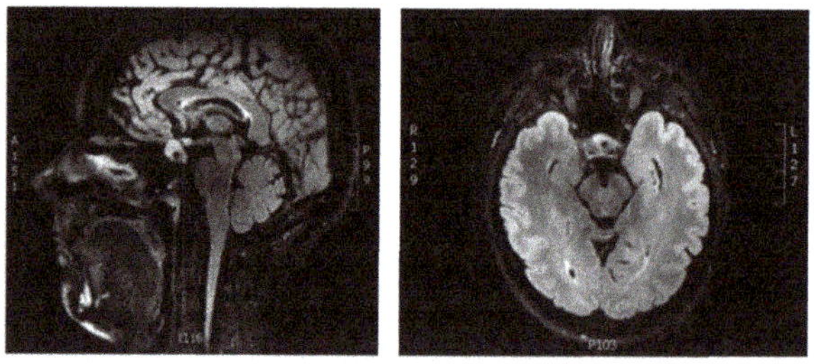

FIGURE 2: Magnetic resonance imaging of cerebrum. Magnetic resonance imaging (MRI) showed signs of recent bleeding into a cystic adenoma comprising 10x10x8 mm placed in sella turcica with close proximity to the chiasma and displacing the pituitary gland to the right.

3. Discussion

Pituitary apoplexy is a rare but acute condition causing severe headache often associated with visual disturbances including ocular palsy, and altered consciousness. The clinical picture resembles that of subarachnoid haemorrhage (SAH) or meningitis, which often delays the diagnosis [1]. Pituitary imaging confirms the diagnosis by revealing a haemorrhagic or necrotic pituitary tumour [12]. Corticotropic deficiency causing adrenal insufficiency must be evaluated and promptly treated, and acute surgery is indicated if the symptoms worsen [1]. The present case of PA is unique owing to its presentation with isolated posterior pituitary dysfunction that transitioned from SIADH into permanent CDI.

It is well known that neurosurgery and brain trauma may cause hyponatremia, which is often attributable to SIADH [13–15]. Furthermore, it is evident that pituitary surgery may elicit a tri-phasic response with acute hypernatremia, transient hyponatremia around postoperative day 7 (between 3 and 11 days), and subsequent development of CDI [16–19].

Table 1

(a) Standard blood test screen at admission

Na^+	126	↓	*(137 - 145)*	*mmol/l*
K^+	3.5		*(3.5 - 4.6)*	*mmol/l*
CRP	1.8		*(<8)*	*mg/l*
Leucocytes	6.4		*(3.5 - 10)*	*10^9/l*
TSH	0.4		*(0.3 - 4.5)*	*10^3 IU/l*
T_3	3.1	↓	*(3.9 - 6.8)*	*pmol/l*
T_4	11.4	↓	*(12 - 21)*	*pmol/l*

(b) Extended blood and urine tests

Prolactin	1375	↑	*(90 - 580)*	*10^3 IU/l*
ACTH	36		*(7 - 64)*	*ng/l*
Cortisol 0 min	541			*nmol/l*
Cortisol 30 min	797		*(> 500)*	*nmol/l*
FSH	23			*IU/l*
LH	6.7			*IU/l*
Estrogen	<15			*pmol/l*
IGF-1	192		*(70-210)*	*μg/l*
Osmolality	241	↓	*(280-300)*	*mmol/kg*
Urine				
U-Osmolality	744		*(300 - 900)*	*mmol/kg*
U-Na^+	140			*mmol/l*

Biochemistry: standard blood test screen and extended blood and urine tests. This table shows selected blood sample concentrations from the standard blood test screening performed on the day of hospital admission and the extended blood test analysis performed on day two of admission. Parenthesis illustrates the normal range. ↓ = below normal range. ↑ = above normal range. *CRP= C reactive protein, TSH = thyroid stimulating hormone, T_3= triiodothyronine, T_4= thyronine, ACTH= adrenocorticotropic hormone, FSH= follicle-stimulating hormone, LH= luteinizing hormone, and IGF-1= insulin-like growth factor 1.*

Our case shows a similar course with SIADH/hyponatremia approximately 5 days following initial symptoms and development of CDI in the ensuing weeks. We therefore speculate that PA may cause sodium disturbances through similar mechanisms as pituitary surgery and brain trauma, which include an acute outburst of ADH from damaged cells in the posterior pituitary gland [14, 15]. This damage may cause subsequent CDI that typically resolves within weeks but occasionally result in permanent CDI [14].

Hyponatremia is the most frequent electrolyte disturbance, especially in hospitalized patients [20], and PA is a rare and often overlooked cause of hyponatremia. Most emergency departments use standard blood test screens at admission, and cerebral CT-scans are also widely used in this setting. Studies have shown that CT only detects 21% of PA, whereas 90% is visualized with MRI [12, 21]. The absence of visual impairment and lack of clear anterior pituitary affection undoubtedly delayed the MRI and hence the final diagnosis in our case.

Pituitary apoplexy remains an important albeit rare differential diagnosis in patients presenting with severe and acutely onset headache, and our case illustrates that PA may masquerade as isolated SIADH and develop into CDI.

Abbreviations

CDI: Central diabetes insipidus
CT: Computed tomography
MRI: Magnetic resonance imaging
PA: Pituitary apoplexy
SAH: Subarachnoid haemorrhage
SIADH: Syndrome of inappropriate antidiuretic hormone secretion.

Disclosure

We confirm that this report is in line with the International Committee of Medical Journal Editors' (ICMJE) recommendations. No human or animal experiments were conducted.

Acknowledgments

The authors would like to thank the Department of Internal Medicine in Horsens for their support. They would also like to thank the patient for allowing them to report this rare medical case.

References

[1] C. Briet, S. Salenave, and P. Chanson, "Pituitary apoplexy," *Endocrinology and Metabolism Clinics of North America*, vol. 44, no. 1, pp. 199–209, 2015.

[2] S. Rajasekaran, M. Vanderpump, S. Baldeweg et al., "UK guidelines for the management of pituitary apoplexy," *Clinical Endocrinology*, vol. 74, no. 1, pp. 9–20, 2011.

[3] D. L. Möller-Goede, M. Brändle, K. Landau, R. L. Bernay, and C. Schmid, "Pituitary apoplexy: re-evaluation of risk factors

for bleeding into pituitary adenomas and impact on outcome," *European Journal of Endocrinology*, vol. 164, no. 1, pp. 37–43, 2011.

[4] F. H. Ebner, T. K. Hauser, and J. Honegger, "SIADH following pituitary adenoma apoplexy," *Neurological Sciences*, vol. 31, no. 2, pp. 217-218, 2010.

[5] D. Agrawal and A. K. Mahapatra, "Pituitary apoplexy and inappropriate ADH secretion," *Journal of Clinical Neuroscience*, vol. 10, no. 2, pp. 260-261, 2003.

[6] K. Morinaga, Y. Inoue, M. Ueda et al., "An interesting case of pituitary apoplexy showing abnormality in water-electrolyte before and after surgery," *Brain And Nerve*, vol. 42, no. 10, pp. 907–911, 1990.

[7] E. A. McAninch and B. W. Kim, "Symptomatic syndrome of inappropriate antidiuretic hormone secretion in pituitary apoplexy: a case report and literature review," *AACE Clinical Case Reports*, vol. 2, no. 2, pp. e100–e105, 2016.

[8] G. Bordo, K. Kelly, N. McLaughlin et al., "Sellar masses that present with severe hyponatremia," *Endocrine Practice*, vol. 20, no. 11, pp. 1178–1186, 2014.

[9] G. Spasovski, R. Vanholder, B. Allolio et al., "Clinical practice guideline on diagnosis and treatment of hyponatraemia," *Nephrology Dialysis Transplantation* , vol. 29, supplement 2, pp. i1–i39, 2014.

[10] P. Gross, "Clinical management of SIADH," *Therapeutic Advances in Endocrinology and Metabolism*, vol. 3, no. 2, pp. 61–73, 2012.

[11] A. Garrahy, C. Moran, and C. J. Thompson, "Diagnosis and management of central diabetes insipidus in adults," *Clinical Endocrinology*, vol. 90, no. 1, pp. 23–30, 2018.

[12] H. S. Randeva, J. Schoebel, J. Byrne, M. Esiri, C. B. T. Adams, and J. A. H. Wass, "Classical pituitary apoplexy: clinical features, management and outcome," *Clinical Endocrinology*, vol. 51, no. 2, pp. 181–188, 1999.

[13] D. K. Kim and K. W. Joo, "Hyponatremia in patients with neurologic disorders," *Electrolytes & Blood Pressure*, vol. 7, no. 2, p. 51, 2009.

[14] C. Capatina, A. Paluzzi, R. Mitchell, and N. Karavitaki, "Diabetes insipidus after traumatic brain injury," *Journal of Clinical Medicine*, vol. 4, no. 7, pp. 1448–1462, 2015.

[15] E. T. Blair, J. S. Clemmer, H. L. Harkey, R. L. Hester, and W. A. Pruett, "Physiologic mechanisms of water and electrolyte disturbances after transsphenoidal pituitary surgery," *World Neurosurgery*, vol. 107, pp. 429–436, 2017.

[16] E. J. Hoorn and R. Zietse, "Water balance disorders after neurosurgery: the triphasic response revisited," *NDT Plus*, vol. 3, no. 1, pp. 42–44, 2010.

[17] S. K. Simon, P. V. Pavithran, A. Asirvatham, R. Ayyadurai, and A. Parasuram, "Disorders of water balance following sellar and suprasellar surgeries: Patterns, determinants and utility of quantitative analysis," *Indian Journal of Endocrinology and Metabolism*, vol. 22, no. 2, pp. 191–195, 2018.

[18] M. Zoli, D. Mazzatenta, and M. Faustini-Fustini, "Transient delayed hyponatremia after transsphenoidal surgery: attempting to enlighten the epidemiology and management of a still-obscure complication," *World Neurosurgery*, vol. 90, pp. 654–656, 2016.

[19] J. F. Cusick, T. C. Hagen, and J. W. Kindling, "Inappropriate secretion of antidiuretic hormone after transsphenoidal surgery for pituitary tumors," *The New England Journal of Medicine*, vol. 311, no. 1, pp. 36–38, 1984.

[20] M. J. Hannon and C. J. Thompson, "The syndrome of inappropriate antidiuretic hormone: prevalence, causes and consequences," *European Journal of Endocrinology*, vol. 162, no. Suppl1, pp. S5–S12, 2010.

[21] P. Goyal, M. Utz, N. Gupta et al., "Clinical and imaging features of pituitary apoplexy and role of imaging in differentiation of clinical mimics," *Quantitative Imaging in Medicine and Surgery*, vol. 8, no. 2, pp. 219–231, 2018.

18

Safety and Efficacy of Insulin and Heparin in the Management of Hypertriglyceridemia-Induced Pancreatitis in a Patient without Diabetes: A Case Report

Luis Tolento Cortes,[1] Jessica Trinh,[1] Mimi Le,[1] Philip Papayanis,[2] Leah Tudtud-Hans,[2] and Lisa Hong[1]

[1]*Loma Linda University Health, School of Pharmacy, 24745 Stewart St, Loma Linda, CA, USA*
[2]*Loma Linda University Health, School of Medicine, 11175 Campus St, Loma Linda, CA, USA*

Correspondence should be addressed to Lisa Hong; lhong@llu.edu

Academic Editor: Osamu Isozaki

Acute pancreatitis (AP) leads to a variety of complications, such as local or systemic inflammatory responses as well as organ failure. While choledocholithiasis and alcohol abuse are two of the most common causes of AP, hypertriglyceridemia causes AP with an incidence rate between 2 and 5%. The management of hypertriglyceridemia-induced pancreatitis (HTGIP) is focused on the lowering of triglyceride (TG) levels, and the efficacy of therapies for the management of HTGIP may vary based on the hypertriglyceridemia etiology. The aim of this article is to report a case of a 43-year-old female with a history of familial hypertriglyceridemia and without diabetes who was admitted for acute pancreatitis with a TG level elevated to 4,435 mg/dL. The patient was treated with a combination of insulin, heparin, atorvastatin, and omega-3-acid ethyl esters, and her TG level was reduced to 880 mg/dL after 9 days of therapy. Despite the successful treatment of the patient, standardization of the approach for the treatment of HTGIP is needed. Future research should aim to identify the appropriateness of insulin therapy specifically in patients without diabetes presenting with hypertriglyceridemia and the dosing associated with optimal safety.

1. Introduction

Pancreatitis is one of the most common gastrointestinal-related disorders, leading to both emergency department visits and hospital readmissions [1]. The prevalence of severe hypertriglyceridemia (triglyceride [TG] levels >500 mg/dL) in adults over the age of 20 years in the United States is approximately 1.7% [2]. Hypertriglyceridemia can have either monogenic or polygenic etiologies, and abnormalities in the LPL, APOC2, APOA5, LMF1, or GPIHBP1 genes can lead to the development of hypertriglyceridemia. Secondary factors include comorbid conditions such as diabetes and obesity. Additionally, lifestyle habits such as alcohol abuse and high-fat diets may also increase the risk of developing hypertriglyceridemia [3, 4]. The mechanism of hypertriglyceridemia-induced pancreatitis (HTGIP) is not well-understood. One theoretical mechanism involves the hydrolysis of triglycerides by pancreatic lipases, which results in the production of free fatty acids (FFA) in the pancreas. This newly hydrolyzed FFA can potentially accumulate in the pancreatic capillary beds. Consequently, the "plugging" of these capillaries may cause ischemia and acidosis. The acidic environment may contribute to the activation of trypsinogen, leading to acinar cell injury and ultimately pancreatitis [5, 6].

Initial management of HTGIP is similar to the management of acute pancreatitis (AP). Therapies tailored to the management of HTGIP involve interventions that can rapidly decrease TG levels. Published reports describe the utilization of agents such as insulin, heparin, fenofibrate, omega-3 fatty acids, and statins, as well as plasmapheresis for TG lowering [7–22]. However, guidance regarding the best practice for pharmacologic treatment in these cases is lacking.

Here we report a case of HTGIP in a patient without diabetes treated with intravenous insulin and subcutaneous heparin. Our case highlights the need for standardization of treatment and close monitoring of adverse events including hypokalemia and hypoglycemia.

2. Case Report

A 43-year-old female with a past medical history of familial hypertriglyceridemia, obesity, hyperlipidemia, hypertension, pituitary adenoma, and a recent hysterectomy presented to the emergency department due to worsening left-sided epigastric abdominal pain with associated nausea and decreased appetite. She denied any fever, chills, chest pain, cough, shortness of breath, diarrhea, or urinary symptoms. Family history was positive for diabetes in both parents. The patient denied any history of smoking, alcohol, or illicit drug use.

Her vital signs demonstrated tachycardia of 119 beats per minute, an elevated blood pressure of 169/111 mmHg, and a respiratory rate of 20 breaths per minute. Physical examination of the abdomen was negative for severe epigastric pain and a left-upper quadrant that was tender to palpation. Laboratory examination revealed serum triglycerides of 4,425 mg/dL, a total cholesterol level of 1,273 mg/dL, high-density lipoprotein <3 mg/dL, lipase of 80 units/L, blood glucose of 256 mg/dL, hemoglobin $A1_C$ of 6.0%, potassium of 3.7 mEq/L, as well as aspartate transaminase (AST) and alanine transaminase (ALT) of 73 and 77 units/L, respectively. Given this clinical presentation, there was suspicion of pancreatitis, but the serum lipase was only mildly elevated. Therefore, a computed tomography (CT) scan was performed. The CT showed mild fat stranding around the pancreas, which is consistent with acute interstitial pancreatitis, hepatic steatosis, and nonobstructive cholelithiasis (Figure 1). Investigation with ultrasonography of the right upper quadrant confirmed no gallstone was obstructing the pancreatic duct. Given the patient's severely elevated TGs, no obstruction seen on imaging, and lack of alcohol use disorder, the patient was diagnosed with pancreatitis secondary to hypertriglyceridemia.

Initial treatment included standard fluid resuscitation and pain management with the oral hydrocodone-acetaminophen combination (5 mg and 325 mg) and intravenous morphine (2 mg). The hospital's endocrinology team was consulted for lipid management, and a continuous infusion of regular insulin was initiated at a rate of 10 units/hour. A 2-bag system consisting of 0.9% sodium chloride alone and 5% dextrose/0.9% sodium chloride (both containing potassium phosphate 20 mmol and potassium acetate 20 mEq) was used in conjunction with insulin. The patient was also treated with omega-3-acid ethyl esters at a dose of 2 grams orally twice daily and atorvastatin 20 mg orally daily as formulary substitutions of home medications icosapent ethyl 2 grams orally twice daily and rosuvastatin 5 mg orally daily with a goal of lowering TG to <500 mg/dL. Subcutaneous heparin at 5,000

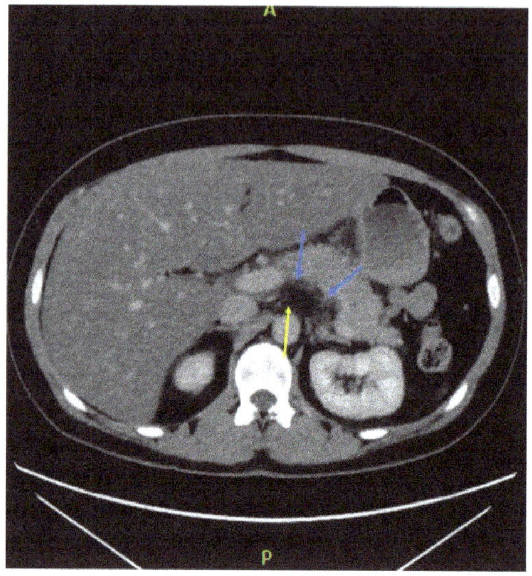

FIGURE 1: CT abdomen. CT illustrates the blurring of the margins of the pancreas (blue arrows) as well as mild retroperitoneal fat stranding (yellow arrows). These findings are due to inflammation of the fat around the pancreas, which is consistent with the diagnosis of acute interstitial pancreatitis.

units every 8 hours was also initiated. The nutrition team was consulted and the patient was maintained on a fat-restricted diet (<30 grams a day). She had 2 days with strict orders to receive nothing by mouth due to severe abdominal pain and her inability to tolerate an oral diet.

On hospital day 2, the serum TG dropped to 2,212 mg/dL and the insulin drip was titrated up to 15 units/hour with a dextrose 10% and 0.45% sodium chloride infusion at a rate of 200 mL/hour. The intravenous insulin continued at 15 units/hour until hospital day 7. During this period, the patient's TG levels continued to downtrend, reaching a low of 863 mg/dL (an 80% decrease from baseline) on hospital day 6. On hospital day 7, the patient's TG increased to 1,112 mg/dL (a 74% reduction from baseline). The insulin infusion rate was changed to a weight-based regimen of 0.2 units/kg/hour (patient weight was 97 kg = approximately 19 units/hour) with continuous dextrose 17.5% (started at 150 mL/hour, then titrated to 200 mL/hour) until hospital day 9. While serum TG decreased to 821 mg/dL in response to the increased insulin, three episodes of hypoglycemia were observed within a 9-hour timeframe during the weight-based insulin infusion. An additional 25-gram ampule of dextrose was given to correct these hypoglycemic events. The last insulin infusion titration to 25 units/hour occurred on hospital day 9 with dextrose 20% running at 200 mL/hour and remained at this rate until the termination of insulin therapy on hospital day 10, when the nadir TG level of 809 mg/dL (81.7% reduction from baseline) was obtained. At this time, the endocrinology team recommended discontinuing insulin therapy, and their rationale was that the TG-reducing effect had likely reached its max. The patient remained on heparin for the rest of her hospitalization for continued thromboprophylaxis until hospital day 12. During this period, the TG increased to 1,415 mg/dL on hospital day 11 and decreased to 1,028 mg/

dL (76% reduction from baseline) without further therapeutic intervention (see Figure 2).

Due to the effect of insulin therapy on serum potassium levels, potassium was assessed and replenished on hospital days 1 to 4 as appropriate. The patient was started on scheduled potassium replacements of 20 mEq on hospital day 5, but still required several additional doses during the admission (see Figure 3), including 100 mEq of supplemental potassium on hospital day 8 to correct hypokalemia.

The patient was discharged home on hospital day 13 and instructed to continue the triglyceride-lowering oral medications as mentioned above, with the addition of 54 mg fenofibrate orally daily. The patient's TG level was 495 mg/dL during a 1-month postdischarge follow-up appointment.

3. Discussion

We report the successful management of a 43-year-old female with a history of familial hypertriglyceridemia without a history of diabetes admitted for acute pancreatitis with the use of continuous insulin infusions and subcutaneous heparin, with serum TG levels falling from 4,425 mg/dL to 809 mg/dL after 8 days of insulin and heparin combination therapy. Triglycerides are normally synthesized in the liver or obtained through exogenous means. Under normal circumstances, these circulating TGs (as chylomicrons and low-density lipoprotein) are metabolized by lipoprotein lipase into FFA. Familial hypertriglyceridemia is polygenic and presents with elevated very low-density lipoprotein (VLDL) levels secondary to impaired catabolism of VLDL. In hypertriglyceridemia, VLDL particles contain a higher percentage of TGs, leading to an increased size of VLDL particles and suboptimal hydrolysis by lipoprotein lipase, which ultimately results in a normal amount of VLDL particles with altered compositions [23].

The role of insulin in the treatment of hypertriglyceridemia is an activation in addition to the synthesis of lipoprotein lipase (LPL). LPL activity is higher in a fed state compared to a fasting state and improves the clearance of TGs from circulation by cleaving TG into FFA, which can be transported into the surrounding tissues for further metabolism or storage. There are also some speculations that insulin may inhibit the re-esterification of FFA into TG [24, 25]. The efficacy of continuous insulin therapy in managing hypertriglyceridemia is referenced in a recent hypertriglyceridemia management article published by the American Family Physician [26]. Success in obtaining significant reductions in TG levels via bolus dosing of insulin has been reported as well [11]. Interestingly, there are no formal recommendations on hypertriglyceridemia management in patients without diabetes.

Heparin has been used in combination with insulin therapy to lower TG levels [27]. The mechanism by which heparin lowers TGs is hypothesized to be due to its ability to release LPL from endothelial cells, preventing LPL from converting to a nonactive unit and decreasing circulating TG. However, there is a concern about rebound hypertriglyceridemia associated with prolonged heparin use due to an imbalance in the production and degradation of LPL [28]. The reported route of heparin administration in the management of hypertriglyceridemia is commonly intravenous, but groups have observed similar efficacy with subcutaneous unfractionated heparin as well as low molecular weight heparin without any reports of bleeding [13, 17].

There is a paucity of data assessing patients without diabetes who present with hypertriglyceridemia. Khan et al. previously reported a successful course of treatment with insulin infusion monotherapy that resulted in a reduction of TG levels from 3,525 mg/dL to 973 mg/dL with only one day of therapy [15]. Gayam et al. also used insulin monotherapy but for a duration of approximately 7 days with a dose of 1–2 units/kg/day (a rate significantly lower than in our case) and observed a reduction in TG levels from >10,000 mg/dL to <300 mg/dL [9]. Another case report by Reed et al. of a patient with familial hypertriglyceridemia and an initial TG level of 3,496 mg/dL demonstrated a decrease in TGs to 426 mg/dL after 3 days of an insulin infusion at 0.07 units/kg/hour [20]. A longer treatment duration of 12 days was necessary in a report by Inayat et al., where insulin monotherapy was administered at a rate of 0.1 units/kg/hour in a patient with prediabetes, resulting in a decrease in TGs from 5,047 mg/dL to under 500 mg/dL [10]. None of these studies discussed the use of heparin, and it is unclear whether subcutaneous heparin was administered in any of the above cases. In three reports where heparin use was described in patients without diabetes, total daily doses were similar to typical doses used for venous thromboembolism prophylaxis [13, 17, 22] and less than or equal to the dose used in our patient case. Interestingly, one reported monotherapy with heparin at 15,000 units/day with a resolution of hypertriglyceridemia (8,500 mg/dL to 408 mg/dL) in 3 days; [22] see (Table 1).

Unlike other studies in patients without diabetes that reported a rapid and substantial correction of TG levels within the first few hours/days of therapy [9, 10, 13, 15, 20, 22], we observed a gradual decrease in TG levels. We did not observe the same magnitude of TG lowering (upwards of 90% reduction in most published cases) despite the use of a higher insulin infusion rate. A maximum reduction of approximately 82% from baseline was observed after 7 days of continuous IV insulin at rates up to 19 units/hr. Notably, a 72% and 80% reduction were also observed on hospital days 4 and 5 at an infusion rate of 15 units/hr, suggestive of a plateau effect. This may be indicative of the need for longer durations of insulin infusions at moderate rates as opposed to aggressive titrations. The observation of a similar TG level reduction from the baseline with less aggressive insulin infusion rates (15 units/hr vs 25 units/hr) may suggest that lower infusion rates of insulin are as efficacious as higher rates in the management of hypertriglyceridemia with a reduced risk for hypoglycemia. In addition to the risk of hypoglycemia, there is a risk of inducing hypokalemia with prolonged/aggressive insulin therapy. In our case, the patient still experienced hypokalemia despite daily potassium supplementation.

Another area of uncertainty was the significance of heparin therapy in the reduction of TG levels. From our

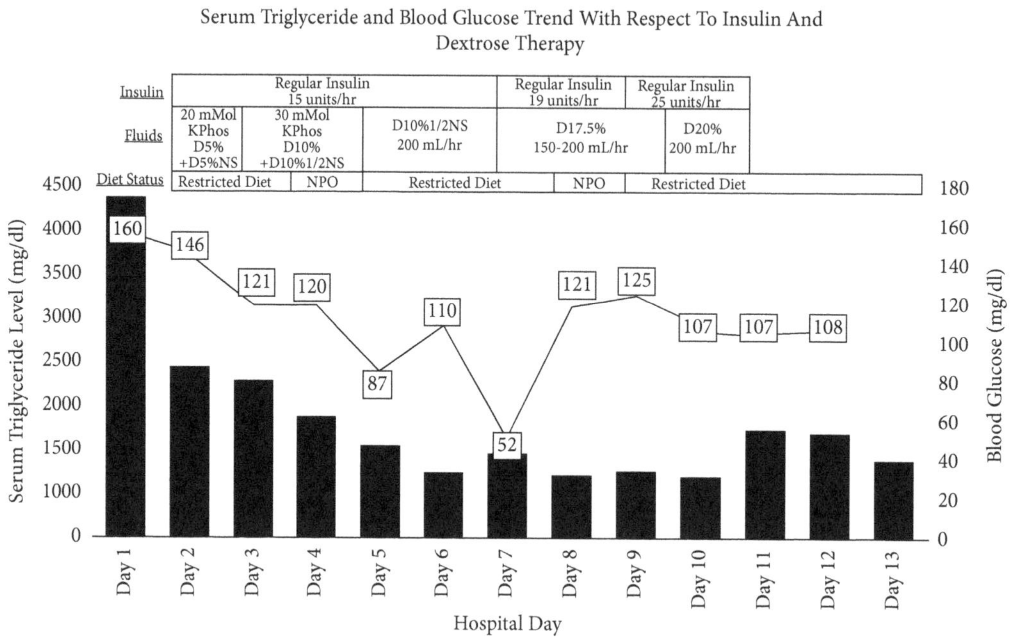

Figure 2: Serum triglycerides and blood glucose during hospital stay.

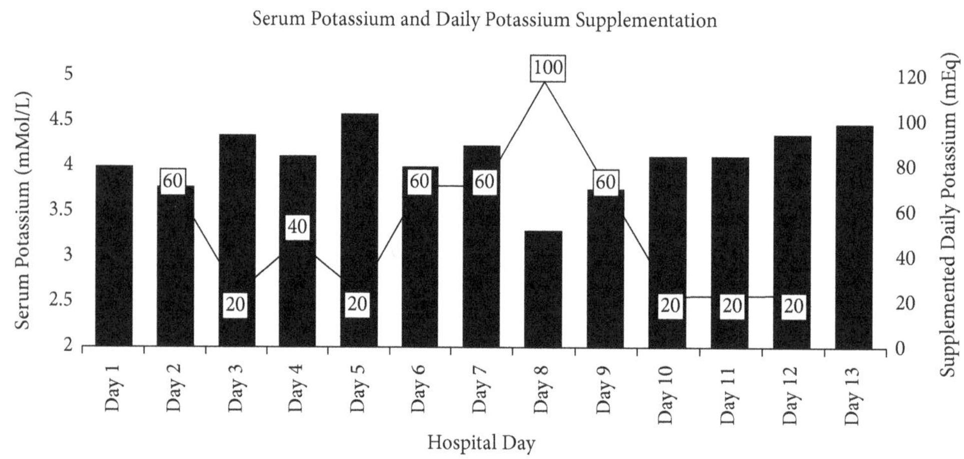

Figure 3: Serum potassium and potassium supplementation.

study, we observed an increase in the serum TG when insulin therapy was discontinued, even though heparin therapy was continued for two days, but it is unclear if the increase observed was attenuated by the use of heparin. Given no reports of increased bleed risk with heparin in this patient population and the often-concurrent indication for thromboprophylaxis, it seems prudent to use subcutaneous heparin at doses to prevent thromboembolism for the potential added benefits in patients with HTGIP.

As the patient received combination therapy, the efficacy of each individual medication is unknown. The patient's lack of adherence to oral TG-lowering agents prior to admission adds even more difficulty in separating the effects of the various treatment components. Though it is reasonable to predict that the reinitiation of omega-3 fatty acid and statin therapy did not contribute significantly to the acute decline in TG levels, we are unable to determine the degree to which they may have assisted with the resolution of hypertriglyceridemia over the hospital course. There is no defined duration of treatment for managing hypertriglyceridemia. Most reports show a fast resolution of symptoms (usually within hours to days), but our patient required more aggressive therapy and we were unable to attain the initial TG goal of <500 mg/dL. While the patient's serum TGs remained around 1,000 mg/dL upon discharge, the "resistance" to conventional treatments was likely multifactorial with a contribution from her history of familial hypertriglyceridemia, obesity, prediabetes, and medication nonadherence prior to admission. The patient reported improved adherence to her medications during a 1-month postdischarge follow-up encounter where her triglycerides were 495 mg/dL.

In this case report, we demonstrate the successful treatment of acute pancreatitis secondary to

Table 1: Studies evaluating insulin and/or heparin for hypertriglyceridemia management in adult patients.

Study	Number of patients (without diabetes)	Age (years)	Gender	Initial TG (mg/dL)	Treatment	Posttreatment TG (mg/dL)	Duration of treatment (days)	Hypo-kalemia	Hypo-glycemia
Monotherapy insulin									
Coskun et al. [8]*	12 (4)	46	8 male 4 female	Mean 1,140	Insulin infusion unspecified rate	Mean 492	Mean 3	No	No
Mikhail et al. [18]	1	38	1 female	10,560	Subcutaneous insulin sliding scale every 4 hours	712	3	No	No
Khan et al. [15]	1 (1)	44	1 female	3,525	Insulin infusion unspecified rate	973	1	No	No
Gayam et al. 2018 [9]	1 (1)	48	1 male	>10,000	Insulin infusion 1–2 units/kg/day	<300	8	No	No
Reed et al. [20]	1 (1)	34	1 female	3,496	Insulin infusion 0.07 units/kg/hour	427	3	No	Yes
Inayat et al. [10]	1 (1)	39	1 male	5,047	Insulin infusion 0.1 units/kg/hour	<500	12	No	No
Monotherapy heparin									
Sleth et al. [22]	1 (1)	28	1 female	8,500	Intravenous heparin 15,000 units/day then subcutaneous tinzaparin 2,500 units/day	408	3 days of heparin	No	No
Combination therapy									
Jain and Zimmerschied [12]	1	54	1 male	10,320	Insulin infusion and intravenous heparin unspecified rates	<2,500	3	No	No
Jain et al. [13]	1 (1)	46	1 male	18,220	Insulin infusion unspecified rate and subcutaneous heparin 10,000 units/day	470	4	No	No
Kuchay et al. [17][$]	4 (1)	36	1 female	1820	Insulin infusion 2–12 units/hour and subcutaneous heparin 60 units/kg every 8 hours	534	3	No	No
Jin et al. [14]*[$]	34	34.6	18 male 16 female	Mean 3,089	Insulin infusion 0.1 units/kg/hour and intravenous heparin 10–15 units/kg/hour	Mean 772	Mean 5	Yes	No
Camargo-Mendoza and Bustos-Calvo [7]	1	30	1 male	6,700	Insulin infusion and heparin 80 unit/kg bolus followed by infusion unspecified rates	454	4	No	No
Patel [19]	1	42	1 female	>5,000	Insulin infusion 0.1 units/kg/hour and intravenous heparin 600 units/hour	423	Unspecified	No	No

*Data from patients without diabetes are not decipherable from the study. [$]No bleeding events were reported in the study.

hypertriglyceridemia in a patient without diabetes with intravenous insulin infusions and subcutaneous heparin, providing additional support for the use of this management strategy among patients without diabetes. The medical management of hypertriglyceridemia-induced acute pancreatitis is more robust in patients with diabetes, but in general, approaches to therapy vary in the literature and are further complicated by the lack of standardization of treatment. Furthermore, research is needed to develop treatment recommendations that differentiate between patients with and without diabetes, especially with regard to the appropriateness and dosing, as well as the duration of insulin, dextrose, potassium, heparin, and combination therapies.

Consent

Written informed consent was obtained from the patient for publication of this case report and any accompanying images.

References

[1] A. F. Peery, S. D. Crockett, C. C. Murphy et al., "Burden and cost of gastrointestinal, liver, and pancreatic diseases in the United States: update 2018," *Gastroenterology*, vol. 156, no. 1, pp. 254–272.e11, 2019.

[2] J. B. Christian, N. Bourgeois, R. Snipes, and K. A. Lowe, "Prevalence of severe (500 to 2, 000 mg/dl) hypertriglyceridemia in United States adults," *The American Journal of Cardiology*, vol. 107, no. 6, pp. 891–897, 2011.

[3] L. S. Santos-Baez and H. N. Ginsberg, "Hypertriglyceridemia-causes, significance, and approaches to therapy," *Frontiers in Endocrinology*, vol. 11, p. 616, 2020.

[4] S. S. Virani, P. B. Morris, A. Agarwala et al., "ACC expert consensus decision pathway on the management of ascvd risk reduction in patients with persistent hypertriglyceridemia: a report of the American college of cardiology solution set oversight committee," *Journal of the American College of Cardiology*, vol. 78, no. 9, pp. 960–993, 2021.

[5] A. D. R. Dixit, V. Dudeja, and A. Saluja, *Role of Trypsinogen Activation in Genesis of Pancreatitis*, Exocrine Pancreas Knowledge Base, Pancreapedia, 2016.

[6] N. Weston, U. Fernando, and V. Baskar, "Hypertriglyceridaemia-induced pancreatitis," *Case Reports*, vol. 2013, no. 1, Article ID bcr2013008722, 2013.

[7] J. P. R. A. D. Camargo-Mendoza and J. S. Bustos-Calvo, "Heparin and insulin in the management of acute hypertriglyceridemic pancreatitis," *Acta Médica Colombiana*, vol. 45, pp. 44–7, 2020.

[8] A. Coskun, N. Erkan, S. Yakan et al., "Treatment of hypertriglyceridemia-induced acute pancreatitis with insulin," *Gastroenterology Review*, vol. 1, pp. 18–22, 2015.

[9] V. Gayam, A. K. Mandal, A. Gill et al., "A rare case of acute pancreatitis due to very severe hypertriglyceridemia (>10 000 mg/dL) successfully resolved with insulin therapy alone: a case report and literature review," *Journal of Investigative Medicine High Impact Case Reports*, vol. 6, 2018.

[10] F. Inayat, F. Zafar, I. Riaz, F. Younus, A. S. Baig, and Z. Imran, "Hypertriglyceridemic pancreatitis: is insulin monotherapy A feasible therapeutic option?" *Cureus*, vol. 10, 2018.

[11] M. A. Jabbar, M. I. Zuhri-Yafi, and J. Larrea, "Insulin therapy for a non-diabetic patient with severe hypertriglyceridemia," *Journal of the American College of Nutrition*, vol. 17, no. 5, pp. 458–61, 1998.

[12] D. Jain and J. Zimmerschied, "Heparin and insulin for hypertriglyceridemia-induced pancreatitis: case report," *The Scientific World Journal*, vol. 9, pp. 1230–2, 2009.

[13] P. Jain, R. R. Rai, H. Udawat, S. Nijhawan, and A. Mathur, "Insulin and heparin in treatment of hypertriglyceridemia-induced pancreatitis," *World Journal of Gastroenterology*, vol. 13, no. 17, pp. 2642–3, 2007.

[14] M. Jin, J. M. Peng, H. D. Zhu et al., "Continuous intravenous infusion of insulin and heparin vs plasma exchange in hypertriglyceridemia-induced acute pancreatitis," *J Dig Dis*, vol. 19, no. 12, pp. 766–72, 2018.

[15] R. Khan, W. Jehangir, K. Regeti, and A. Yousif, "Hypertriglyceridemia-induced pancreatitis: choice of treatment," *Gastroenterology Research*, vol. 8, no. 3-4, pp. 234–6, 2015.

[16] S. K. Kota, S. K. Kota, S. Jammula, S. V. S. Krishna, and K. D. Modi, "Hypertriglyceridemia-induced recurrent acute pancreatitis: a case-based review," *Indian Journal of Endocrinology and Metabolism*, vol. 16, no. 1, pp. 141–3, 2012.

[17] M. S. Kuchay, K. J. Farooqui, T. Bano, M. Khandelwal, H. Gill, and A. Mithal, "Heparin and insulin in the management of hypertriglyceridemia-associated pancreatitis: case series and literature review," *Arch Endocrinol Metab*, vol. 61, no. 2, pp. 198–201, 2017.

[18] N. Mikhail, K. Trivedi, C. Page, S. Wali, and D. Cope, "Treatment of severe hypertriglyceridemia in nondiabetic patients with insulin," *The American Journal of Emergency Medicine*, vol. 23, no. 3, pp. 415–7, 2005.

[19] A. D. Patel, "Hypertriglyceridemia-induced acute pancreatitis treatment with insutin and heparin," *Indian Journal of Endocrinology and Metabolism*, vol. 16, no. 4, pp. 671–2, 2012.

[20] J. M. Reed, B. M. Hogan, N. Nasser-Ghodsi, and C. G. Loftus, "Management of hypertriglyceridemia-induced acute pancreatitis in a nondiabetic patient," *Mayo Clinic Proceedings: Innovations, Quality & Outcomes*, vol. 5, no. 2, pp. 520–4, 2021.

[21] Y. Rodriguez Santana, A. Nimo Roman, I. Garcia Saez, J. M. Lopez Alvarez, E. Consuegra Llapur, and R. Gonzalez Jorge, "Treatment of severe hypertriglyceridemia with continuous insulin infusion," *Case Reports in Critical Care*, vol. 2011, Article ID 293917, 3 pages, 2011.

[22] J. C. Sleth, E. Lafforgue, R. Servais et al., "A case of hypertriglycideremia-induced pancreatitis in pregnancy: value of heparin," *Annales Françaises d'Anesthesie et de Reanimation*, vol. 23, no. 8, pp. 835–7, 2004.

[23] I. Cruz-Bautista, A. Huerta-Chagoya, H. Moreno-Macias et al., "Familial hypertriglyceridemia: an entity with distinguishable features from other causes of hypertriglyceridemia," *Lipids in Health and Disease*, vol. 20, no. 1, p. 14, 2021.

[24] C. N. Sadur and R. H. Eckel, "Insulin stimulation of adipose tissue lipoprotein lipase. Use of the euglycemic clamp technique," *Journal of Clinical Investigation*, vol. 69, no. 5, pp. 1119–25, 1982.

[25] R. J. Havel, "Pathogenesis, differentiation and management of hypertriglyceridemia," *Advances in Internal Medicine*, vol. 15, pp. 117–54, 1969.

[26] R. C. Oh, E. T. Trivette, and K. L. Westerfield, "Management of hypertriglyceridemia: common questions and answers," *American Family Physician*, vol. 102, no. 6, pp. 347–54, 2020.

[27] R. Garg and T. Rustagi, "Management of hypertriglyceridemia induced acute pancreatitis," *BioMed Research International*, vol. 2018, Article ID 4721357, 12 pages, 2018.

[28] B. Nasstrom, G. Olivecrona, T. Olivecrona, and B. G. Stegmayr, "Lipoprotein lipase during continuous heparin infusion: tissue stores become partially depleted," *The Journal of Laboratory and Clinical Medicine*, vol. 138, no. 3, pp. 206–13, 2001.

19

Cushing Syndrome in a Pediatric Patient with Topical Steroid Overuse

Sandip Kuikel,[1] **Sunil Aryal**,[1] **Rupesh Shingh Basnyat**,[1] **and Suman Rimal**[2]

[1]*Shishuwa Hospital, 33700 Pokhara, Nepal*
[2]*Department of Internal Medicine, Tribhuvan University Institute of Medicine, 44600 Kathmandu, Nepal*

Correspondence should be addressed to Sandip Kuikel; kuikelsandip@iom.edu.np

Academic Editor: Osamu Isozaki

Cushing syndrome is a state of hypercortisolism from exogenous or endogenous exposure to glucocorticoids resulting in various clinical manifestations. In this case report, we present a case of a 15-month-old child who presented with cushingoid facies due to over-the-counter misuse of a very potent topical steroid (clobetasol 0.05%) for suspected scabies. Laboratory measurement of urinary free cortisol level was low, and 8 : 00 am basal cortisol level was measured, which was decreased, which confirmed the diagnosis of Cushing syndrome due to exogenous source. Over-the-counter topical steroids should not be used, and one should always consult a registered medical practitioner before using such products. Physicians when prescribing topical steroids should warn patients about the potential side effects of prolonged use of topical steroids.

1. Introduction

Cushing syndrome is a state of hypercortisolism from exogenous or endogenous exposure to glucocorticoids resulting in various clinical manifestations [1]. The most common manifestations of Cushing syndrome include obesity, moon face, hirsutism, facial plethora, muscle weakness, and glucose intolerance [2]. Causes of Cushing syndrome include exogenous administration of glucocorticoids, hypersecretion of adrenocorticotropic hormone (ACTH) from pituitary or other sources, and hypersecretion of cortisol from adenomas of the adrenal gland [3]. Cushing syndrome is a very rare condition in the pediatric age group, and its incidence is about 2–5 new cases per million per year [4]. Cushing syndrome due to exogenous administration of glucocorticoids is common; however, topical preparation resulting in Cushing syndrome is a rare phenomenon [5]. In this case report, we present the case of a 15-month-old child who presented with cushingoid facies due to over-the-counter misuse of a very potent topical steroid (clobetasol 0.05%) for suspected scabies.

2. Case Report

A 15-month-old child was brought to the outpatient department of our center with the chief complaint of swelling of the face with growth of excess facial hair. The mother also gives a history of excessive weight gain of the child evidenced by tightening of clothes and facial puffiness (Figure 1). The mother was breastfeeding the child and at the same time consumed prednisolone 5 mg once daily for the treatment as a maintenance dose of IgA nephropathy. The mother had been applying over-the-counter very potent topical steroid (clobetasol 0.05%) (Figure 2) for treatment of some dermatological conditions of the patient. The topical steroid was not prescribed, but was used as it used to relieve the symptoms of itching in the patient. The family history was suggestive of scabies as every member of the family had itchiness in the hands and groin region.

The child was born at home assisted by a midwife, and there were no complications at the time of delivery. The birth weight was not taken, but the mother states the child's birth weight was comparable to other newborns in her family.

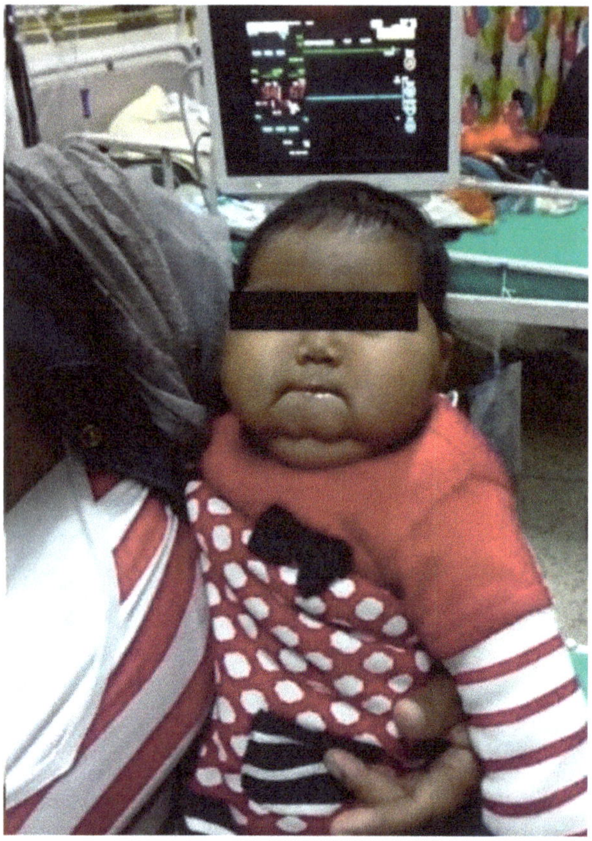

Figure 1: Moon facies of the child.

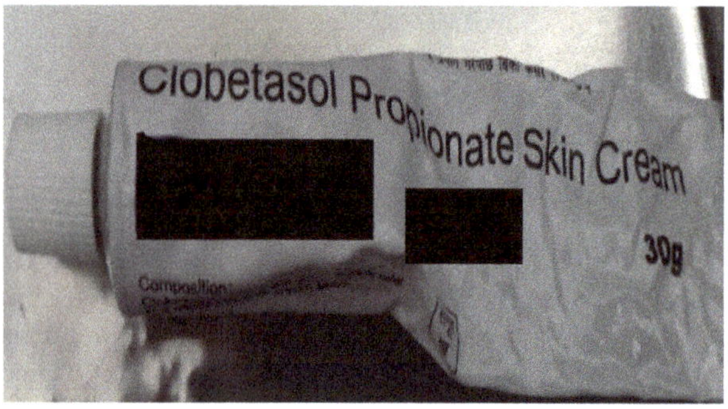

Figure 2: Very potent topical steroid used by the patient.

Developmental history was normal, and the growth of infants was comparable to others of the same age. There were no parental concerns regarding the growth and development of the child, but exact documentation of the child's height and weight had not been done.

On physical examination, the patient was 14 kg (above 97th percentile) and the height of the patient was 40 cm (between 25th and 50th percentile). The patient had prominent facial hairs with moon facies. Blood pressure was raised for the corresponding height and age. There were no purple striae or facial plethora. Other system examinations were normal for the child's age. Routine blood tests were within the normal range including raised random blood sugar. The thyroid function test was normal.

In the background of the mother consuming prednisolone while breastfeeding and use of topical corticosteroids, the literature review was done which showed the safety of prednisolone in breastfeeding mothers, but there were reported cases of Cushing syndrome caused due to application of topical steroids for a long time. So, a provisional diagnosis of Cushing syndrome due to topical steroids was made. Laboratory measurement of 24-hour urinary free cortisol level was low; however, 8:00 am basal cortisol level was measured, which was decreased. This confirmed the diagnosis of Cushing syndrome due to an exogenous source of corticosteroids. Telemedicine consultation was done for the patient as the patient was too poor to afford treatment in the higher center. So, the patient was discharged with permethrin lotion for the treatment of scabies and discontinuation of topical steroids. Maintenance of steroid was done with 15 mg of oral prednisolone syrup in tapering doses over 45days.

On follow-up in 45 days, the moon face of the patient was persistent; however, local effects of topical steroids were reduced, and after three months, all the features of Cushing syndrome subsided. The patient is now on a regular follow-up to record the growth of the child. Recording of height for age, weight for age, and weight for height are being done and plotted in the World Health Organization (WHO) growth chart. This will help assess the residual effect, if any, of the erroneous use of steroids.

3. Discussion

Cushing syndrome is a rare condition in children; iatrogenic Cushing syndrome due to exogenous administration of steroids can be the cause, but topical steroid leading to Cushing syndrome is very unusual [6–9]. The recognition of Cushing syndrome by the treating physician is important for early diagnosis and treatment. Late-night salivary cortisol measurement, dexamethasone suppression test, and 24-hour urinary free cortisol determination are performed for the diagnosis of Cushing syndrome, followed by a stepwise evaluation to find out the cause [10]. Exogenous overuse of corticosteroids can be diagnosed based on classic signs of Cushing syndrome, and the confirmation of a decreased 8:00 am basal cortisol associated with low ATCH levels can be indicative of the diagnosis [3].

Siklar et al. described Cushing syndrome in a 9-month-old girl caused by long-term topical clobetasol propionate application. The patient was found to have severe adrenal suppression [6]. A similar phenomenon was described in a 72-year-old woman who developed manifestations of Cushing syndrome after long-term topical clobetasol propionate ointment for psoriasis. Shortly after tapering the dose of topical steroids, she developed signs of adrenal insufficiency (provoked by a urinary tract infection) requiring intravenous administration of hydrocortisone [7]. Ohnishi et al. [8], Ermis et al. [9], Al-Khenaizan et al. [11], Tiwari et al. [12], and Alkhuder et al. [13] described cases with a similar phenomenon to our case. Our patient had the use of a very potent topical steroid, and due to the presence of moon face with weight gain and laboratory finding of low

8 : 00 am basal cortisol, the diagnosis of Cushing syndrome due to exogenous steroid was confirmed. The family history of itching of the whole body more on axilla and groin suggested the diagnosis of scabies. Prolonged use of topical corticosteroids may cause Cushing syndrome, whereas suppression of the hypothalamic-pituitary-adrenal axis is less pronounced as reported in previous case reports [6–9]. The ACTH level and ACTH stimulation test as being normal rules out the suppression of HPA axis, thus not mandating the requirement of maintenance and tapering dose of steroid.

Topical steroids are frequently prescribed in the management of various dermatological conditions like dermatitis, lichen planus, psoriasis, pruritus ani, pemphigus, and vitiligo [14]. When used in these conditions, patients should be counseled about the potential side effects of topical steroids such as striae, purpura, telangiectasia, ulceration, easy bruising, rosacea, and hirsutism [15]. In a country like ours, where there is a misuse of topical steroids either by patients or by a medical practitioner, there can be a frequent occurrence of these potential side effects [16]. Though being rare, Cushing syndrome due to topical steroids in this situation can be observed as in our case.

When presented with the complaint of excessive weight gain, changes in a facial structure like moon face, excessive hair growth, and abdominal stria, Cushing syndrome should be suspected. It is often near impossible to extract the history of steroid use leading to Cushing syndrome in a setting like ours where most of the patients are just literate (able to read and write names only). So, in these cases, urinary free cortisol should be measured, and if the concentration is low, Cushing syndrome due to exogenous cause is suggested. Then, 8 : 00 am basal cortisol level should be measured, and if the level is low, the diagnosis of Cushing syndrome due to exogenous administration of glucocorticoids is confirmed [3]. Although the random blood sugar level was within normal range, the use of a glucose tolerance test is advised in such cases as the glucose metabolism is often disturbed in cases with excess corticosteroid resulting in hyperglycemia [17].

In our case, the topical steroid was not the drug of choice for the treatment of scabies but was permethrin. Inadvertent long-term use of topical steroids can cause thinning of the skin on the applied site, and steroids can permeate through this thinned out skin causing a systemic adverse effect like Cushing syndrome. Management of this kind of Cushing syndrome includes cessation of causative drugs and administration of corticosteroids in physiological dosage and gradually tapers it until the hypothalamic-pituitary-adrenal (HPA) axis normalizes [18]. In a low-resource setting like ours, the patency of the HPA axis could not be checked by the ACTH stimulation test, so assuming the axis was suppressed, we put the patient on an oral steroid for maintenance at 1 mg/kg dose tapering it over 45 days.

This manuscript reports a rare phenomenon of occurrence of Cushing syndrome with topical steroids. Some similar reported cases of Cushing syndrome due to exogenous topical steroid use can be found in a review of the literature. They provide gross ideas on the presentation, diagnosis, establishment of the integrity of the HPA axis, and treatment of such cases [6–9, 11–13]. However, early detection and management in a low-resource setting, with people just literate to read and write, is often difficult as described in this case. Because of limited resources, laboratory tests such as ACTH stimulation tests to evaluate the patency of the HPA axis could not be done in our case, and it is a limitation of this manuscript.

4. Conclusion

Topical steroids can cause various side effects. Over-the-counter topical steroids should not be used, and one should always consult a registered medical practitioner before using such products. Physicians when prescribing topical steroids should warn patients about the potential side effects of prolonged use of topical steroids. The patient should be advised to firmly apply topical steroids in thin layers and avoid exceeding the daily dose, and these preparations should only be used for a short course.

4.1. Patient Perspective. This manuscript draws the attention of patients toward the possible systemic side effects of potent topical steroids and the need for use as recommended by a registered practitioner only.

Ethical Approval

Informed expressed consent was acquired from the patient for the publication of photographic and clinical data of the patient.

References

[1] A. Lacroix, R. A. Feelders, C. A. Stratakis, and L. K. Nieman, "Cushing's syndrome," *The Lancet*, vol. 386, no. 9996, pp. 913–927, 2015.

[2] L. K. Nieman, "Cushing's syndrome: update on signs, symptoms and biochemical screening," *European Journal of Endocrinology*, vol. 173, no. 4, pp. M33–M38, 2015.

[3] S. T. Sharma, L. K. Nieman, and R. A. Feelders, "Cushing's syndrome: epidemiology and developments in disease management," *Clinical Epidemiology*, vol. 7, pp. 281–293, 2015.

[4] C. A. Stratakis, "Cushing syndrome in pediatrics," *Endocrinology and Metabolism Clinics of North America*, vol. 41, no. 4, pp. 793–803, 2012.

[5] S. Manubolu and O. Nwosu, "Exogenous Cushing's syndrome secondary to intermittent high dose oral prednisone for presumed asthma exacerbations in the setting of multiple emergency department visits," *Journal of Clinical and Translational Endocrinology: Case Reports*, vol. 6, pp. 4–8, 2017.

[6] Z. Siklar, I. Bostanci, O. Atli, and Y. Dallar, "An infantile cushing syndrome due to misuse of topical steroid," *Pediatric Dermatology*, vol. 21, no. 5, pp. 561–563, 2004.

[7] E. M. Abma, R. Blanken, and L. J. M. De Heide, "Cushing's syndrome caused by topical steroid therapy for psoriasis," *The Netherlands Journal of Medicine*, vol. 60, no. 3, pp. 148–150, 2002.

[8] T. Ohnishi, T. Suzuki, S. Watanabe, and H. Takahashi, "Erythrodermic psoriasis associate with hyperuricemia and iatrogenic Cushing's syndrome due to topical corticosteroid therapy," *International Journal of Dermatology*, vol. 35, no. 5, pp. 379-380, 1996.
[9] B. Ermis, R. Ors, A. Tastekin, and B. Ozkan, "Letters to the editors: 1," *Clinical Endocrinology*, vol. 58, no. 6, pp. 795-796, 2003.
[10] A. R. Lila, V. Sarathi, V. S. Jagtap, T. Bandgar, P. Menon, and N. S. Shah, "Cushing's syndrome: stepwise approach to diagnosis," *Indian Journal of Endocrinology and Metabolism*, vol. 15, no. Suppl4, p. S317, 2011.
[11] S. Al-Khenaizan and I. Al Alwan, "Topical steroid-induced Cushing syndrome," *Annals of Saudi Medicine*, vol. 28, no. 4, pp. 300–302, 2008.
[12] A. Tiwari, M. Goel, P. Pal, and P. Gohiya, "Syndrome in the pediatric age group: a rare case report," *Indian Journal of Endocrinology and Metabolism*, vol. 17, no. 1, pp. S257–S258, 2013.
[13] L. Alkhuder and H. Mawlawi, "Infantile iatrogenic cushing syndrome due to topical steroids," *Case Reports in Pediatrics*, vol. 2019, Article ID 2652961, 4 pages, 2019.
[14] A. Mehta, N. Nadkarni, S. Patil, K. Godse, M. Gautam, and S. Agarwal, "Topical corticosteroids in dermatology," *Indian Journal of Dermatology Venereology and Leprology*, vol. 82, no. 4, pp. 371–378, 2016.
[15] A. Coondoo, M. Phiske, S. Verma, and K. Lahiri, "Side-effects of topical steroids: a long overdue revisit," *Indian Dermatology Online Journal*, vol. 5, no. 4, pp. 416–425, 2014.
[16] V. Dey, "Misuse of topical corticosteroids: a clinical study of adverse effects," *Indian Dermatology Online Journal*, vol. 5, no. 4, pp. 436–440, 2014.
[17] C. Scaroni, M. Zilio, M. Foti, and M. Boscaro, "Glucose metabolism abnormalities in cushing syndrome: from molecular basis to clinical management," *Endocrine Reviews*, vol. 38, no. 3, pp. 189–219, 2017.
[18] P. Igaz, K. Rácz, M. Tóth, E. Gláz, and Z. Tulassay, "Treatment of iatrogenic Cushing's syndrome: questions of glucocorticoid withdrawal," *Hungarian Medical Journal*, vol. 1, no. 1, pp. 63–72, 2007.

20

A Case of Growth Hormone use in Dyggve–Melchior–Clausen Syndrome

Ravi Upadhyay,[1] **Claire Ruane**,[1] **Rachel Umans**,[1] **Beth A. Pletcher**,[2] **Aditi Khokhar**,[2] and **Kristin Wong**[1]

[1]*Departments of Medicine and Pediatrics, Rutgers University New Jersey Medical School, Newark, NJ, USA*
[2]*Department of Pediatrics, Rutgers University New Jersey Medical School, Newark, NJ, USA*

Correspondence should be addressed to Kristin Wong; kgw22@njms.rutgers.edu

Academic Editor: Michaël R. Laurent

Short stature has many causes including genetic disease, skeletal dysplasias, endocrinopathies, familial short stature, and nutritional deficiencies. Recombinant growth hormone (rGH) therapy may be employed to improve stature based on the underlying etiology and growth velocity. Skeletal dysplasia in Dyggve–Melchior–Clausen (DMC) syndrome tends to be progressive, typically with hip involvement, and ultimately leads to bilateral dislocation of the hip joints. Here, we present a pediatric patient with short stature treated with rGH therapy, complicated by the development of debilitating, bilateral hip pain, and found to have DMC syndrome. Our patient had limited range of motion at several joints including the hips after receiving 6 months of rGH therapy. Given the timing of the patient's rGH therapy and the progression of her disease, it is difficult to determine if there were any benefits and instead, is concerning for worsening of her skeletal dysplasia with rGH therapy use. Consequently, patients with severe short stature should have a thorough workup for genetic causes like DMC syndrome, before initiating rGH therapy to determine any potential benefits or harms of treatment.

1. Introduction

Short stature is defined as a height of 2 standard deviations (SDs) or more below the mean height for children of that age and sex in a given population. Extreme cases of short stature, such as height standard deviations below 2.5 or 3, account for approximately 0.6 and 0.1% of the general population, respectively, and are usually associated with syndromic conditions such as skeletal dysplasias [1]. After a thorough workup, she was diagnosed with Dyggve–Melchior–Clausen (DMC) syndrome, a rare autosomal recessive genetic disorder. This syndrome is associated with short stature, intellectual disability, and a host of skeletal abnormalities which can affect the hips, vertebrae, and extremities [2]. Short stature is a universal feature of the disease with presentation typically after 5 years of age [3]. Recombinant growth hormone (rGH) therapy may be considered in patients with certain genetic diseases and idiopathic short stature, but in patients with severe short statures, especially those with skeletal disproportion and other developmental abnormalities, a thorough workup, including investigation of possible endocrine and genetic causes, is warranted to identify any underlying condition that should preclude treatment. In this case report, we present a pediatric patient who had progressive, severe bilateral hip pain after treatment of her short stature with rGH.

2. Case Presentation

A 12-year-old Hispanic girl, with a past medical history of short stature and microcephaly, presented to the ambulatory clinic to establish care. Physically, her mother reported that the patient had always been "small for her age." She was noted to have growth delays and was followed by pediatric endocrinology beginning at 7 years of age in Honduras. At age 10.5 years, she was started on rGH therapy (dose unknown). Therapy was discontinued after 6 months on noting a disproportionate growth of limbs relative to the torso. She

Table 1: Laboratory analysis.

Laboratory results on presentation	
Thyroid stimulating hormone	3.4 uu/ml
Free T4	1.0 ng/dl
Parathyroid hormone	31 pg/ml
Calcitriol	54.7 pg/ml
ESR	17 mm/hr
CRP	<1 mg/l
Lead	<1 ug/dl
HIV antibody/antigen screen	Nonreactive
Phosphorus	4.3 mg/dl
Alkaline phosphatase	233 u/l
Complete blood count	
White blood cell count	8.4×10^3/ul
Hemoglobin	13.7 g/dl
Hematocrit	41.1%
Platelet count	298×10^3/ul
Creatinine kinase	126 u/l

also reported that the patient had severe pain in the bilateral thighs, knees, and posterior calves with inability to walk. The pain gradually worsened over the prior four months and was also associated with a regression in her gross motor skills, including her ability to jump and ride a bike. The patient's gross motor milestones were otherwise appropriate until her recent difficulties ambulating.

Developmentally, the patient began to exhibit speech and language delays beginning at the age of 18 months. She was not able to use 2-word phrases until 4 or 5 years of age. She also reported a history of fine motor delays, being unable to tie her shoes or print her name. Her emotional and cognitive abilities were also delayed and the patient had never learned to name colors, recite the alphabet, or participate in elaborate play.

Birth history revealed that the patient was born full-term via a repeat cesarean section to nonconsanguineous Honduran parents after an uneventful pregnancy. There were no complications during delivery; the patient was noted to have microcephaly at birth, but no other abnormalities were identified. The mother was only able to reproduce a viral test report showing Rubeola IgG+ and IgM−. Upon social history, the patient had immigrated from Honduras 5 months prior to presentation and had no other significant exposures or risks. Her family history was also noncontributory to the patient's condition, and she had two healthy siblings. There was no family history of learning or intellectual disabilities nor neurological, growth, or genetic disorders.

Physical examination on presentation revealed a short (height 121.9 cm, <1%, $Z = -3.80$; weight 30.8 kg, 5%, $Z = -1.63$; BMI 20.75 kg/m^2, 80%, $Z = 0.83$; head circumference 49.5 cm, < 1%; midparental height 160 cm, 6%) and an alert, social, and friendly girl who looked younger than the stated age. Her vital signs were within normal limits for age. At 12 years, she was able to speak in simple phrases and name some objects but was unable to name letters or numbers, count fingers, or write her name. She was unable to answer simple questions and could follow only very simple commands. She had a short neck, broad chest, kyphosis with no scoliosis, brachydactyly with broad feet and hands, and

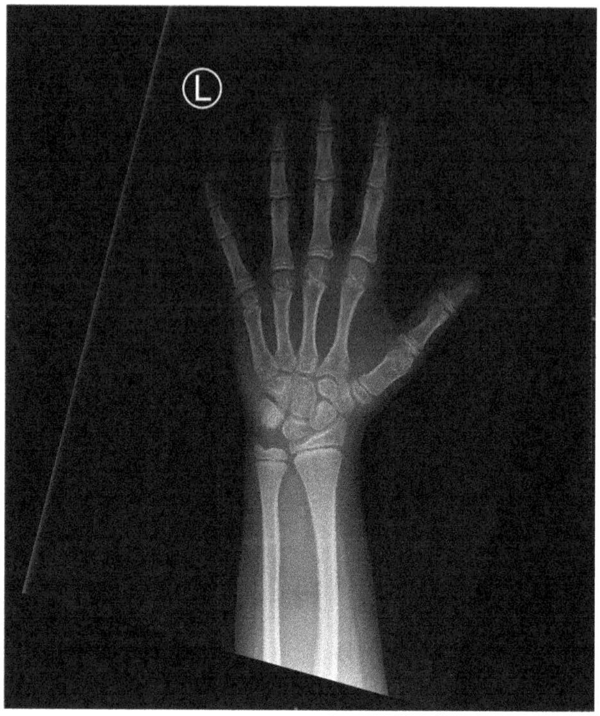

Figure 1: PA radiograph of the left hand for bone age evaluation. A radiograph of the left hand is depicted. The patient's chronological age at the time of the evaluation was 12 years and 2 months. According to the second edition of Greulich and Pyle, the patient's bone age is 11 years. Also noted is a short first metacarpal bone. The remaining bones have normal morphology. There is normal bone mineral density.

Tanner 2 breast development. Lower extremity exam revealed severe genu valgum, tenderness over bilateral posteromedial knees, and generalized, diffuse lower extremity tenderness, with a limited active range of motion due to pain; no pain elicited on passive movement. Bilateral hip flexor strength was 4/5 (limited by pain), while it was 5/5 in all the other major muscle groups. Clumsy fine motor movements were noted in the upper extremities with normal tone, intact sensation, and normal reflexes. No spasticity, atrophy, tremors, ataxia, or dysmetria were found. Her gait was notable for genu valgum, intoeing, and asymmetric step with limping greater on the right than the left side. She was able to take only a few steps without support.

The patient was referred to genetics, endocrinology, neurology, developmental pediatrics, and orthopedics. Laboratory workup including thyroid-stimulating hormone, lead level, hepatitis panel, and human immunodeficiency virus testing was all normal (Table 1). Her bone age was consistent with her chronological age. Her chromosomal microarray, however, showed normal dosage with a single large region of homozygosity on the long arm of chromosome 18, which increased concerns for an autosomal recessive condition. Radiographic imaging revealed a shortened 1st metacarpal bone of the left hand, diminished height of the cervical vertebrae along with a dysmorphic appearance (Figures 1 and 2), exaggerated lumbar lordosis, severe subluxation of bilateral femoral heads with

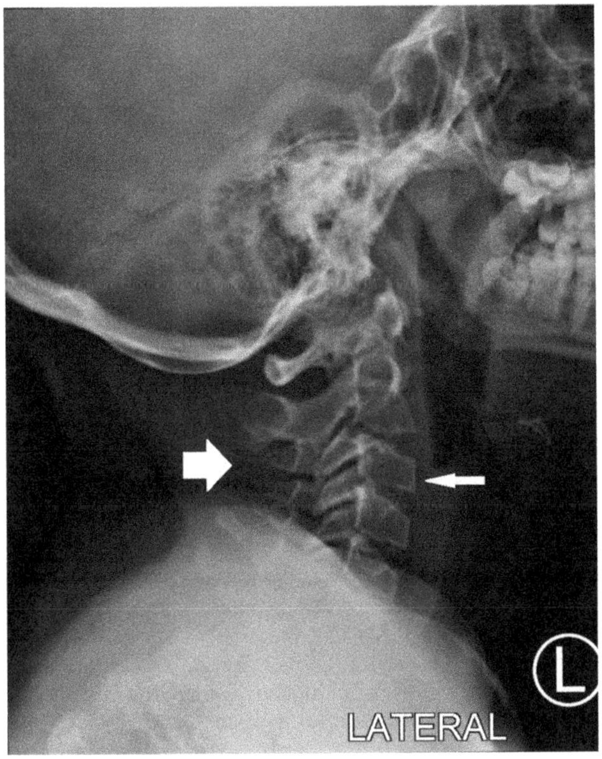

Figure 2: The cervical spine visualized to the C5 level. The vertebrae are diminished in height and dysmorphic in appearance (thick arrow). There is anterior wedging (thin arrow).

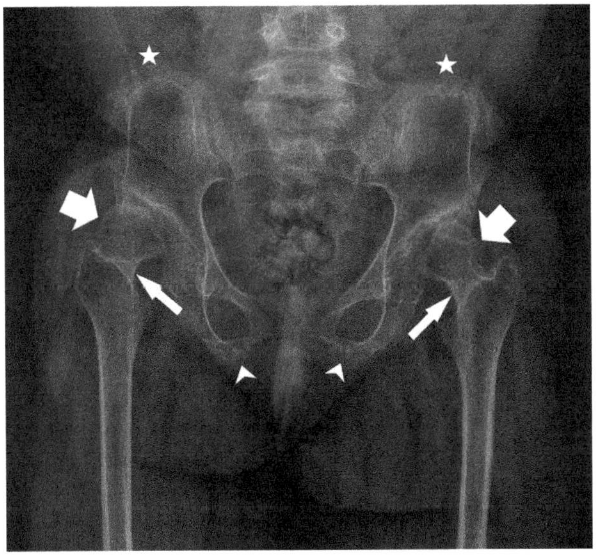

Figure 3: Pelvic and hip abnormalities associated with DMC syndrome. The pelvis with both hips is depicted. Both femoral heads are essentially dislocated/severely subluxated from the shallow, dysplastic acetabulum with resultant formation of a pseudoacetabulum superior and lateral to the native acetabulum bilaterally (thick arrow). Both femoral heads are deformed and small in size (thick arrow). There is premature growth plate fusion at the proximal femoral epiphyses (thin arrow). The iliac rest margins appear deformed (star). The ischial bones and inferior pubic rami are hypoplastic as well (arrowhead). There is decreased bone mineral density throughout, and the bones appear gracile.

dysplastic acetabulae and pseudoacetabulum formation (Figure 3), deformed iliac crests with hypoplasia of inferior pubic rami (Figure 3), and bowing of the right femur. Magnetic resonance imaging of the brain depicted partial agenesis of the corpus callosum and distal body of the splenium but was otherwise unremarkable. Subsequent genetic testing included an Invitae Skeletal Dysplasia Panel which revealed a homozygous missense mutation in a highly conserved region of the DYM gene (c 1244A⟶T, p.His415Leu in exon 11), with algorithms predicting this to be a pathogenic mutation. This particular mutation has not been seen in population databases but has been seen in patients with DMC syndrome. Written informed consent for publication of this case report was provided by the parent.

3. Discussion

Our case revolves around a 12-year-old girl with short stature, developmental delays, and skeletal dysplasia who was eventually diagnosed with DMC syndrome and had bilateral femoral head subluxation which was preceded by a 6-month course of rGH therapy in Honduras. DMC syndrome is a rare progressive genetic disorder which is characterized by intellectual disability, microcephaly, short stature, and progressive spondyloepimetaphyseal dysplasia, with skeletal deformities such as shallow acetabular roofs, lace-like iliac crests, and small femoral heads [3]. Approximately 100 cases have been described in the literature to date. The genetic syndrome is caused by mutations in the dymeclin (DYM) gene on the long arm of chromosome 18 which encodes a protein that is necessary for normal skeletal development and brain function [4]. The exact mechanism of the osteochondrodysplasia requires further elucidation, but DYM deficient murine models suggest that disorganized chondrocyte ossification is the result of impaired vesicular trafficking to and from the Golgi complex [5].

According to one study, age at presentation can vary with a reported range of 3 to 17 years, although delays in motor and intellectual development tend to be identified in the first few years of life [3]. The very specific lace-like appearance of the iliac crests and double-humped vertebral bodies become evident by 3-4 years of age [6]. Interestingly, one study found that subluxation of the hips is not a universal feature of the disease [3]. When present, progressive hip deformities in patients with DMC syndrome invariably lead to bilateral hip subluxation and eventual bilateral dislocation of the hip joint. The pain associated with changes at the hip is ultimately managed surgically although this can be delayed until late adolescence in some cases [7]. At the time of our initial evaluation, our patient already had limited range of motion at several joints including the hips. Radiographic studies revealed severe subluxation at the hips bilaterally along with bowing of the right femur. Our patient falls within the reported age range for skeletal dysplasia progression described in patients with DMC syndrome, but it is not known if prior rGH therapy could have precipitated or worsened hip subluxation in this case given the close timing of events.

Histochemical analysis of iliac crest growth plates in patients with DMC syndrome has revealed that a defect in endochondral ossification may cause skeletal dysplasia [8, 9]. Studies thus far have not evaluated the GH axis in patients with this syndrome, and the role of rGH therapy in this disorder has not been studied either. Our patient received daily rGH injections for six months before it was self-discontinued by the family on noting disproportionate limb growth, and she presented within a year of treatment with debilitating hip pain and gait abnormalities. To the best of our knowledge, this is the first reported case of rGH therapy use in a patient with DMC syndrome.

It is interesting to note that rGH therapy in other syndromes with skeletal dysplasias have had mixed results. On occasion, DMC syndrome can be misdiagnosed as a mucopolysaccharidosis (MPS) due to similar radiologic and clinical features [10]. Recombinant growth hormone therapy has shown some benefit in patients with MPS with reversion of growth deceleration, although controlled clinical trials are lacking [11, 12]. One clinical trial demonstrated efficacy of rGH therapy in patients with achondroplasia with only modest clinical impact, but not in patients with endochondral ossification abnormalities, such as spondyloepiphyseal dysplasia congenita, a disorder that shares features of skeletal dysplasia with DMC disease [13]. Therefore, it is difficult to ascertain whether rGH treatment was of any benefit to our patient, or if it accentuated the patient's skeletal dysplasia or precipitated her hip subluxation. Recombinant growth hormone therapy has indeed been associated with several orthopedic complications including scoliosis and slipped capital femoral epiphysis [14]. Adult height is severely reduced in DMC syndrome with a height range of 115–127 cm [15]. It will be interesting to see what the postpubertal height of this patient will be and whether it will be outside of the range of final height typically seen in this disorder. In our patient with severe short stature, skeletal disproportion, and developmental abnormalities, a thorough genetic workup was likely indicated prior to initiation of rGH therapy. Further studies are needed involving patients with DMC in order to determine the indications of use and possible adverse effects of rGH therapy in this rare genetic disorder.

Authors' Contributions

All authors have provided substantial contributions to the conception and design, acquisition and interpretation of data, and/or the drafting and revisions for intellectual content. All authors have provided final approval for publication and agree to be accountable for all aspects of the work.

References

[1] M. Grunauer and A. A. L. Jorge, "Genetic short stature," *Growth Hormone & IGF Research*, vol. 38, pp. 29–33, 2018.

[2] Rare Disease Database, "Dyggve Melchior Clausen syndrome," 2021, https://rarediseases.org/rare-diseases/dyggve-melchior-clausen-syndrome/.

[3] M. S. Aglan, S. A. Temtamy, E. Fateen, A. M. Ashour, K. Eldeeb, and G. A. Hosny, "Dyggve-Melchior-Clausen syndrome: clinical, genetic, and radiological study of 15 Egyptian patients from nine unrelated families," *Journal of Children's Orthopaedics*, vol. 3, no. 6, pp. 451–458, 2009.

[4] N. E. A. Gaboon, A. Parveen, K. A. Ahmad et al., "A novel homozygous frameshift variant in DYM causing dyggve-melchior-clausen syndrome in Pakistani patients," *Frontiers in Pediatrics*, vol. 8, p. 383, 2020.

[5] A. B. Osipovich, J. L. Jennings, Q. Lin, A. J. Link, H. E. Ruley, and H. Earl Ruley, "Dyggve-Melchior-Clausen syndrome: chondrodysplasia resulting from defects in intracellular vesicle traffic," *Proceedings of the National Academy of Sciences*, vol. 105, no. 42, pp. 16171–16176, 2008.

[6] V. Paupe, T. Gilbert, M. Le Merrer, A. Munnich, V. Cormier-Daire, and V. El Ghouzzi, "Recent advances in Dyggve-Melchior-Clausen syndrome," *Molecular Genetics and Metabolism*, vol. 83, no. 1-2, pp. 51–59, 2004.

[7] E. Nectoux, B. Hocquet, D. Fron, A. Mezel, A. Paris, and B. Herbaux, "Unpredictability of hip behavior in Dyggve-Melchior-Clausen syndrome: a mid-term assessment of siblings," *Orthopaedics and Traumatology: Surgery & Research*, vol. 99, no. 6, pp. 745–748, 2013.

[8] W. A. Horton and C. I. Scott, "Dyggve-Melchior-Clausen syndrome. A histochemical study of the growth plate," *The Journal of Bone and Joint Surgery*, vol. 64, no. 3, pp. 408–415, 1982.

[9] B. Engfeldt, T.-H. Bui, O. Eklöf et al., "Dyggve-melchior-clausen dysplasia," *Acta Paediatrica*, vol. 72, no. 2, pp. 269–274, 1983.

[10] A. Coëslier, O. Boute-Bénéjean, A. Moerman, D. Fron, and S. Manouvrier-Hanu, "Dyggve-Melchior-Clausen syndrome: differential diagnosis of mucopolysaccharidosis type IV or Morquio disease," *Archives of Pediatrics*, vol. 8, no. 8, pp. 838–842, 2001.

[11] L. E. Polgreen and B. S. Miller, "Growth patterns and the use of growth hormone in the mucopolysaccharidoses," *Journal of Pediatric Rehabilitation Medicine*, vol. 3, no. 1, pp. 25–38, 2010.

[12] A. Cattoni, S. Motta, N. Masera, S. Gasperini, A. Rovelli, and R. Parini, "The use of recombinant human growth hormone in patients with Mucopolysaccharidoses and growth hormone deficiency: a case series," *Italian Journal of Pediatrics*, vol. 45, no. 1, p. 93, 2019.

[13] H. Kanazawa, H. Tanaka, M. Inoue, Y. Yamanaka, N. Namba, and Y. Seino, "Efficacy of growth hormone therapy for patients with skeletal dysplasia," *Journal of Bone and Mineral Metabolism*, vol. 21, no. 5, pp. 307–310, 2003.

[14] R. K. Haidar, M. P. Nasrallah, A. H. Der-Boghossian, and I. B. Ghanem, "Orthopedic complications related to growth hormone therapy in a pediatric population," *Journal of Pediatric Orthopaedics B*, vol. 20, no. 1, pp. 57–61, 2011.

[15] V. Kenis, A. Baindurashvili, E. Melchenko, F. Grill, and A. Al Kaissi, "Management of progressive genu varum in a patient with Dyggve-Melchior-Clausen syndrome," *GMS German Medical Science*, vol. 9, 2011.

21

A Case of Severe Acute Kidney Injury Exacerbated by Canagliflozin in a Patient with Type 2 Diabetes

Kimya Hassani-Ardakania,[1] Mark L. Lipman,[2] Denny Laporta,[3] and Oriana Hoi Yun Yu[4,5]

[1]*Department of Medicine, Jewish General Hospital, McGill University, Montreal, H3T 1E2, Canada*
[2]*Division of Nephrology, Department of Medicine, Jewish General Hospital, Montreal, H3T 1E2, Canada*
[3]*Division of Adult Critical Care, Department of Medicine, Jewish General Hospital, Montreal, H3T 1E2, Canada*
[4]*Centre for Clinical Epidemiology, Lady Davis Institute, Jewish General Hospital, Montreal, H3T 1E2, Canada*
[5]*Division of Endocrinology, Department of Medicine, Jewish General Hospital, Montreal, H3T 1E2, Canada*

Correspondence should be addressed to Oriana Hoi Yun Yu; hoi.yu@mcgill.ca

Academic Editor: John Broom

Background. Sodium glucose cotransport (SGLT)-2 inhibitors are the newest class of antihyperglycemic agents used as second- or third-line treatment in the management of type 2 diabetes. Although the use of SGLT-2 inhibitors has not been shown to cause nephrotoxicity, there have been case reports of SGLT-2 inhibitor use being associated with acute kidney injury. *Case Presentation.* A 72-year-old woman with a history of type 2 diabetes and no known chronic renal insufficiency presented to the emergency room with a 3-day history of nausea, vomiting, and increased somnolence. She was found to have potassium level of 7.4 (normal: 3.5-5.5) mmol/L and a markedly elevated creatinine level at 1154 (normal: 45-95) μmol/L. Imaging of the abdomen and pelvis did not reveal any findings of obstruction. Urine microscopy showed many granular casts. In the absence of other causes for her clinical presentation, the patient was diagnosed with acute kidney injury secondary to ischemic acute tubular necrosis, with canagliflozin use likely an important contributing factor. *Conclusions.* Physicians should inform patients to stop the use of SGLT-2 inhibitors when patients are unable to maintain hydration or during acute illness. Use of SGLT-2 inhibitors in managing type 2 diabetes should be done with caution among more vulnerable populations, including individuals with cognitive impairment and the elderly.

1. Introduction

Sodium glucose cotransporter-2 (SGLT-2) inhibitors, including canagliflozin, empagliflozin, and dapagliflozin, are the newest antihyperglycemic agents approved for treatment of type 2 diabetes. The EMPA-REG trial [1] and a subsequent post hoc analysis of renal outcomes among patients with chronic renal insufficiency reported that empagliflozin reduced cardiovascular outcomes and slowed progression of kidney disease, respectively [2]. Similarly, the CANVAS trial demonstrated that patients treated with canagliflozin had a lower risk of cardiovascular events and renal outcomes [3]. The DECLARE-TIMI trial showed a decrease in the risk of acute kidney injury (AKI) associated with the use of dapagliflozin treatment [4].

More recently, the CREDENCE trial [5] found a significantly decreased risk of renal outcomes which were a composite of end stage renal disease, a doubling of creatinine levels, or death from cardiovascular or renal causes associated with the use of low dose canagliflozin (100mg daily) compared to placebo among patients with diabetes and albuminuric chronic kidney disease (with an estimated glomerular filtration rate of 30 to <90 ml per minute per 1.73m^2 of body surface area and urinary albumin [milligrams]-to-creatinine [grams] ratio of >300 to 5000). While these large trials have demonstrated positive impact of SGLT-2 inhibitors on renal function, findings from clinical trials are not necessarily reflective of the realities of clinical practice. Indeed, several case reports have linked acute renal injury to use of SGLT-2 inhibitors including one recent report of acute renal injury with biopsy proven acute tubular necrosis (ATN) associated with the use of dapagliflozin [6]. As a result, the United States Food and Drug Administration (FDA) strengthened the warning on the risk of AKI associated with canagliflozin and dapagliflozin following assessment of these cases [7].

The following case illustrates an example of AKI that was exacerbated or potentially caused by the use of SGLT-2 inhibitors in a patient that was unable to maintain adequate hydration during a viral illness. This case emphasizes the importance of physicians to inform patients to stop the use of SGLT-2 inhibitors during acute illness.

2. Case Presentation

A 72-year-old female was admitted to the intensive care unit for AKI and severe shock. Her medical history included type 2 diabetes mellitus, Alzheimer's disease, hypertension, dyslipidemia, gastroesophageal reflux disease, and obstructive sleep apnea. The patient had no history of underlying chronic kidney disease.

During the three-day period before admission to the hospital, the patient was feeling unwell and increasingly somnolent, had significantly decreased oral intake, and was vomiting. She denied any fever, night sweats, or sick contacts. There was no history of diarrhea. Her medications included valsartan, metoprolol, rosuvastatin, aspirin, canagliflozin, sitagliptin, metformin, insulin degludec and aspart, donepezil, citalopram, gabapentin, and pantoprazole. Canagliflozin 300mg prescribed once daily was initiated approximately 18 months prior to presentation and was added to the antihyperglycemic agents that are listed. Otherwise, her medications were not changed during the 18 months prior to her presentation to the emergency room. She was not using herbal products or any other over-the-counter medications and did not ingest alcohol.

At presentation, the patient was somnolent, responding only to painful stimuli. Vital signs at presentation were the following: blood pressure 97/36 mmHg, heart rate 76 beats/min, respiratory rate 28 breaths/min, temperature 37.2°C, and SaO2 97% on nasal prongs. Physical examination was otherwise unremarkable. A Foley catheter was inserted which revealed minimal urine output. A point-of-care venous blood gas showed the following results: pH 7.00 (normal 7.35-7.45), pCO2 29 (normal 37-43 mmHg), bicarbonate 7 (normal 22-26 mmol/L), lactate 11.9 (normal 0.5-2.5 mmol/L), sodium 122 (normal 134-144 mmol/L), potassium 7.4 (normal: 3.5-5.5 mmol/L), and anion gap 48 mmol/L. There was an absence of ketones in the urinary dipstick. Laboratory evaluation revealed markedly elevated creatinine level at 1154 (normal: 45-95 μmol/L). A complete blood count was unremarkable except for an elevated white blood cell count with a result of 24.5 x 10^9/L (normal: 4-11x10^9/L). Blood cultures did not result in any growth obtained at the time of presentation. A CT scan of the abdomen and pelvis did not show any evidence of hydronephrosis or hydroureter. Urine microscopy showed many granular casts. In the absence of other causes for her clinical presentation, the patient was diagnosed with AKI secondary to ischemic ATN, with canagliflozin use likely an important contributing factor in the presence of a possible viral infection that led to the nausea and vomiting.

She was immediately started on renal replacement therapy. She initially received continuous veno-venous hemofiltration (CVVH) and was subsequently converted to intermittent hemodialysis (IHD) when she became hemodynamically stable. The patient was anuric when the CVVH was initiated; however during the third week of her admission, the patient was noted to have a small quantity of urine output. Her renal function recovered gradually after 8 weeks of IHD (Figure 1).

3. Discussion

SGLT-2 inhibitors can cause kidney function decline through different mechanisms including volume depletion due to excessive diuresis, decrease in transglomerular pressure, and renal medullary hypoxic injury caused by increased distal tubular transport [9]. These effects become further amplified in the setting of volume depletion and underlying renal impairment [10]. Therefore, SGLT-2 inhibitors could induce AKI from prerenal failure caused by increased diuresis and ATN has also been described to occur secondary to renal hypoxic injury induced by the use of these agents [9, 11].

The FDA has raised concerns for AKI associated with SGLT-2 inhibitor use. More recently, an analysis of the FDA adverse event report system database found that patients with type 2 diabetes on SGLT-2 inhibitors were at a significantly greater risk of AKI compared to those who were not treated with SGLT-2 inhibitors [10]. Among the SGLT-2 inhibitors, canagliflozin was associated with the highest proportion of renal failure. Interestingly, cases of renal failure with SGLT-2 inhibitors were four times more likely to report concomitant use of angiotensin converting enzyme (ACE) inhibitors, angiotensin II receptor blockers (ARBs), and diuretics, compared to cases with SGLT-2 inhibitors reporting other adverse events [10].

A meta-analysis of 55 randomized clinical trials, performed in 2013, demonstrated that canagliflozin and dapagliflozin use was associated with an increased risk of AKI compared to use of non-SGLT-2 inhibitor antihyperglycemic agents [12]. The findings from this systematic review and meta-analysis showed that patients with moderate renal impairment had a higher incidence of renal adverse events when treated with canagliflozin or dapagliflozin. Furthermore, patients with normal to mild renal impairment had a higher incidence of renal adverse events if they were treated with the higher dose of canagliflozin (i.e., 300mg daily). However, three subsequent large randomized control trials studying cardiovascular outcomes associated with the use of empagliflozin [1], canagliflozin [3], and dapagliflozin [4] found no increased risk of AKI among individuals treated with SGLT2 inhibitors compared to placebo. In fact, the DECLARE-TIMI58 trial, which studied dapagliflozin, found a decreased risk of renal events among patients treated with dapagliflozin compared to patients treated with placebo (hazard ratio [HR]: 0.69; 95% confidence interval [CI]: 0.55–0.87) [4]. More recently, the CREDENCE trial studied adverse renal outcomes among patients with type 2 diabetes

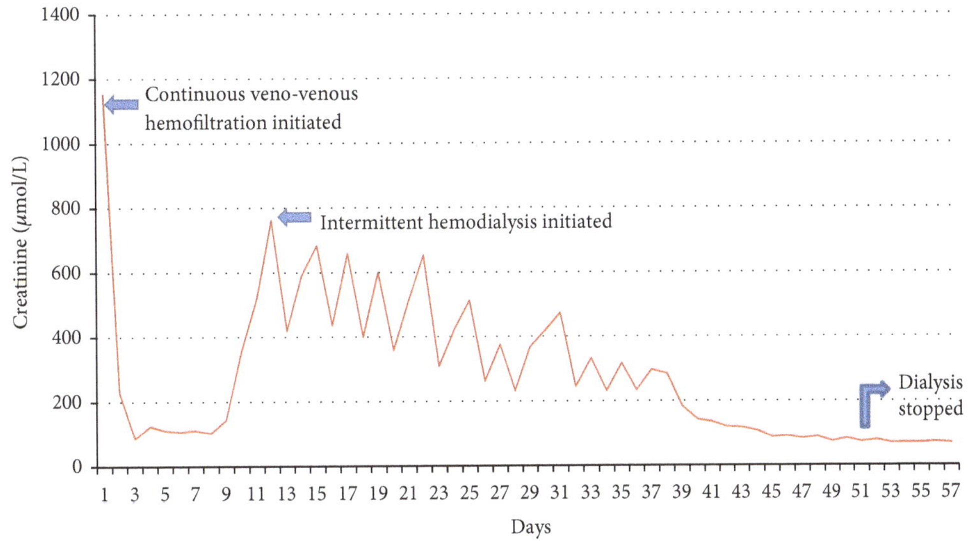

FIGURE 1: Graph showing creatinine levels from time of presentation until resolution of acute kidney injury.

Sulfonylureas
Angiotensin converting enzyme (ACE) inhibitors
Diuretics, direct renin inhibitors

Metformin
Angiotensin receptor blockers
Nonsteroidal anti-inflammatory (NSAIDS) drugs
Sodium glucose cotransporter-2 inhibitors

FIGURE 2: Sick day medication list. Figure adapted from Diabetes Canada [8].

and albuminuric chronic kidney disease and found that low dose canagliflozin (100mg daily) was associated with lower risk of adverse renal outcomes defined by a composite of end stage renal disease, a doubling of creatinine levels, or death from cardiovascular or renal causes (HR: 0.66; 95% CI: 0.53-0.81) [5]. These findings are further supported by real-world data from the Mount Sinai chronic kidney disease registry and the Geisinger Health System cohort that assessed the risk of AKI associated with the use of SGLT-2 inhibitors compared to use of non-SGLT-2 inhibitor antihyperglycemic agents using propensity-score matched analyses [13]. However, the authors acknowledge that SGLT-2 inhibitor use may be associated with AKI among high-risk individuals, which were not studied in this observational study cohort.

In this case report, we believe that canagliflozin played an important causative role in our patient's AKI in addition to her acute viral illness, poor oral intake, and concomitant use of valsartan. Unfortunately, it is difficult to determine whether the AKI was caused by a prerenal mechanism as urinary sodium levels were not obtained at presentation. However, the microscopic urinary analysis showed many granular casts, which suggested that the AKI was caused by ATN. To our knowledge, this is the second case report of AKI secondary to ATN that was associated with the use of SGLT-2 inhibitor [6].

In conclusion, this case report illustrates an example of canagliflozin use contributing to AKI in the event of an acute illness. Given the efficacy of SGLT-2 inhibitors and their cardiovascular benefits, their usage in patients with type 2 diabetes is well justified. However, given that there are plausible mechanisms linking SGLT-2 inhibitors to AKI, especially when having concomitant use of ACE inhibitors, ARBs, diuretics, or other nephrotoxic medications such as nonsteroidal anti-inflammatory drugs, amphotericin, and radiocontrast media [9], it is important to consider this adverse effect when prescribing SGLT-2 inhibitors. Moreover, usage of SGLT-2 inhibitors should be done with caution in elderly patients [14] and in patients with cognitive impairment as they may not be able to maintain hydration or remember to stop SGLT-2 inhibitors in the event of acute illness. Finally, given that SGLT-2 inhibitor use can exacerbate volume depletion via its diuretic effects, resulting in renal function decline during illness, guidelines from Diabetes

Canada have integrated SGLT-2 inhibitors as one of the class of medications that should be stopped during acute illness (Figure 2) [8]. As SGLT-2 inhibitors are becoming more frequently prescribed due to the metabolic and cardiovascular benefits in the treatment of type 2 diabetes, it is important for clinicians to inform their patients of the potential side effects to decrease the complications associated with the use of these agents.

Abbreviations

SGLT-2: Sodium glucose cotransporter-2
AKI: Acute kidney injury
ATN: Acute tubular necrosis
FDA: Food and Drug Administration
CVVH: Continuous veno-venous hemofiltration
IHD: Intermittent hemodialysis
ACE: Angiotensin converting enzyme
ARB: Angiotensin II receptor blockers.

Disclosure

Dr. Oriana Hoi Yun Yu holds a Chercheur-Clinicien Junior 1 Award from the FRQS.

Authors' Contributions

All authors were involved in the preparation, writing, and reviewing of the case report.

References

[1] B. Zinman, C. Wanner, J. M. Lachin et al., "Empagliflozin, cardiovascular outcomes, and mortality in type 2 diabetes," *The New England Journal of Medicine*, vol. 373, no. 22, pp. 2117–2128, 2015.

[2] C. Wanner, S. E. Inzucchi, J. M. Lachin et al., "Empagliflozin and progression of kidney disease in type 2 diabetes," *The New England Journal of Medicine*, vol. 375, no. 4, pp. 323–334, 2016.

[3] B. Neal, V. Perkovic, K. W. Mahaffey et al., "Canagliflozin and cardiovascular and renal events in type 2 diabetes," *The New England Journal of Medicine*, 2017.

[4] S. D. Wiviott, I. Raz, M. P. Bonaca et al., "Dapagliflozin and cardiovascular outcomes in type 2 diabetes," *The New England Journal of Medicine*, vol. 380, no. 4, pp. 347–357, 2019.

[5] V. Perkovic, M. J. Jardine, B. Neal et al., "Canagliflozin and renal outcomes in type 2 diabetes and nephropathy," *The New England Journal of Medicine*, 2019.

[6] C. Pleros, E. Stamataki, A. Papadaki et al., "Dapagliflozin as a cause of acute tubular necrosis with heavy consequences: a case report," *CEN Case Reports*, vol. 7, no. 1, pp. 17–20, 2018.

[7] "FDA Drug Safety Communication: FDA strengthens kidney warnings for diabetes medicines canagliflozin (Invokana, Invokamet) and dapagliflozin (Farxiga, Xigduo XR)," 2018, https://www.fda.gov/Drugs/DrugSafety/ucm505860.htm.

[8] Diabetes Canada, "Sick day medication list," *Canadian Journal of Diabetes*, vol. 42, no. S316, 2018.

[9] A. Szalat, A. Perlman, M. Muszkat, M. Khamaisi, Z. Abassi, and S. N. Heyman, "Can SGLT2 inhibitors cause acute renal failure? plausible role for altered glomerular hemodynamics and medullary hypoxia," *Drug Safety*, vol. 41, no. 3, pp. 239–252, 2018.

[10] A. Perlman, S. N. Heyman, I. Matok, J. Stokar, M. Muszkat, and A. Szalat, "Acute renal failure with sodium-glucose-cotransporter-2 inhibitors: Analysis of the FDA adverse event report system database," *Nutrition, Metabolism & Cardiovascular Diseases*, vol. 27, no. 12, pp. 1108–1113, 2017.

[11] S. N. Heyman, M. Khamaisi, S. Rosen, C. Rosenberger, and Z. Abassi, "Potential hypoxic renal injury in patients with diabetes on SGLT2 inhibitors: Caution regarding concomitant use of NSAIDs and iodinated contrast media," *Diabetes Care*, vol. 40, no. 4, pp. e40–e41, 2017.

[12] D. Vasilakou, T. Karagiannis, E. Athanasiadou et al., "Sodium-glucose cotransporter 2 inhibitors for type 2 diabetes: a systematic review and meta-analysis," *Annals of Internal Medicine*, vol. 159, no. 4, pp. 262–274, 2013.

[13] G. N. Nadkarni, R. Ferrandino, A. Chang et al., "Acute kidney injury in patients on SGLT2 inhibitors: A propensity-matched analysis," *Diabetes Care*, vol. 40, no. 11, pp. 1479–1485, 2017.

[14] A. J. Scheen, "SGLT2 inhibition: Efficacy and safety in type 2 diabetes treatment," *Expert Opinion on Drug Safety*, vol. 14, no. 12, pp. 1879–1904, 2015.

22

A Novel Variant in the Calcium-Sensing Receptor Associated with Familial Hypocalciuric Hypercalcemia and Low-to-Normal PTH

Sachin K. Majumdar,[1,2] Tess Jacob,[2] Allen Bale,[3] Allison Bailey,[3] Jeffrey Kwon,[2] Terence Hughes,[4] Andrea L. Barbieri,[3] William Laskin,[3] Paul Cohen,[3] and Tobias John Eric Carling[5]

[1]*Department of Endocrinology, Bridgeport Hospital, Yale New Haven Health System, Bridgeport, CT, USA*
[2]*Department of Internal Medicine, Bridgeport Hospital, Yale New Haven Health System, Bridgeport, CT, USA*
[3]*Department of Pathology, Yale University School of Medicine, New Haven, CT, USA*
[4]*Department of Radiology, Bridgeport Hospital, Yale New Haven Health System, Bridgeport, CT, USA*
[5]*Section of Endocrine Surgery, Department of Surgery, Yale University School of Medicine, New Haven, CT, USA*

Correspondence should be addressed to Sachin K. Majumdar; psmaju@bpthosp.org

Academic Editor: Lucy Mastrandrea

Familial hypocalciuric hypercalcemia (FHH) is considered a relatively benign condition characterized by mild elevations in serum calcium and relatively low urinary calcium excretion. It results from an elevated set point in serum calcium arising from variants in the calcium-sensing receptor (CaSR) gene but also AP2S1 and GNA11 genes, which encode for adaptor-related protein complex 2 and G11 proteins, respectively. The manifestations of FHH can vary and sometimes overlap with primary hyperparathyroidism making the diagnosis challenging. *Case Presentations.* We report a mother and daughter with a novel heterozygous variant in the CaSR gene resulting in a serine to leucine substitution at position 147 (S147L) of the CaSR. Both patients had mild hypercalcemia, relatively low urinary calcium excretion, elevated calcitriol, and low-to-normal intact PTH. The proband (daughter) presented with symptoms associated with hypercalcemia and was incidentally found to have a bony lesion suspicious for osteitis fibrosa cystica, and she was also diagnosed with sarcoidosis. Subtotal parathyroidectomy revealed normal-weight parathyroid glands comprised of 50–80% parathyroid epithelial cells, which has been documented as within the spectrum of normal. Her mother had no symptoms, and no intervention was pursued. *Conclusion.* We report a novel variant in the CaSR associated with FHH in two patients with similar biochemical features yet differing clinical manifestations. While the relationship of the bony findings and parathyroid histology with this variant remains unclear, these cases enrich our knowledge of CaSR physiology and provide further examples of how varied the manifestations of FHH can be.

1. Introduction

The calcium-sensing receptor (CaSR) is present in all vertebrates where its principal function is to regulate serum calcium concentration by modulating parathyroid hormone and urinary calcium excretion [1]. A number of variants in the CaSR have been reported in humans associated with disorders of calcium balance, particularly familial hypocalciuric hypercalcemia (FHH), where the setpoint for serum calcium concentration is altered resulting in elevated serum calcium and relatively low renal calcium excretion [2]. Were it not for the inclusion of calcium in routine laboratory testing, most patients with mild primary hyperparathyroidism (PHPT) and FHH would not be identified given their largely asymptomatic nature, yet when mild hypercalcemia is detected, it is appropriate to exclude FHH, given that surgical management is rarely necessary. However, the phenotypes of FHH differ in their degree of calcium and PTH concentrations and even symptomatology, based on the particular variant in the CaSR, and can overlap clinically with PHPT [3–5]. Herein, we report two patients with FHH and a novel variant in the CaSR associated with low to normal PTH, elevated calcitriol, and symptoms associated with hypercalcemia that resolved after surgical parathyroidectomy in one patient.

2. Case Report

A 26-year-old woman of Korean and Irish descent was evaluated for chronic hypercalcemia and complaints of fatigue, body and joint aches, and dental pain for ~4 years. She had no history of kidney stones or other medical problems except for multiple dental caries. Her mother had been treated for tuberculosis in Korea, and her maternal aunt had neck surgery in Korea at ~age 70 reportedly for a parathyroid problem. Physical examination revealed a BMI of 23.3, BP 114/68, P 68, weight 63.6 kg, and absence of dental or jaw lesions and was otherwise unremarkable.

Laboratory studies 4 years prior to presentation revealed calcium levels of 10.3 mg/dL (8.4–10.2 mg/dL) and 10.8 mg/dL, phosphorus 2.4 mg/dL (2.5–4.5 mg/dL), 25 vit D 22 ng/dL (10 to 100 nM), albumin 4.4 g/L (3.4–5.4 g/dL), chloride 106 mM (96–106 mM), and creatinine 0.63 mg/dL (0.52–1.04 mg/dL). She underwent extensive evaluation over 2 years with results of blood and urine studies shown in Table 1 (daughter). Studies revealed mildly elevated calcium and calcitriol and low normal PTH. PPD and chest X-ray were negative, and urine testing favored FHH; however, she refused genetic testing citing the literature on the Internet, suggesting that PHPT is often misdiagnosed as FHH. CT imaging was performed to assess kidney stones, which were absent but, instead, showed a ~3 cm indeterminate lesion of the left iliac wing. It appeared benign on MRI (Figure 1(a)), and subsequent biopsy revealed results consistent with osteitis fibrosis cystica (Figures 1(b)–1(d)). This prompted concern for an atypical case of PHPT with low PTH levels. Further testing revealed low normal values for PTH by dilution, mid-molecule PTH, and PTHrp (Table 1). Dual-energy X-Ray absorptiometry (DXA-Hologic) revealed bone densities and Z scores of 0.717 (Z – 1.2), 0.81 (Z – 2.1), 0.797 (Z – 1.2), and 0.346 (Z – 1.4), in g/cm^2, at the femoral neck, spine, hip, and ultra distal forearm, respectively. Parathyroid Tc-99 sestamibi revealed equivocal tracer retention in the right thyroid lobe, yet neck ultrasonography revealed several lymph nodes but no parathyroid adenoma. A 4D CT scan of the neck showed mild prominence of the parathyroid glands and unexpected bilateral mediastinal and hilar lymphadenopathy.

Pulmonary lymph node biopsy revealed noncaseating granulomas consistent with sarcoidosis. A two-month trial of prednisone, 60 mg/d tapered to 20 mg/d, resulted in a normalization of calcitriol, 61 pg/mL and 37 pg/mL (18–72 pg/mL), at weeks 4 and 6, respectively, but no change in calcium, 10.9 mg/dL and 10.8 mg/dL, or PTH, 13 pg/mL and 16 pg/mL (10–65 pg/mL), respectively. Subsequent CT scanning of the chest revealed resolution of lymphadenopathy, and given the combination of elevated calcium, normal PTH, and low urine calcium, suspicion for FHH remained. The bone pathology was reviewed extensively and remained curious, yet its interpretation was not strictly limited to osteitis fibrosis cystica. At this time, she refused further medical evaluation and sought consultation from an endocrine surgeon.

The case was presented and discussed at a multidisciplinary treatment conference, and the patient was counselled by the endocrine surgeon that parathyroid surgery was unproven in this scenario but could be considered based on her symptoms and she requested to proceed with parathyroidectomy [6]. She underwent a subtotal parathyroidectomy with intraoperative PTH measurements, with a drop from 32 pg/mL to 9 pg/mL, 10 minutes after subtotal resection, leaving a remnant of approximately 20 mg of the left lower parathyroid gland. Intraoperatively, the parathyroid glands appeared minimally hyperplastic, and upon histologic review, they were each composed of 50–80% parathyroid epithelial cells with the rest composed of adipose tissue. Final pathology demonstrated that the left and right upper and left lower parathyroid glands weighed 20, 16, and 15 mg, respectively; two appeared histologically normal and one was hypercellular (Figures 1(g) and 1(h)). She developed postoperative hypoparathyroidism, with calcium 7.2 to 9.1 mg/dL and PTH < 3 to 5 pg/mL, but was maintained on calcitriol and reported an overall improvement in well-being and resolution of fatigue and body aches.

The patient referred her mother since she was noted to have hypercalcemia based on further inquiry. Her mother, a 62-year-old Korean woman with a history of treated tuberculosis, hypertension, and hyperlipidemia had mild asymptomatic hypercalcemia. Her calcium levels from 1997 to 2014 ranged from 10.2 mg/dL to 11.3 mg/dL, and further testing revealed similar findings to her daughter (Table 1, mother). CT imaging of the chest and abdomen did not reveal kidney stones or evidence of sarcoidosis, and the neck US revealed a thyroid nodule found to be benign on FNA. Surgery was discouraged, and she agreed to genetic testing revealing a novel heterozygous variant in the calcium-sensing receptor gene (CaSR) resulting in a serine to leucine substitution at position 147 (S147L). After this, her daughter agreed to testing which revealed the same heterozygous variant in the CaSR.

On follow-up, the probands bony lesion was rebiopsied, 3 years after the initial biopsy and 1.5 years after surgery, revealing woven bone deposition and peritrabecular fibrosis, and it has been stable on imaging over 5.5 years. Repeat DXA (Hologic) 5.5 years after her initial one, and 3.5 years after parathyroid surgery, revealed increased bone density and Z scores of 0.798 (Z – 0.3), 0.927 (Z – 1.1), and 0.870 (Z – 0.5) in g/cm^2 at the femoral neck, spine and hip, respectively, although the study was performed at a different location. Three years postoperatively, she continues to report a resolution in symptoms since her surgery, particularly in fatigue and mental clarity, yet remains hypoparathyroid (calcium 7.8 mg/dL; PTH 4 pg/mL) and on treatment with calcitriol and calcium. She had an uncomplicated pregnancy resulting in a healthy male child whose calcium so far has not been tested. Her mother remains asymptomatic.

Table 1: Range of values displayed when numerous results are available.

Measure	Reference	Daughter	Mother
Calcium	8.4–10.2 mg/dL	10.1.–11.1	10.2–11.3
Ionized calcium	4.4–5.5 mg/dL	5.7	5.8–6.0
Creatinine	0.52–1.04 mg/dL	0.54–0.69	0.5–0.61
Chloride/phosphate ratio		33–41	35
Phosphorus	2.5–4.5 mg/dL	2.1–3.4	3.1–3.3
Magnesium	1.6–2.3 mg/dL	2.2–2.4	2.2
Intact PTH	10–65 pg/mL	13–24	12–42
25-OH vit D	Variable ng/dL	20–22	25–42
1,25-OH vit D	18–72 pg/mL	72–94	67–81
24 hour urine calcium (grams creatinine/24 h)		103 (1.27 g Cr), 105 (1.65 g Cr)	84 (1 g Cr) 90 (1.02 g Cr)
Ca/Cr clearance ratio		0.004	0.004
PTH by dilution		24, 24 (1 : 2), 27 (1 : 4)	
Midmolecule PTH	10–25 nLmeq/mL	11	10
ACE	9–67 U/L	34	38
Alk phos-bone specific	4.7–17.8 mcg/L	8.9	
CTX	64–640 pg/mL	239	

ACE, angiotensin converting enzyme; PPD, purified protein derivative; PTH, parathyroid hormone; CTX, collagen type 1 C-telopeptide.

3. Discussion

We report a novel variant in the CASR gene (TCA > TTA: hg19chr2:121976182, NM_000388) resulting in a serine to leucine substitution at position 147 (S147L) associated with FHH and low to normal PTH. The initial evaluation of the proband was complicated by the presence of sarcoidosis, a bony lesion suspicious for osteitis fibrosa cystica, as well as symptoms of fatigue and bony pains. Interestingly, she reported resolution of her symptoms and improvement in mental clarity after subtotal parathyroidectomy and was satisfied with surgery despite being maintained on calcium and calcitriol. However, her mother was asymptomatic despite sharing similar biochemical findings.

Studies identify Serine 147 as an important site for calcium sensing; for example, in one structural study, a serine to alanine (S147A) substitution resulted in a 4-fold decrease in maximal response to calcium in vitro [7, 8]. The general findings in these two patients fit well within the spectrum of previously reported FHH phenotypes where other variants are associated with low to normal PTH concentrations and elevated calcitriol [9, 10]. Examination of the probands parathyroid tissue revealed 50–80% parathyroid epithelial cells in each gland. The significance of these findings is unclear, as autopsy studies have documented large variations in intraparathyroidal adipose tissue in normal patients at autopsy [11]. Sarcoid may have contributed to her elevations in calcitriol, yet in the mother, calcitriol was elevated without evident sarcoid and therefore may be a feature of this variant.

The proband's unexpected bone lesion in the iliac wing revealed pathology suggestive of osteitis fibrosis cystica and complicated the evaluation. While the CaSR is present in cartilage and bone and contributes to skeletal homeostasis, the bone pathology reported in rare variants of FHH is associated with excess PTH rather than being independent of it [12, 13]. This lesion was stable over 5 years on imaging, and repeat biopsy results were less specific suggesting that the finding may be unrelated yet parathyroidectomy may have altered its characteristics. Symptoms associated with hypercalcemia in the proband appeared real given their resolution after parathyroidectomy and absence after several years of follow-up. This is consistent with prior reports describing overlapping symptoms in FHH and PHPT. In an early description of 15 kindreds with FHH, affected members reported significantly more frequent fatigue, weakness, headaches, and arthralgia, in comparison to those unaffected [3, 14]. Given the absence of symptoms in the mother, we cannot argue that this particular variant is associated with symptom development, rather it may be a consequence of the inherent differences individuals possess in susceptibility to hypercalcemia-associated symptoms, perhaps independently of the cause.

In summary, these cases support experimental evidence that serine 147 is an important site on the CaSR for calcium sensing and that the S147L substitution is associated with clinical and biochemical features of FHH. This adds to the database of known variants in the CaSR providing further insight into genotype phenotype relationships in humans and supports the notion that FHH is quite variable biochemically and clinically, and can overlap with PHPT. Also, given that symptoms might occur in individuals with mild hypercalcemia and FHH, attempts to normalize the serum calcium either medically or surgically may occasionally be indicated.

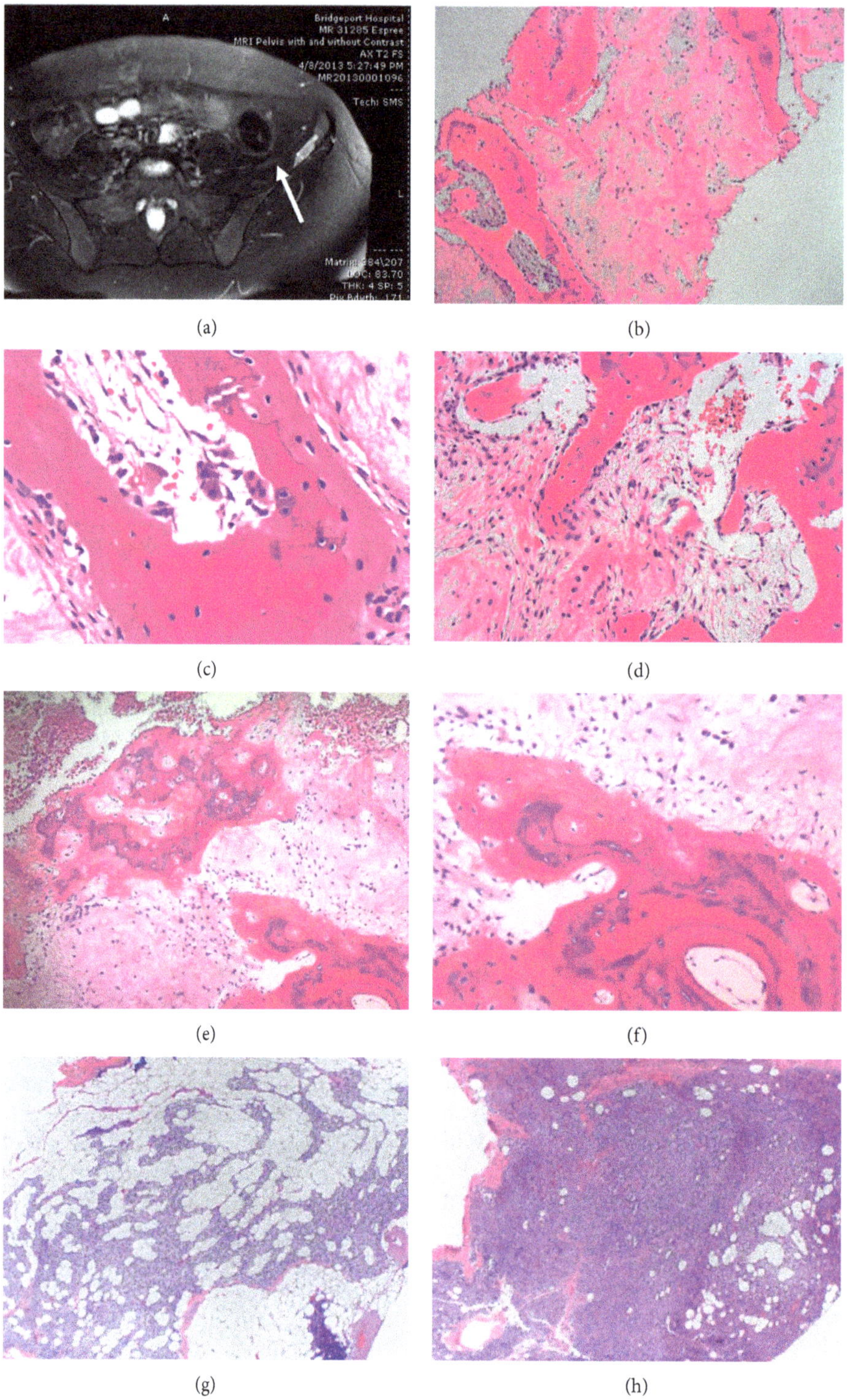

FIGURE 1: Bone imaging and bone and parathyroid histology. (a–f) Bone. (a) Initial MRI in 2013 showing bony lesion on the left iliac wing (bright area, white arrow) and (b–d) bone biopsy from 2013 reported as consistent with osteitis fibrosa cystica. Woven bone with marrow fibrosis (b), multinucleated osteoclasts with bone resorption (c), and osteoblastic rimming of new woven bone (d). (e) Repeat biopsy showing woven bone and peritrabecular fibrosis, with magnified portion (f). (g, h) Parathyroid. (g) Left lower parathyroid partial resection H&E stain, the specimen weighed 20 mg and measured 0.4 cm. Parenchyma was approximately 50% parathyroid epithelial cells (predominantly chief cells) and 50% adipocytes. (h) Right upper parathyroid gland biopsy, H&E stain, the specimen weighed 16 mg and measured 0.6 cm. Compared to that in (g), the parathyroid parenchyma is composed of approximately 80% parathyroid epithelial cells (predominantly chief cells) and 20% adipocytes. The amount of cellularity may be seen in normal parathyroid tissue or in hyperplasia. An additional biopsy of the left upper parathyroid gland was performed and was within normal limits based on weight and cellularity (not shown).

Additional Points

Summary. The clinical and biochemical features of FHH are described in a mother and daughter harboring a novel variant in the CaSR. The daughter (proband) had symptomatic hypercalcemia reversed by surgery and an unusual bony lesion, while her mother was asymptomatic and required no intervention. These cases illustrate the clinical variability of FHH and its occasional overlap with PHTP.

Disclosure

This case was presented as an abstract and poster presentation at the Endocrine Society meeting in Chicago, 2018.

Authors' Contributions

Dr. Majumdar worked up the cases and wrote the manuscript. All authors contributed to review and revision of the manuscript. Dr. Jacob contributed to case evaluation, Dr. Bale and Allison Bailey did genetic testing, and Dr. Kwon assisted in the diagnosis and evaluation of sarcoidosis. Dr. Hughes performed biopsy of the bony lesion. Dr. Barbieri reviewed parathyroid pathology and authored the pathology descriptions. Dr's. Laskin and Cohen reviewed the bone pathology and authored its description. Dr. Carling performed subtotal parathyroidectomy, reviewed the index patient, and contributed expertise from a surgical perspective.

References

[1] A. L. Herberger and C. A. Loretz, "Vertebrate extracellular calcium-sensing receptor evolution: selection in relation to life history and habitat," *Comparative Biochemistry and Physiology Part D: Genomics and Proteomics*, vol. 8, no. 1, pp. 86–94, 2013.

[2] https://databases.lovd.nl/shared/variants/CASR, 2018.

[3] S. J. Marx, "Familial hypocalciuric hypercalcemia as an atypical form of primary hyperparathyroidism," *Journal of Bone and Mineral Research*, vol. 33, no. 1, pp. 27–31, 2018.

[4] T. Carling, E. Szabo, M. Bai et al., "Familial hypercalcemia and hypercalciuria caused by a novel mutation in the cytoplasmic tail of the calcium receptor," *Journal of Clinical Endocrinology & Metabolism*, vol. 85, no. 5, pp. 2042–2047, 2000.

[5] L. F. Starker, T. Åkerström, W. D. Long et al., "Frequent germline mutations of the MEN_1, CASR and $HRPT_2/CDC_{73}$ genes in young patients with clinically non-familial primary hyperparathyroidism," *Hormones & Cancer*, vol. 3, no. 1-2, pp. 44–51, 2012.

[6] E. Szabo, P. Hellman, E. Lundgren, T. Carling, and J. Rastad, "Parathyroidectomy in familial hypercalcemia with clinical characteristics of primary hyperparathyroidism and familial hypocalciuric hypercalcemia," *Surgery*, vol. 131, no. 3, pp. 257–263, 2002.

[7] H. Bräuner-Osborne, A. A. Jensen, P. O. Sheppard, P. O'Hara, and P. Krogsgaard-Larsen, "The agonist-binding domain of the calcium-sensing receptor is located at the amino-terminal domain," *Journal of Biological Chemistry*, vol. 274, no. 26, pp. 18382–18386, 1999.

[8] J. Hu and A. M. Spiegel, "Structure and function of the human calcium-sensing receptor: insights from natural and engineered mutations and allosteric modulators," *Journal of Cellular and Molecular Medicine*, vol. 11, no. 5, pp. 908–922, 2011.

[9] S. E. Christensen, P. H. Nissen, P. Vestergaard, and L. Mosekilde, "Familial hypocalciuric hypercalcaemia," *Current Opinion in Endocrinology & Diabetes and Obesity*, vol. 18, no. 6, pp. 359–370, 2011.

[10] P. H. Nissen, S. E. Christensen, L. Heickendorff, K. Brixen, and L. Mosekilde, "Molecular genetic analysis of the calcium sensing receptor gene in patients clinically suspected to have familial hypocalciuric hypercalcemia: phenotypic variation and mutation spectrum in a Danish population," *The Journal of Clinical Endocrinology & Metabolism*, vol. 92, no. 11, pp. 4373–4379, 2007.

[11] D. R. Dufour and S. Y. Wilkerson, "The normal parathyroid revisited," *Human Pathology*, vol. 13, no. 8, pp. 717–721, 1982.

[12] D. Glotzman and G. N. Hendy, "The calcium-sensing receptor in bone—mechanistic and therapeutic insights," *Nature Reviews. Endocrinology*, vol. 11, no. 5, pp. 298–307, 2015.

[13] B. Wu, O. Wang, Y. Jiang, M. Li, X. Xing, and W. Xia, "Atypical skeletal manifestations of rickets in a familial hypocalciuric hypercalcemia patient," *Bone Research*, vol. 5, no. 17001, pp. 1-8, 2017.

[14] S. J. Marx, M. F. Attie, M. A. Levine, A. M. Spiegel, R. W. Downs, and R. D. Lasker, "The hypocalciuric or benign variant of familial hypercalcemia: clinical and biochemical features in fifteen kindreds," *Medicine*, vol. 60, no. 6, pp. 397–412, 1981.

23

Bilateral Leydig Cell Hyperplasia: A Rare Cause of Postmenopausal Hirsutism

S. Pathmanathan,[1] **S. D. N. De Silva**,[1] **M. Sumanatilleke**,[1] **D. Lokuhetty**,[2] **and U. V. V. Ranathunga**[2]

[1]*Diabetes and Endocrinology Unit, National Hospital of Sri Lanka, Colombo, Sri Lanka*
[2]*Department of Pathology, Faculty of Medicine, University of Colombo, Colombo, Sri Lanka*

Correspondence should be addressed to S. D. N. De Silva; neomalde@gmail.com

Academic Editor: Toshihiro Kita

Background. Postmenopausal hirsutism could be due to a myriad of causes, including ovarian and adrenal tumours, ovarian hyperthecosis, exogenous androgens, and Cushing's syndrome. We report a patient who was found to have a rare cause of postmenopausal hirsutism. *Case Presentation.* A 64-year-old postmenopausal woman with a history of hypertension, thyrotoxicosis, and poorly controlled diabetes on multiple oral hypoglycaemic agents presented with gradual onset progressive excessive hair growth without any virilizing features. On examination, she did not have Cushingnoid features or clitoromegaly. Her hirsutism was quantified with Ferriman–Gallwey score which was 9. Her biochemical evaluation showed elevated testosterone levels with normal DHEAS, ODST, 17-OHP, and prolactin. Low-dose dexamethasone suppression test did not suppress testosterone more than 40%. Contrast-enhanced CT of the adrenal and pelvis did not show any adrenal or ovarian mass lesions. Transvaginal ultrasound scan showed bilateral prominent ovaries only. Combined adrenal and ovarian venous sampling was carried out to localize the source of excess androgen, but only the left adrenal vein was successfully cannulated which showed suppressed testosterone level compared to periphery. The patient underwent total abdominal hysterectomy and bilateral salphingo oophorectomy, and her testosterone level normalized postoperatively. Her glycaemic control improved. Histology showed evidence of bilateral diffuse ovarian Leydig cell hyperplasia. *Conclusion.* Evaluation of postmenopausal hirsutism needs careful history and examination followed by biochemical evaluation and imaging. While adrenal and ovarian venous sampling can help to arrive at a diagnosis, it is a technically demanding procedure with low success rates even at centers of excellence. Therefore, in such situations, bilateral oophorectomy may be the best course of action which will give the histological confirmation of the diagnosis. Successful treatment of hyperandrogenism can result in improvement of glycaemic control. Bilateral diffuse Leydig cell hyperplasia is a rare but important cause of postmenopausal hirsutism.

1. Background

Postmenopausal androgen excess can present as hirsutism or frank virilization. Proper evaluation and management of this clinical entity is of paramount importance to improve the quality of life and psycho-social well-being of these patients. [1].

We report a case of postmenopausal hirsutism due to bilateral ovarian diffuse Leydig cell hyperplasia which is quite a rare entity.

2. Case presentation

A 64-year-old lady presented with a 5-year history of hirsutism. She entered menopause at the age of 45 years. She initially noted excessive hair growth involving the upper lips, chin, arms, and legs at the age of 59 years. There was progression of symptoms since the age of 61 years. However, there was no associated frontal balding, enlarged muscle mass or deepening of voice. She attained menarche at the age of 12 years and had regular menstrual cycles until menopause. She did not have any subfertility or excessive hair growth during her reproductive period suggestive of polycystic ovarian syndrome. She is a diagnosed patient with type II diabetes mellitus for 12 years and was on maximum doses of three oral hypoglycaemic agents without any evidence of micro- or macrovascular complications. Deterioration of glycaemic control has been noted for the past 1 year. She is also a diagnosed patient with hypertension for 12 years and thyrotoxicosis due to Graves' disease for 2 years, on medical therapy with satisfactory control. She had delivered 4 children through normal vaginal delivery without any significant obstetric or neonatal complications. She was not on any androgenic drugs. She is a nonsmoker, and there was no significant family history of any malignancy.

On examination, her weight was 76 kg and height was 160 cm, and body mass index was 29.68 kg/m^2. She had dark, coarse, terminal hair in androgen dependent areas with a Ferriman–Gallwey score of 9 (upper lip: 3; chin: 3; abdomen: 1; arm: 1; thighs: 1). There was no frontal balding or clitoromegaly. She did not have acanthosis nigricans, acne, or Cushingnoid features. She was clinically euthyroid with a pulse rate of 68 beats per minute and blood pressure of 130/80 mmHg.

Biochemical evaluation showed increased serum fasting testosterone levels (measured by the fully automated immunoassay analyzer ADVIA Centaur XP). Follicle-stimulating hormone (FSH) and luteinizing hormone (LH) levels were in the expected range for postmenopausal women. Basal 17-hydroxyprogesterone (17-OHP) level and dehydroepiandrosterone sulphate (DHEAS) level were normal. Hyperandrogenism was confirmed by repeating serum testosterone which was 176 ng/dL. Fasting blood sugar was 212 mg/dL, and HbA1c was 12.1 mmol/L (Table 1).

Table 1: Relevant hormonal evaluation of the patient.

Investigation	Value	Reference range
Total testosterone	123 ng/dL	14–76 (adult female)
FSH	31.92 IU/L	23–116.3 (postmenopausal)
LH	26.33 IU/L	15.9–54 (postmenopausal)
Prolactin	5.8 mU/L	48–430 (postmenopausal)
9.00 am cortisol (ODST)	24 nmol/L	<50
DHEAS	1 μmol/L	0.8–4.9
17-OHP	5.8 nmol/L	<6 excludes 21OHD
SHBG	53.3 mmol/L	13.5–71.4

FSH: follicle-stimulating hormone; LH: luteinizing hormone; ODST: overnight dexamethasone suppression test; DHEAS: dehydroepiandrosterone sulphate; 17-OHP: 17-hydroxyprogesterone; SHBG: sex hormone binding globulin, 21OHD: 21-hydroxylase deficiency.

To evaluate the source of excess testosterone, we measured dexamethasone suppressed testosterone level and carried out ovarian and adrenal imaging studies. Serum testosterone level was checked after oral dexamethasone 0.5 mg 6 hourly for 48 hours. Serum testosterone level got suppressed by 36.9% (basal serum testosterone 176 ng/dL and after dexamethasone 111 ng/dL). Studies have shown that the majority of patients with nontumerous hyperandrogenism normalizes testosterone or suppress by more than 40% after low dose dexamethasone suppression [2]. Therefore, the possibility of an androgen secreting tumour was considered in our patient. Although nonsuppression of testosterone is thought to indicate an ovarian source, no studies of hyperandrogenism in postmenopausal women have been reported using this approach.

Transvaginal ultrasound scan showed prominent ovaries (right ovary: 3.5 cm * 2.1 cm; left ovary: 3.4 cm * 2.2 cm), and her endometrial thickness was 6 mm which is slightly above normal for postmenopausal women. Contrast-enhanced CT scan of the abdomen and pelvis showed normal bilateral adrenal glands and a left adenexial cystic lesion suggestive of a simple ovarian cyst. Her CA-125 level was 4.5 U/mL (normal < 30.2). At this point, we were not able to exclude an adrenal source of androgen excess reliably. Thus, bilateral oophorectomy could be a futile surgery if hyperandrogenism did not resolve after surgery due to a missed small adrenal tumour. Therefore, we decided it would be worthwhile going ahead with combined adrenal and ovarian venous sampling to confirm the source of androgen excess prior to surgery. Biochemical confirmation of successful catheterization of the ovarian veins was based on an estradiol ratio >2 and that of adrenal veins when the cortisol ratio was >2. A testosterone ratio of >2 was considered to imply a source of androgen production [3]. Unfortunately, only the left adrenal vein fulfilled the biochemical criteria for successful catheterization and the testosterone ratio of the left adrenal vein to femoral vein was 0.6, thus excluding the left adrenal gland as the possible source of testosterone excess.

Although we could not definitively exclude the right adrenal gland as the possible source of excess androgen considering the negative imaging, we decided to refer her to surgery and she underwent total abdominal hysterectomy and bilateral salphingo oophorectomy. Total abdominal hysterectomy was done because her endometrial thickness was marginally high in the initial evaluation, and at her age, benefit of the procedure was considered to be more than any risk or adverse event. There were no surgical complications. On pathological examination, the right and left ovaries measured $40 \times 30 \times 17$ mm and $50 \times 30 \times 23$ mm, respectively. Both ovaries revealed a smooth outer surface and a homogenously tan white cut surface. There was no evidence of haemorrhage, cyst formation, or necrosis. Histological examination of bilateral ovaries revealed Leydig cells diffusely scattered within the normal appearing ovarian stroma (Figures 1 and 2). Cell clusters did not form large aggregated nodules leading to either significant ovarian enlargement or shape distortion. There was no evidence of nuclear atypia or increased mitotic activity. Similar cell clusters were also seen in the hilus. Androgen receptor immunostaining did not reveal any theca cells. Sertoli cells were not seen. On postsurgery day 1, total testosterone level came down to 15.27 ng/dL (normal range: 14–76). Her fasting blood sugar level was 85 mg/dL, and we were able to reduce the doses of oral hypoglycaemic agents. In 3 months of follow-up, her hirsutism showed a marked improvement.

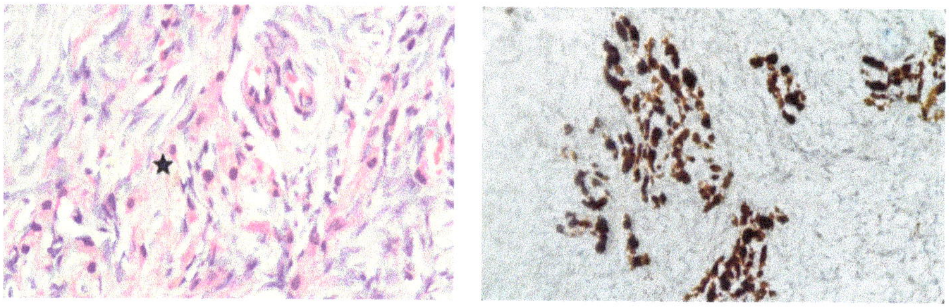

(a) (b)

Figure 1: Histology of right ovary showing small clusters of Leydig cells, which has oval round nuclei with inconspicuous nucleoli and moderate eosinophilic cytoplasm (a, asterix, H&E, 400x). The Leydig cells display strong cytoplasmic staining with Calretinin (b, 400x). Histological appearance of the left ovary was similar.

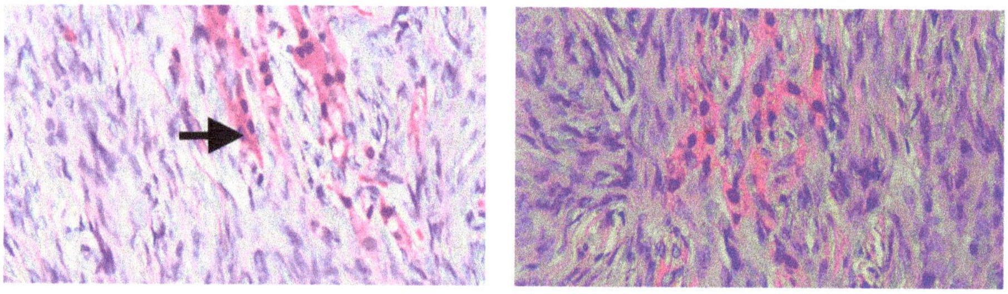

(a) (b)

Figure 2: Rod-like structure resembling a Reinke crystal (a, arrow, H&E, 400x). Leydig cells with cytoplasmic vacuolation and brown lipofuschin pigment (b, H&E, 400x).

3. Discussion

In this postmenopausal lady with clinical and biochemical hyperandrogenism with clear postmenopausal onset and normal menstruation and fertility prior to menopause, normal ODST, and no history of exogenous androgen exposure, only 3 differential diagnoses remain [4]: androgen-secreting adrenal tumours, androgen-secreting ovarian tumours (Sertoli–Leydig cells, granulosa-theca cells, hilus cells), and ovarian hyperthecosis/leydig cell hyperplasia.

Imaging studies like transvaginal ultrasound scan and contrast-enhanced CT can help in differentiation. If the imaging studies are negative, the following investigations can help in differentiation.

(1) High DHEAS levels will support a diagnosis of adrenal tumour. However, in a study of 478 women with hyperandrogenism, 10 patients had DHEAS level more than 16.3 μmol/L, and none of them were found to have an adrenal tumour [5].

(2) Low dose dexamethasone suppression of serum testosterone can differentiate ovarian and adrenal neoplasms from nonneoplastic hyperandrogenism as testosterone level is suppressed by more than 40% in the latter but not in the former [2].

(3) Combined ovarian and adrenal venous sampling is a technically challenging procedure and therefore is not routinely recommended. Even in centers of excellence where the procedure is done by an experienced radiologist, the success rate of venous catheterization has been quite low: all four veins in 27%, three veins in 65%, and two veins in 87% [3].

(4) Ovarian androgen synthesis depends on LH stimulation while adrenal does not. Therefore, suppression of LH with GnRH analogues (GnRH-analog suppression test) leads to a reduction of testosterone level by more than 50%, if the ovary is the source of androgen excess. However, this test does not differentiate between ovarian hyperthecosis and virilizing ovarian tumours [6].

There are 3 main options for the management of nontumerous hyperandrogenism such as ovarian hyperthecosis or Leydig cell hyperplasia.

(1) Anti-androgen-cyproterone acetate is a competitive inhibitor of testosterone at the level of androgen receptors.

(2) As described above, GnRH analogues suppress LH, thus leading to suppression of ovarian androgen production.

(3) Bilateral oophorectomy is the definitive treatment. Adrenal tumours are almost always visible on contrast-enhanced adrenal protocol CT. Therefore, if the

adrenal CT is negative, bilateral oophorectomy may be the best therapeutic option.

Leydig cell hyperplasia is a rare cause of postmenopausal hirsutism. Review of the literature yielded only about 10 reported patients with this condition [7–14].

In postmenopausal women, the ovarian stroma is a source of testosterone [15]. However, ovarian hilar cells, which are morphologically indistinguishable from testicular Leydig cells, also secrete testosterone in the postmenopausal ovary. Hilar cells are predominantly seen in the ovarian hilum. Sometimes these cells can extend to the ovarian medullary stroma and such cells are called "Leydig cells of non-hilar type" [11]. Leydig cells are present in more than 80% of all female ovaries. These Leydig cells can undergo hyperplasia or can transform into a tumour. Distinction between the two entities is based on the histopathology depending on the pattern and size of the cell clusters. Hyperplasia is usually nodular but widely separated and diffuse. A nodule more than 1 cm is considered a tumour.

Etiopathogenesis of Leydig cell hyperplasia is not well defined. However, it could be due to autonomous origin or central stimulation due to high LH levels seen in postmenopausal women [12].

Ovarian stroma has two types of cells: female type granulosa and theca cells and male type Sertoli and Leydig cells. Ovarian hyperthecosis is a morphologic alteration of ovarian stromal cells so that they resemble luteneized theca cells. There are ample case reports of this entity [16]. In our patient, even though ovarian hyperthecosis comes in to the differential diagnosis, diffusely proliferating Leydig cells among normal stromal cells were favoured on histomorphology. Even though few Leydig cells were seen in the ovarian hilar region, there was no associated hyperplasia. This pattern of diffuse Leydig cell hyperplasia within the normal stroma has been described only in a very few patients previously.

High testosterone levels are associated with a lower risk of type 2 diabetes mellitus in men and a higher risk in women [17]. Possible physiological mechanism of testosterone-induced increased insulin resistance in women is testosterone-induced serine phosphorylation of insulin receptor substrate-1 (IRS-1). IRS-1 is a signaling protein which couples insulin receptor to the phosphoinositide-3-kinase (PI3K) signaling cascade, which is important in bringing about the biologic actions of insulin. Serine phosphorylation of IRS-1 leads to uncoupling of insulin receptor and PI3K, thus leading to insulin resistance [18]. This may be the explanation for the deterioration of glycaemic control of our patient with hyperandrogenism and improvement of glycaemic control after surgery.

4. Conclusions

Bilateral ovarian diffuse Leydig cell hyperplasia is a rare but important cause of postmenopausal hirsutism. Successful treatment of hyperandrogenism in postmenopausal women can lead to reduced insulin resistance and improved glycaemic control.

Abbreviations

17-OHP: 17-Hydroxyprogesterone
CA-125: Cancer antigen 125
CT: Computed tomography
DHEAS: Dehydroepiandrosterone sulphate
DL: Dyslipidaemia
DM: Diabetes mellitus
FSH: Follicle-stimulating hormone
HbA1c: Haemoglobin A1C
LH: Luteinizing hormone
ODST: Overnight dexamethasone suppression test
SHBG: Sex hormone binding globulin.

Consent

Written informed consent was obtained from the patient herself for publication of patient details and identifying images.

Authors' Contributions

SDND was a part of the treating team and did the literature search and wrote the manuscript, SP was the primary physician who managed the patient and reviewed the manuscript. MS reviewed the manuscript and contributed to literature analysis. DL was the reporting pathologist and contributed to writing the manuscript, providing images and reviewing the manuscript. UVVR contributed to pathological examination, image editing, and writing the manuscript. All authors read and approved the final manuscript.

Acknowledgments

This work was supported by the University Gynaecology and Obstetrics Unit of De Soysa Hospital for women.

References

[1] M. S. Rothman and M. E. Wierman, "How should postmenopausal androgen excess be evaluated?" *Clinical Endocrinology*, vol. 75, no. 2, pp. 160–164, 2011.

[2] G. A. Kaltsas, A. M. Isidori, B. P. Kola et al., "The value of the low-dose dexamethasone suppression test in the differential diagnosis of hyperandrogenism in women," *Journal of Clinical Endocrinology & Metabolism*, vol. 88, no. 6, pp. 2634–2643, 2003.

[3] G. A. Kaltsas, J. J. Mukherjee, B. Kola et al., "Is ovarian and adrenal venous catheterization and sampling helpful in the investigation of hyperandrogenic women?" *Clinical Endocrinology*, vol. 59, no. 1, pp. 34–43, 2003.

[4] M. Alpañés, J. M. González-Casbas, J. Sánchez, H. Pián, and H. F. Escobar-Morreale, "Management of postmenopausal virilization," *Journal of Clinical Endocrinology & Metabolism*, vol. 97, no. 8, pp. 2584–2588, 2012.

[5] W. Waggoner, L. R. Boots, and R. Azziz, "Total testosterone and DHEAS levels as predictors of androgen-secreting neo-

plasms: a populational study," *Gynecological Endocrinology*, vol. 13, no. 6, pp. 394–400, 1999.

[6] M.-M. Pascale, M. Pugeat, M. Roberts et al., "Androgen suppressive effect of GnRH agonist in ovarian hyperthecosis and virilizing turnours," *Clinical Endocrinology*, vol. 41, no. 5, pp. 571–576, 1994.

[7] I. Taliaferro, "Ovarian hilus cell (Leydig cell) hyperplasia associated with masculinization," *Archives of Internal Medicine*, vol. 91, no. 5, p. 675, 1953.

[8] D. J. MacRae, M. P. Willmott, A. A. A. Ismail, and D. N. Love, "Androgen patterns in a case of hilar cell hyperplasia of the ovary," *BJOG: An International Journal of Obstetrics and Gynaecology*, vol. 78, no. 8, pp. 741–745, 1971.

[9] A. R. Mclellan, A. Mowat, J. Cordiner et al., "Hilus cell pathology and hirsutism," *Clinical Endocrinology*, vol. 32, no. 2, pp. 203–212, 1990.

[10] H. C. Taylor, I. Pillay, and S. Setrakian, "Diffuse stromal leydig cell hyperplasia: a unique cause of postmenopausal hyperandrogenism and virilization," *Mayo Clinic Proceedings*, vol. 75, no. 3, pp. 288–292, 2000.

[11] F. S. M. Ali, S. E. R. S. Stanaway, H. D. Zakhour, G. Spearing, and D. Bowen-Jones, "A case of hirsutism due to bilateral diffuse ovarian Leydig cell hyperplasia in a post-menopausal woman," *European Journal of Internal Medicine*, vol. 14, no. 7, pp. 432-433, 2003.

[12] M. Hofland, S. Cosyns, P. De Sutter, C. Bourgain, and B. Velkeniers, "Leydig cell hyperplasia and Leydig cell tumour in postmenopausal women: report of two cases," *Gynecological Endocrinology*, vol. 29, no. 3, pp. 213–215, 2013.

[13] J. M. Mehta, J. L. Miller, A. J. Cannon, S. K. Mardekian, L. C. Kenyon, and S. A. Jabbour, "Ovarian leydig cell hyperplasia: an unusual case of virilization in a postmenopausal woman," *Case Reports in Endocrinology*, vol. 2014, pp. 1–4, 2014.

[14] M. Tutzer, I. Winnykamien, J. Davila Guardia, and C. Castelo-Branco, "Hyperandrogenism in post-menopausal women: a diagnosis challenge," *Gynecological Endocrinology*, vol. 30, no. 1, pp. 23–25, 2014.

[15] R. H. Fogle, F. Z. Stanczyk, X. Zhang, and R. J. Paulson, "Ovarian androgen production in postmenopausal women," *Journal of Clinical Endocrinology & Metabolism*, vol. 92, no. 8, pp. 3040–3043, 2007.

[16] S. S. Braithwaite, E. B. Balis, and T. D. Avila, "Postmenopausal virilization due to ovarian stromal hyperthecosis," *Journal of Clinical Endocrinology & Metabolism*, vol. 46, no. 2, pp. 295–300, 1978.

[17] E. L. Ding, Y. Song, V. S. Malik, and S. Liu, "Sex differences of endogenous Sex hormones and risk of type 2 diabetes," *JAMA*, vol. 295, no. 11, p. 1288, 2006.

[18] M. C. Allemand, B. A. Irving, Y. W. Asmann et al., "Effect of testosterone on insulin stimulated IRS1 ser phosphorylation in primary rat myotubes-A potential model for PCOS-related insulin resistance," *PLoS One*, C. Zhang, Ed., vol. 4, no. 1, Article ID e4274, 2009.

24

ACTH-Independent Cushing's Syndrome Associated with Left Adrenocortical Oncocytoma of Uncertain Malignant Potential

Giuseppe S. Sica,[1] **Leandro Siragusa**,[1] **Bruno Sensi**,[1] **Vittoria Bellato**,[1] **Pierangela Floris**,[2] **Valentina Rovella**,[2] **Alessandro Mauriello**,[3] **Monia Di Prete**,[3] **Rossana Telesca**,[3] **Valerio Ciavoni**,[2] **Carmine Cardillo**,[4] **Nicola Di Daniele**,[2] **and Manfredi Tesauro**[2]

[1]*Department of Surgery, University of Rome "Tor Vergata", 00133 Rome, Italy*
[2]*Department of Systems Medicine, University of Rome "Tor Vergata", 00133 Rome, Italy*
[3]*Department of Experimental Medicine, University of Rome "Tor Vergata", 00133 Rome, Italy*
[4]*Department of Internal Medicine, Universitá Cattolica del Sacro Cuore, Rome 00168, Italy*

Correspondence should be addressed to Giuseppe S. Sica; sigisica@gmail.com

Academic Editor: Osamu Isozaki

Adrenocortical oncocytomas are rare and mostly nonfunctioning neoplasms. We report the case of a 27-year-old woman diagnosed with an ACTH-independent Cushing's syndrome due to left adrenal oncocytoma. She underwent laparoscopic adrenalectomy. Histopathological examination revealed an oncocytoma of uncertain malignant potential with a low Ki-67 proliferation index, inhibin A positivity, and chromogranin A negativity. Electron micrographs confirmed adrenal oncocytoma cells, characterized by the presence of a large amount of mitochondria. The postoperative course was uneventful, and the patient experienced a progressive regression of Cushing-related symptoms. Periodical follow-ups with MRI and cortisol dosage are required due to the neoplasm's uncertain malignant potential. Considerations on the diagnosis, pathology findings, clinical remarks, and interventions are made.

1. Introduction

Adrenocortical oncocytic neoplasms (ACONs) are an epithelial subtype of adrenal tumours, firstly reported by Kakimoto et al. in 1986 [1]. Oncocytomas have distinctive histopathological features, as they are characterized by large cells with a wide granular eosinophilic cytoplasm, related to numerous swollen mitochondria [2, 3]. The adrenal gland is a very uncommon location for oncocytomas, which are usually found in different sites, such as kidneys, thyroid, parathyroid, pituitary, and salivary glands [3, 4]. These tumours are usually incidentalomas, unwittingly detected during radiological investigations performed for other medical reasons. Nevertheless, up to 35% are capable of synthesizing hormones such as aldosterone and cortisol, originating visible clinical manifestations [5]. Indeed, the virilisation and feminization syndromes due to sexual hormone hypersecretion are well described in the literature, as well as Cushing's and Conn's syndromes due to primary hypercortisolism and hyperaldosteronism, respectively. However, adrenocortical oncocytomas generally do not have particular radiological features but large dimensions for which the diagnosis is rarely made before surgery and pathology examination [6–8]. We, hereby, report a case of a 27-year-old woman undergoing left laparoscopic adrenalectomy at our institution, for endogenous Cushing's syndrome, due to an adrenocortical mass, which was also an oncocytoma of uncertain malignant potential.

2. Case Report

2.1. Clinical Presentation, Diagnosis, and Treatment. A 27-year-old Caucasian woman was referred to our Emergency Department due to the acute onset of severe hypertension

(190/110). She reported one year of insomnia caused by recurring sleep hyperhidrosis. Apart from that, she had neither relevant medical history nor any previous surgical history. She was a regular cigarette smoker, with a body mass index of 21, who followed a vegan diet. Physical examination revealed a full-moon face, a mild buffalo hump, and a light hypotrophy of proximal limb muscles. In addition, dermatologic signs showed thin skin with the tendency to bruise, purple striae, thickened hair, and facial seborrheic dermatitis. There were no signs of virilisation nor did she report menstrual irregularities. Initially, hormonal studies showed a slightly elevated basal cortisol level (21.4 mg/dL, reference range 3.7–19.4 mg/dL); however, D4-androstenedione, progesterone, aldosterone, testosterone, and adrenaline urinary catabolites levels were normal. After performing an overnight suppression test with 1 mg of dexamethasone, basal serum cortisol was increased to 19.90 μg/dL. Hormonal test results are summarized in Tables 1 and 2. An abdominal ultrasound was performed, highlighting a bilateral adrenal gland hypertrophy. Magnetic resonance imaging (MRI) with paramagnetic contrast showed a 23 mm nodular mass of the left adrenal gland cortex with regular and well-defined margins and early arterial postcontrast enhancement. Following the diagnosis of ACTH-independent Cushing's syndrome, the patient was referred for surgery. The patient underwent laparoscopic left adrenalectomy: firstly, a medial to lateral approach and no-touch technique was chosen to dissect and divide the left adrenal vein. There was no intraoperative rebound and no need for blood arterial pressure adjustment. There were no postoperative complications, and the young woman was sent home on the second postoperative day following ACTH and cortisol blood determination as well as 24 h urinary free cortisol testing.

2.2. Pathology Examination. The surgical specimen underwent histopathological examination: it consisted of adipose tissue containing a tan-brown neoplasm, with regular and smooth margins, of 2.7 × 2 cm in size, largely replacing the normal adrenal gland parenchyma (Figure 1). Microscopically, the nodule was composed of more than 90% of an encapsulated proliferation of oncocytes (cells with large eosinophilic and granular cytoplasm, pleomorphic nuclei, and prominent nucleoli) in a diffuse architectural pattern (Figure 2(a) and inset). The tumour only focally showed capsular infiltration (Figures 2(a) and 2(b)). Immunohistochemical tests revealed that the tumour cells were negative for chromogranin A (Figure 2(c)) and positive for inhibin A, a specific marker of adrenocortical origin (Figure 2(d)). Specific mitochondrial immunohistochemical techniques (mES-13; SDHA/SDHB) would have been helpful to prove that the eosinophilic aspect of the cells are indeed mitochondria accumulated in the cytoplasm, but unfortunately, we do not have it available. Electron micrographs confirmed adrenal oncocytoma cells, characterized by the presence of a large amount of mitochondria (Figure 3). Although neither necrosis nor vascular invasion was detected, one mitosis per 50 high-power fields was counted, thus resulting in a Ki-67 proliferation index lower than 5%. Based on the Lin–Weiss–Bisceglia (LWB) grading scale—reported by the WHO for oncocytic neoplasm of the adrenal gland [9]—a final diagnosis of oncocytoma of uncertain malignant potential was established.

2.3. Postoperative Outcome. Postoperatively, the patient began glucocorticoid and mineralocorticoid replacement therapies with cortisone 21-acetate 18, 75 mg per day, which were gradually tapered. One month after surgery, the patient had already experienced a progressive regression of Cushing-related symptoms and a relative normalization of blood pressure levels, as confirmed by a blood pressure Holter. She was advised to undergo quarterly ACTH cortisol dosage and referred for follow-up to our oncological team.

3. Discussion

ACONs are a rare epithelial subtype of adrenal tumours firstly reported by Kakimoto in 1986 [1]. More than 2/3 of ACONs are nonfunctioning or clinically silent. Functioning ACONs are reported with a frequency of 17–34%, of which less than 6% are cortisol-secreting. Moreover, although 41% of ACONs are of uncertain malignant potential, the functioning forms of these range between 22 and 29% [5, 8].

While renal oncocytomas have radiological features suggesting preoperative diagnosis, such as the central scarring, the same is not true for adrenal oncocytomas. Benign adrenal oncocytomas may be distinguished from lipid-rich adenomas on CT scan due to the fact that the latter show low attenuation on CT scan (<10 Hounsfield-HU), whereas the malignant oncocytic neoplasm can demonstrate features similar to adrenocortical carcinomas (ACCs), including larger size, internal necrosis, and lower percentage enhancement washout [10].

An ultrasound-guided biopsy is safe but rarely performed as it is frequently inconclusive and is difficult to use for the discrimination between kidney-originated tumours and adrenal tumours [11, 12]. Indeed, in all reported cases of ACONs, the diagnosis was always made at the histopathological examination. Immunohistochemical tests show positivity for inhibin A (69%), melan-A (85%), synaptophysin (74%), vimentin (80%), mitochondrial antibody mES-13 (100%), calretinin (78%), neuron-specific enolase (94%), and cytokeratin AE1/AE3 (52%); they show negativity for chromogranin A (91%) and S100 protein (96%) [5].

In the last edition of the WHO classification of endocrine neoplasms, the LWB-specific criteria was reported in order to classify ACONs as malignant when at least one major criterion was present, such as a high mitotic rate (>5 mitoses per 50 high-power fields), atypical mitoses, and venous invasion. ACONs of uncertain malignant potential are classified as such in the presence at least one of the minor criteria: large size (more than 10 cm), necrosis, and capsular and sinusoidal invasion [8, 13, 14]. In the case at hand, we found a minimal capsular invasion, and the neoplasm was classified as of uncertain malignant potential. The reticulin algorithm, reported by Volante et al. [15], was not used

Table 1: Laboratory tests.

		Before hospitalization	First visit	Overnight suppression test	2 days postsurgery	A month later surgery	Normal range
Plasma sodium	mEq/L	146	143		137	141	136–145
Plasma potassium	mEq/L	5.10	4.30		4.50	4.50	3.50–5.10
Plasma basal cortisol	μg/dl	**28.4**	21.40	19.90	1.10	0.9	4.4–22.0
Plasma ACTH	pg/ml	**<5**	**<5**		**<5**	**<5**	0.0–46.00
24 h urinary free cortisol	mcg/24 h	**434.70**	**356.4**		2.5		0–100
24 h urinary sodium	mMol/24 h	78.30	**250.80**				40–220
24 h urinary potassium	mMol/24 h	75.60	**132.00**				25–125

Laboratory tests are conducted to determine the etiology of Cushing's syndrome showed modest increase in basal cortisol with abolition of its circadian rhythm and ACTH levels constantly and markedly suppressed. Bold values represent lab tests out of range and the ones useful in diagnosing ATCH-independent Cushing's syndrome.

Table 2: Other hormonal tests.

		Patient	Normal range
Metanephrine	mcg/24 h	292.00	64-303
Normetanephrine	mcg/24 h	345.00	163-530
Urinary aldosterone	mcg/24 h	<9.7	2.5–20
DHEA-S	mcg/dl	**15.20**	18.00–391
Total testosterone	ng/dl	8.20	13.84–53.35
Delta-4 androstenedione	ng/ml	0.56	0.3–3.3
Thyroid stimulating hormone	uU/ml	1.35	0.50–6.5
Free T3	pg/ml	2.88	1.3–3.6
Free T4	pg/ml	1.30	0.8–2.0
FSH	ng/ml	5.01	5.00–35.0
Prolactin	ng/ml	24.10	5.00–25
LH	mIU/ml	4.99	
17-Beta estradiol	pg/ml	37.86	
Progesterone	ng/ml	1.47	

Bold values are the ones out of range.

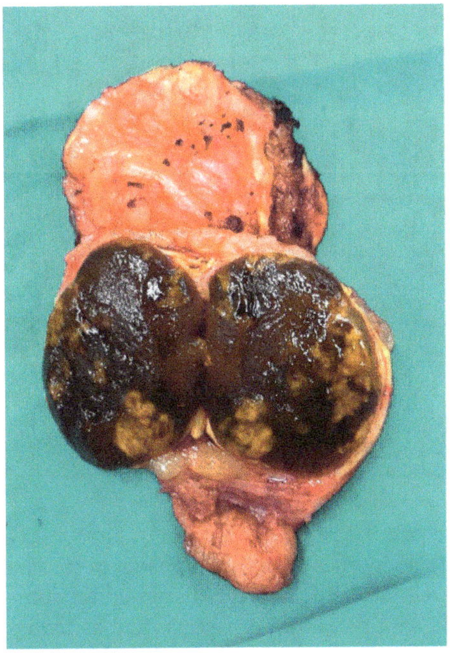

Figure 1: Macroscopic specimen: tan-brown neoplasm with regular and smooth borders largely replacing the normal adrenal gland parenchyma, which is recognizable at the margin of the specimen.

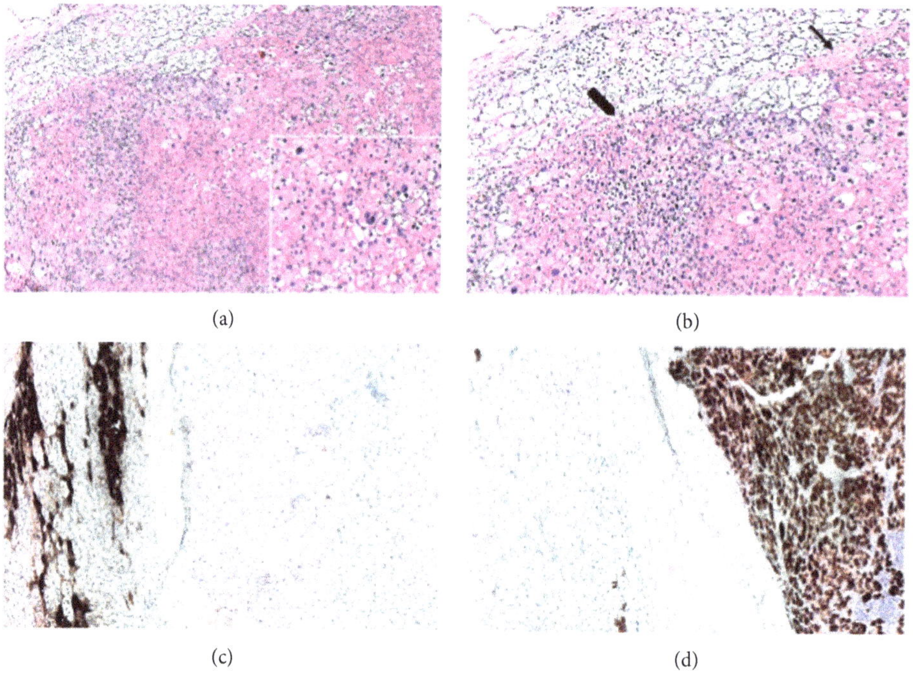

Figure 2: Histopathological features and immunohistochemical findings: (a) encapsulated diffuse proliferation of large cells with focal capsular invasion. Inset: the cells show pleomorphic nuclei, prominent nucleoli, and wide eosinophilic and granular cytoplasm. (b) At higher magnification, capsular invasion is shown in detail (the arrow signs a thin fibrous capsule dividing the neoplasm from the cortex of the adrenal gland, while the thick arrow shows the focal infiltration of the adrenal parenchyma by the tumour). (c) The neoplastic cells resulted negative for chromogranin A (positive internal control: adrenal medulla). (d) The neoplastic cells resulted strongly and diffusely positive for inhibin A (internal control: adrenal cortex, mild and sparse positivity). (a, b) Haematoxylin-eosin stain. (c) Chromogranin A. (d) Inhibin A. Original magnification: (a) 40x, inset 200x; (b) 200x, (c, d) 100x.

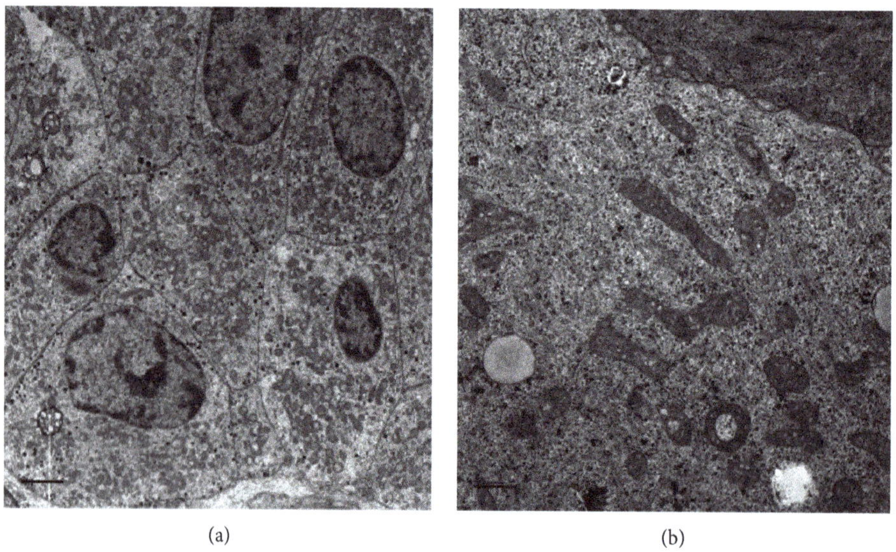

Figure 3: Electron microscopy findings: (a) electron micrographs show adrenal oncocytoma cells, characterized by the presence of large amount of mitochondria (scale bar represents 2 μm). (b) high magnification displays ultrastructural details of crista-type mitochondria (scale bar represents 0.2 μm).

because although useful in discriminating adenomas from carcinomas, it does not determine the eventual malignant potential of adenomas with uncertain malignant potential as considering mitosis >5/10 HPF without taking account of features such as necrosis or vascular invasion. The case hereby reported had a Weiss score <3, and the presence of a disrupted reticulin framework would not be sufficient to be classified as malignant.

ACONs preferably arise from the left gland, with an M/F ratio of 1 : 2 and an average age of 44. The ACON reported retains an uncertain malignant potential since the capsule was focally infiltrated, but it was certainly a smaller lesion (2.7 × 2 cm) when compared to the average size of 10 cm for the commonly found borderline ACONs.

Prognostic factors still need to be validated because of the low number of patients reported in literature. However, males appear to be more frequently associated with malignant ACONs, whereas younger patients are more commonly affected by smaller benign ACONs compared to borderline and malignant ones [5].

Currently, ACONs of uncertain malignant potential appear to have an 88% probability of a 5-year survival rate, with only two recurrences reported in literature out of 57 cases. Although malignant potential is classified by the LWB criteria, there are still no formal guidelines regulating the follow-up. Surely, borderline and malignant ACONs should undergo periodic MRI/CT scan. Ipsilateral adrenalectomy is usually indicated for the uncertain nature of the mass and to resolve the concomitant symptomatology. Laparoscopy seems to achieve similar rates of R0 resection of open surgery for ENSAT I and II ACC and for masses smaller than 10 cm. Laparoscopic adrenalectomy is feasible, safe, and offers all the advantages of the minimally invasive surgical technique [16–19].

4. Conclusions

Functioning and cortisol-secreting ACONs are very rare entities, but they can certainly be responsible of ACTH-independent Cushing's syndrome. Surgical excision is indicated, and the laparoscopic approach appears to be feasible and safe in most instances. Since borderline ACONs are of uncertain malignant potential, a proper follow-up is warranted.

References

[1] S. Kakimoto, Y. Yushita, T. Sanefuji et al., "Non-hormonal adrenocortical adenoma with oncocytoma-like appearances," *Hinyokika Kiyo Acta Urologica Japonica*, vol. 32, no. 5, pp. 757–763, 1986.

[2] H. Sasano, T. Suzuki, T. Sano, T. Kameya, N. Sasano, and H. Nagura, "Adrenocortical oncocytoma," *The American Journal of Surgical Pathology*, vol. 15, no. 10, pp. 949–956, 1991.

[3] A. Chang and S. J. Harawi, "Oncocytes, oncocytosis, and oncocytic tumors," *Pathology Annual*, vol. 27, no. Pt 1, pp. 263–304, 1992.

[4] G. Tallini, "Oncocytic tumours," *Virchows Archiv*, vol. 433, no. 1, pp. 5–12, 1998.

[5] J. J. Kanitra, J. C. Hardaway, T. Soleimani, T. J. Koehler, M. K. McLeod, and S. Kavuturu, "Adrenocortical oncocytic neoplasm: a systematic review," *Surgery*, vol. 164, no. 6, pp. 1351–1359, 2018.

[6] Y. Hong, Y. Hao, J. Hu, B. Xu, H. Shan, and X. Wang, "Adrenocortical oncocytoma 11 case reports and review of the literature," *Medicine*, vol. 96, no. 48, p. e8750, 2017.

[7] H. Peynirci, B. Taskıran, N. Dik, Ö. Saraydaroğlu, and C. Ersoy, "Oncocytic neoplasms; rare adrenocortical tumours—a report of eleven patients," *Endokrynologia Polska*, vol. 69, no. 6, pp. 682–687, 2018.

[8] D. D. Wong, D. V. Spagnolo, M. Bisceglia, M. Havlat, D. McCallum, and M. A. Platten, "Oncocytic adrenocortical neoplasms-a clinicopathologic study of 13 new cases emphasizing the importance of their recognition," *Human Pathology*, vol. 42, no. 4, pp. 489–499, 2011.

[9] M. Bisceglia, O. Ludovico, A. Di Mattia et al., "Adrenocortical oncocytic tumors: report of 10 cases and review of the literature," *International Journal of Surgical Pathology*, vol. 12, no. 3, pp. 231–243, 2004.

[10] M. Khan, E. M. Caoili, M. S. Davenport et al., "CT imaging characteristics of oncocytic adrenal neoplasms (OANs): comparison with adrenocortical carcinomas," *Abdominal Imaging*, vol. 39, no. 1, pp. 86–91, 2014.

[11] E. Cham, W. Watkin, R. Goldschmidt, and L. Liu, "Fine needle aspiration cytology of adrenocortical oncocytic neoplasm," *Acta Cytologica*, vol. 54, no. 4, pp. 627–634, 2010.

[12] P. Rossi, P. Sileri, P. Gentileschi et al., "Percutaneous liver biopsy using an ultrasound-guided subcostal route," *Digestive Diseases and Sciences*, vol. 46, no. 1, pp. 128–132, 2001.

[13] I. Marafini, I. Monteleone, D. Di Fusco et al., "TNF-α producing innate lymphoid cells (ILCs) are increased in active celiac disease and contribute to promote intestinal atrophy in mice," *PLoS One*, vol. 10, no. 5, 2015.

[14] E. Duregon, M. Volante, S. Cappia et al., "Oncocytic adrenocortical tumors," *The American Journal of Surgical Pathology*, vol. 35, no. 12, pp. 1882–1893, 2011.

[15] M. Volante, E. Bollito, P. Sperone et al., "Clinicopathological study of a series of 92 adrenocortical carcinomas: from a proposal of simplified diagnostic algorithm to prognostic stratification," *Histopathology*, vol. 55, no. 5, pp. 535–543, 2009.

[16] B. Carnaille, "Adrenocortical carcinoma: which surgical approach?" *Langenbeck's Archives of Surgery*, vol. 397, no. 2, pp. 195–199, 2012.

[17] G. S. Sica, E. Iaculli, L. Biancone et al., "Comparative study of laparoscopicvsopen gastrectomy in gastric cancer management," *World Journal of Gastroenterology*, vol. 17, no. 41, pp. 4602–4606, 2011.

[18] G. Sgourakis, S. Lanitis, A. Kouloura et al., "Laparoscopic versus open adrenalectomy for stage I/II adrenocortical carcinoma: meta-analysis of outcomes," *Journal of Investigative Surgery*, vol. 28, no. 3, pp. 145–152, May 2015.

[19] P. Sileri, G. Sica, P. Gentileschi et al., "Ischemic preconditioning protects intestine from prolonged ischemia," *Transplantation Proceedings*, vol. 36, no. 2, pp. 283–285, 2004.

25

A Case of Von Hippel–Lindau Disease with Bilateral Pheochromocytoma and Ectopic Hypersecretion of Intact Parathyroid Hormone in an Adolescent Girl

Rym Belaid, Ibtissem Oueslati, Melika Chihaoui, Meriem Yazidi, Wafa Grira, and Fatma Chaker

Department of Endocrinology, La Rabta University Hospital, Faculty of Medicine, University of Tunis El Manar, Tunis, Tunisia

Correspondence should be addressed to Ibtissem Oueslati; ouesibtissem@gmail.com

Academic Editor: Takeshi Usui

Von Hippel–Lindau disease is an autosomal dominant inherited syndrome predisposing to a variety of highly vascularised tumors in different organs. Although bilateral pheochromocytoma was reported in patients with von Hippel–Lindau disease, the coexistence of primary hyperparathyroidism is not a common condition. We report an observation of a primary hyperparathyroidism secondary to an ectopic secretion of intact parathyroid hormone in a 17-year-old girl with von Hippel–Lindau disease and bilateral pheochromocytoma. She presented with a newly diagnosed diabetes mellitus and a severe arterial hypertension. Blood tests disclosed hypercalcemia with increased intact PTH level. Cervical ultrasound and sestamibi scintigraphy were normal. Twenty-four-hour urinary normetanephrine level was highly elevated pointing to a catecholamine-secreting tumor. The abdominal computed tomography showed bilateral adrenal masses. MIBG scintigraphy exhibited a high accumulation of the tracer in both adrenal tumors. Genetic testing revealed a mutation of the VHL gene. The patient underwent a bilateral adrenalectomy. The postoperative outcome was marked by normalization of blood pressure, blood glucose, calcium, and PTH levels. In our case, the elevation of intact PTH and its spontaneous normalization after surgical treatment of pheochromocytomas confirms its ectopic secretion.

1. Introduction

Pheochromocytomas are uncommon neuroendocrine tumors that arise from chromaffin cells of the adrenal medulla and produce excessive amounts of catecholamines: epinephrine, norepinephrine, and dopamine [1]. Although most pheochromocytomas are sporadic, more than 25% are associated with an inherited mutation, and this frequency can be as high as 55%, if diagnosed before 18 years of age [2]. In childhood, pheochromocytomas are mostly due to genetic causes including von Hippel–Lindau (VHL) disease, multiple endocrine neoplasia type 2 (MEN2), hereditary pheochromocytoma paraganglioma syndrome, and rarely neurofibromatosis type 1 [3]. Compared to adults, VHL disease is reported to be the most frequent genetic disorder causing pheochromocytomas in children [4]. While bilateral pheochromocytomas were reported in patients with VHL disease, the coexistence of primary hyperparathyroidism is not a common condition [5].

Herein, we report a case of a VHL disease with bilateral pheochromocytoma and an ectopic secretion of intact parathyroid hormone in an adolescent girl.

2. Presentation of Case

A 17-year-old girl was referred to our department for the investigation of a newly diagnosed diabetes mellitus and a severe arterial hypertension. She was the first child of consanguineous parents. Her past medical history was unremarkable. Her family history was notable for type 2 diabetes and dyslipidemia but no history of pheochromocytoma, paraganglioma, unexplained sudden death, or condition that may lead to thinking about VHL disease was reported.

As symptoms, the patient complained of headaches, palpitations, diaphoresis, and hot flashes since one month. She reported also asthenia and body weight loss of five kilograms in two weeks.

On examination, she had a body weight of 50 kg, a body height of 154 cm, a body mass index of 21.1 kg/m^2, a blood pressure of 200/100 mmHg without orthostatic hypotension, a regular pulse of 120 bpm, and a large abdominal café-au-lait spot (Figure 1). Thyroid, abdominal, and neurological examinations were normal.

Twenty-four-hour blood pressure monitoring confirmed the diagnosis of hypertension and the presence of peaks of 230/110 mmHg. Electrocardiogram showed a sinus tachycardia. Capillary glucose level was 2.68 g/l without ketosis.

Fundoscopy showed grade 3 hypertensive retinopathy without any other abnormalities.

The results of biological investigations are shown in Table 1.

The diagnosis of clinically suspected pheochromocytoma was confirmed by the dosage of urinary methoxylated derivatives at 5 times the upper limit of normal. In addition, the diagnosis of diabetes mellitus, dyslipidemia, and primary hyperparathyroidism were made.

The abdominal computed tomography (CT) showed two adrenal masses: the first on the right measuring 35 × 55 × 70 mm with a spontaneous density of 30 HU heterogeneously enhanced in the arterial time showing areas of necrosis with an absolute washout of 40%, the second on the left measuring 24 × 27 mm with the same characteristics as the first one (Figure 2). There were neither other localizations nor lymph nodes. Metaiodobenzylguanidine (MIBG) scintigraphy exhibited a high accumulation of the tracer in both adrenal tumors with no other localization. Cervical ultrasound and 99mTc-sestamibi scintigraphy were normal. Cardiac ultrasound was normal.

The diagnosis of multiple endocrine neoplasia type 2a was highly suspected, and the patient underwent a molecular investigation. DNA analysis did not find a RET proto-oncogene mutation. However, it showed a missense mutation c.191G > C (p.Arg64Pro) in exon 1 of the VHL gene on chromosome 3. The diagnosis of bilateral pheochromocytoma in the setting of VHL disease was established. Abdominal CT scan and craniospinal magnetic resonance imaging with contrast did not show any cysts or other tumors.

The patient was treated with an alpha blocker, prasozine, a calcium channel blocker, a beta blocker, and insulin at a daily dose of 1.4 units/kg. She underwent a bilateral adrenalectomy in two steps. The pathological examination confirmed bilateral adrenal pheochromocytomas. Replacement therapy with hydrocortisone was initiated after surgery.

The postoperative outcome was determined by the spontaneous normalization of blood pressure, blood glucose, calcium, and PTH levels. The patient remained asymptomatic with no evidence of local recurrence or distant metastasis during the 12 months of follow-up. The family screening for VHL has not been performed yet.

3. Discussion

VHL disease is a dominantly inherited familial cancer syndrome caused by a germline mutation in the VHL tumor suppressor gene and predisposing to a variety of benign and malignant neoplasms most frequently retinal, central nervous system and spinal hemangioblastomas, renal cell carcinoma (RCC), pheochromocytoma, and pancreatic tumors [6, 7]. While central nervous system and retinal hemangioblastomas are the earliest expressions of the VHL syndrome, pheochromocytoma may be the first manifestation of the disease especially in children and adolescents as it was the case of our patient [6–8]. The frequency of pheochromocytoma in VHL syndrome is about 10 to 20% [6].

Families with VHL disease have been divided into two subtypes: VHL type 1 and VHL type 2, based on the likelihood of developing a pheochromocytoma. The presence of pheochromocytoma defines types 2 VHL disease. This latter is subdivided based on the risk of developing RCC. Type 2A and 2B families have a low and high incidence of RCC, respectively, whereas VHL type 2C kinds are characterized by the development of pheochromocytoma without any other manifestations of the disease [7]. However, late onset of other attacks is possible, and a follow-up, even spaced, is required [9].

Genotype-phenotype correlations have been documented for this disorder, and specific mutations are associated with the appearance of tumors in certain organs. While most type 2 families were reported to be more likely carrying a missense mutation in the VHL gene, most type 1 families are affected by truncating or deletion mutations [10]. In our case, the presence of pheochromocytomas and the missense mutation in VHL gene suggested type 2 VHL disease. Moreover, the mutation found in our patient, p.Arg64Pro, has been described in patients with isolated pheochromocytoma, associated with RCC or with pancreatic neuroendocrine tumor [11–13]. However, our patient did not present any sign of RCC or pancreatic neuroendocrine tumor during the 12 months of follow-up. This evaluation may be early in our case as RCC and pancreatic neuroendocrine tumors in patients with VHL disease generally appear at more advanced ages (around 25–35 years) [7].

Pheochromocytoma in VHL disease tends to be seen at a younger age and is more frequently multifocal, as in our patient and may be extra-adrenal [14, 15]. In most published cases, the mean age at presentation was about 30 years, but very young cases have been described, the youngest before 5 years [7, 10]. In addition, VHL-associated pheochromocytomas are less likely to be associated with symptoms or biochemical evidence of catecholamines production compared with those occurring in patients without VHL [16, 17]. In a report of the National Institute of Health about 64 patients with VHL disease and pheochromocytomas, a total of 106 tumors were identified. Of these, 12% originated outside the adrenal gland, and 35% of the patients were asymptomatic, without hypertension or evidence of

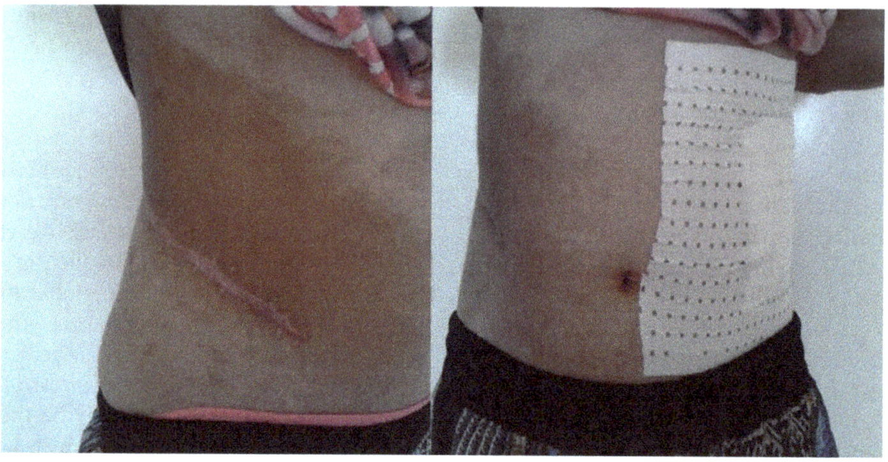

Figure 1: A large abdominal café-au-lait spot.

Table 1: Biological parameters before and after surgery.

	Before surgery	After surgery	Reference ranges
Fasting glucose level (mmol/l)	16.39	4.78	4.12–5.55
Glycated hemoglobin (%)	10.12	5.91	≤5.6
Total cholesterol (mmol/l)	11.83	5.23	3.1–5.18
Triglycerides (mmol/l)	2.43	1.21	0.57–1.71
Natremia (mmol/l)	135	140	135–145
Kalemia (mmol/l)	3.3	4	3.6–5
Creatinine (mg/L)	6	6	4–13
Calcium (mg/L)	111.2	98	88–105
Phosphate (mg/L)	44	36	27–45
Albumin (g/l)	47.22	—	35–52
Intact PTH* (μg/L)	182	54	11–62
TSH (mUI/L)	0.625	—	0.12–3.4
FT4 (ng/dl)	1.31	—	0.71–1.85
Calcitonin (ng/L)	2.70	—	<10.00
24 h-urine NMN (μg/24)	3150	570	30–600
24 h-urine MN (μg/24)	40.2	12	20–345
24 h-urine sodium (mmol/24 h)	88.5	—	
24 h-urine potassium (mmol/24 h)	60	—	
24 h-urine calcium (mg/24 h)	200	—	
24 h-proteinuria (g/24)	0.3	—	<0.3

PTH: parathormone, TSH: thyroid stimulating hormone, FT4: free-T4, NMN: normetanephrines, MN: metanephrines. *The intact PTH dosage was made using 3rd generation chemiluminescence immunoassay.

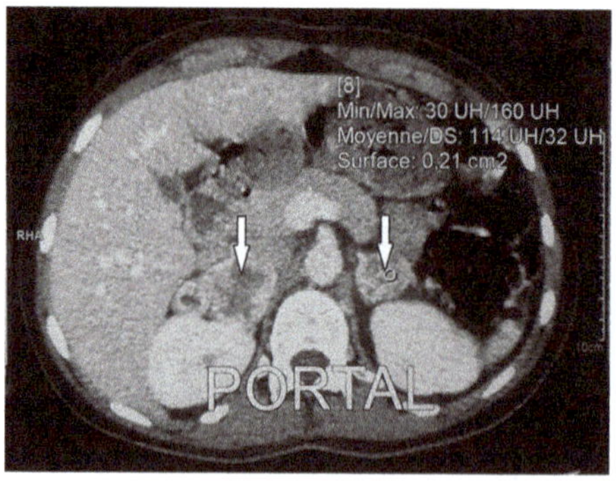

Figure 2: Abdominal computed tomography showing the two adrenal masses (two white arrows).

increased catecholamines production [15]. This was not the case of our patient who had sustained severe hypertension associated with the classic symptoms of pheochromocytoma (palpitation, sweating, and hot flashes), hypokalemia, and a secondary diabetes mellitus. In our case, as reported in the literature [16, 17], a remarkable remission of diabetes mellitus and an improvement of lipid profile were noticed after tumor removal confirming the secondary character of these two metabolic disorders. In fact, catecholamine excess affects insulin secretion, decreased glucose uptake in the peripheral tissues, and increased insulin resistance leading to impaired fasting glucose or overt diabetes mellitus [18]. Moreover, the increase in catecholamine production may be responsible for decreased inhibition of lipolysis by insulin and decreased activity of lecithin-cholesterol acyltransferase, an enzyme which breaks down free cholesterol [1].

The risk of malignancy is low. Less than 5% of all pheochromocytomas in VHL disease are malignant [7]. In our case, neither distant metastasis nor lymph nodes were found, but a long term follow-up should be carried out.

Measurement of plasma or urinary metanephrines and normetanephrines is the gold standard in diagnosing pheochromocytoma and can also provide important diagnostic information [1]. In fact, in a study carried out by Eisenhofer et al. [14], comparing the clinical and biochemical characteristics of pheochromocytomas in multiple endocrine neoplasia type 2 versus the VHL syndrome and including 19 and 30 patients with these disorders, respectively, VHL patients almost exclusively produced normetanephrines. So, a high normetanephrines-to-metanephrines ratio is expected in patients with VHL disease, as was found in our patient. Furthermore, in comparison with MEN2 tumors, VHL tumors had lower total tissue contents of catecholamines and expression of tyrosine hydroxylase (TH), the rate-limiting enzyme in catecholamine synthesis. They also had much lower expression of phenylethanolamine N-methyltransferase (PNMT, the enzyme that converts norepinephrine to epinephrine) and tissue stores of epinephrine [14]. Regarding the histopathological features, VHL-associated pheochromocytomas are characterized by a thick vascular tumor capsule and are in contrast to MEN 2 not associated with adrenal medullar hyperplasia [19].

While bilateral pheochromocytomas were reported in patients with VHL disease, the coexistence of primary hyperparathyroidism as in our case is not a common condition [5]. Hypercalcemia associated with pheochromocytoma has been documented and is thought to be caused by several mechanisms. First, elevated catecholamines can activate the PTH receptor resulting in catecholamine-induced osteoclastic bone resorption, but in contrast to our case, the PTH level is not elevated [20]. Secondly, hypercalcemia can be due to the production of PTH-related peptide (PTH-rp) by the tumor which was doubtless not the case in our patient as the level of intact PTH was elevated [21]. Furthermore, intact PTH in our case was quantified using a 3rd generation chemiluminescence immunoassay which does not recognize PTH-rp.

Third, parathyroid adenoma can be a part of multiple endocrine neoplasia that was, however, rarely reported in VHL disease [5]. The negativity of the topographic investigations and the spontaneous normalization of intact PTH after surgical treatment are against this hypothesis. Finally, although the exact physiopathological mechanism is not clear, the fact that both serum calcium and PTH levels were elevated before surgery and became normal after the removal of the pheochromocytomas strongly suggests that the tumor itself was secreting PTH or a substance that stimulates excessive PTH secretion by the parathyroid glands. Only few cases of ectopic hormonal secretion by pheochromocytoma such as adrenocorticotropic hormone (ACTH), calcitonin, parathyroid hormone (PTH), vasoactive intestinal peptide (VIP), and growth hormone-releasing hormone (GHRH) were reported [22, 23]. Unfortunately, immunohistochemistry assay for PTH in the tumor tissue was not available to clarify this question in our case.

4. Conclusion

This report highlights the rare case of ectopic intact PTH secretion by a bilateral pheochromocytoma in an adolescent girl with VHL disease. We consider that controlling calcium and PTH after adrenalectomy is useful if the topographic assessment of primary hyperparathyroidism is negative.

To the best of our knowledge, our patient is the second youngest reported childhood VHL case in the literature, presenting with a bilateral pheochromocytoma secreting ectopic intact PTH. Genetic testing and a meticulous follow-up are necessary for the diagnosis of the associated comorbidities in VHL disease.

Acknowledgments

The authors thank Professor Anne Barlier (Laboratory of Molecular Biology, Hospital La Conception, Marseille, France) for her help in molecular study.

References

[1] J. W. M. Lenders, Q.-Y. Duh, G. Eisenhofer et al., "Pheochromocytoma and paraganglioma: an endocrine society clinical practice guideline," *The Journal of Clinical Endocrinology & Metabolism*, vol. 99, no. 6, pp. 1915–1942, 2014.

[2] E. Sbardella, T. Cranston, A. M. Isidori et al., "Routine genetic screening with a multi-gene panel in patients with pheochromocytomas," *Endocrine*, vol. 59, no. 1, pp. 175–182, 2018.

[3] S. G. Waguespack, T. Rich, E. Grubbs et al., "A current review of the etiology, diagnosis, and treatment of pediatric pheochromocytoma and paraganglioma," *The Journal of Clinical Endocrinology & Metabolism*, vol. 95, no. 5, pp. 2023–2037, 2010.

[4] M. Barontini, G. Levin, and G. Sanso, "Characteristics of pheochromocytoma in a 4- to 20-year-old population," *Annals of the New York Academy of Sciences*, vol. 1073, no. 1, pp. 30–37, 2006.

[5] T. Arao, Y. Okada, T. Tanikawa et al., "A case of von Hippel-Lindau disease with bilateral pheochromocytoma, renal cell carcinoma, pelvic tumor, spinal hemangioblastoma and primary hyperparathyroidism," *Endocrine Journal*, vol. 49, no. 2, pp. 181–188, 2002.

[6] A. N. A. V. D. Horst-Schrivers, W. J. Sluiter, R. C. Kruizinga et al., "The incidence of consecutive manifestations in Von Hippel-Lindau disease," *Familial Cancer*, vol. 18, no. 3, pp. 369–376, 2019.

[7] R. R. Lonser, G. M. Glenn, M. Walther et al., "von Hippel-Lindau disease," *The Lancet*, vol. 361, no. 9374, pp. 2059–2067, 2003.

[8] A. D. Çakır, H. Turan, A. Aykut, A. Durmaz, O. Ercan, and O. Evliyaoğlu, "Two childhood pheochromocytoma cases due to von Hippel-Lindau disease, one associated with pancreatic neuroendocrine tumor: a very rare manifestation," *Journal of Clinical Research in Pediatric Endocrinology*, vol. 10, no. 2, pp. 179–182, 2018.

[9] S. P. Rednam, A. Erez, H. Druker et al., "Von hippel-lindau and hereditary pheochromocytoma/paraganglioma syndromes: clinical features, genetics, and surveillance recommendations in childhood," *Clinical Cancer Research*, vol. 23, no. 12, pp. e68–e75, 2017 15.

[10] G. F. C. Fagundes, J. Petenuci, D. M. Lourenco et al., "New insights into pheochromocytoma surveillance of young patients with VHL missense mutations," *Journal of the Endocrine Society*, vol. 3, no. 9, pp. 1682–1692, 2019.

[11] F. Hes, R. V. D. Luijt, A. Janssen et al., "Frequency of Von Hippel-Lindau germline mutations in classic and non-classic Von Hippel-Lindau disease identified by DNA sequencing, Southern blot analysis and multiplex ligation-dependent probe amplification," *Clinical Genetics*, vol. 72, no. 2, pp. 122–129, 2007.

[12] T. Krauss, A. M. Ferrara, T. P. Links et al., "Preventive medicine of von Hippel-Lindau disease-associated pancreatic neuroendocrine tumors," *Endocrine-Related Cancer*, vol. 25, no. 9, pp. 783–793, 2018.

[13] E. Wittström, M. Nordling, and S. Andréasson, "Genotype-phenotype correlations, and retinal function and structure in von Hippel-Lindau disease," *Ophthalmic Genetics*, vol. 35, no. 2, pp. 91–106, 2014.

[14] G. Eisenhofer, M. M. Walther, T.-T. Huynh et al., "Pheochromocytomas in von Hippel-Lindau syndrome and multiple endocrine neoplasia type 2 display distinct biochemical and clinical phenotypes," *The Journal of Clinical Endocrinology & Metabolism*, vol. 86, no. 5, pp. 1999–2008, 2001.

[15] M. M. Walther, R. Reiter, H. R. Keiser et al., "Clinical and genetic characterization of pheochromocytoma in von Hippel-Lindau families: comparison with sporadic pheochromocytoma gives insight into natural history of pheochromocytoma," *Journal of Urology*, vol. 162, no. 3, pp. 659–664, 1999.

[16] J. Cha, M. Khurram, L. Gellert, P. Epstein, N. Baregamian, and C. Hendrickson, "Case of reversible diabetes mellitus in the setting of benign Pheochromocytoma," *Journal of Clinical and Translational Endocrinology: Case Reports*, vol. 10, pp. 1–3, 2018.

[17] M. L. Good, P. Malekzadeh, S. M. Ruff et al., "Surgical resection of pheochromocytomas and paragangliomes is associated with lower cholesterol levels," *World Journal of Surgery*, vol. 44, no. 2, pp. 552–560, 2020.

[18] B. Mesmar, S. Poola-Kella, and R. Malek, "The physiology behind diabetes mellitus in patients with pheochromocytoma: a review of the literature," *Endocrine Practice*, vol. 23, no. 8, pp. 999–1005, 2017.

[19] O. Mete, A. S. Tischler, R. D. Krijger et al., "Protocol for the examination of specimens from patients with pheochromocytomas and extra-adrenal paragangliomas," *Archives of Pathology & Laboratory Medicine*, vol. 138, no. 2, pp. 182–188, 2014.

[20] N. O. Atuk, T. McDonald, T. Wood et al., "Familial Pheochromocytoma, Hypercalcemia, and von Hippel-Lindau Disease: a ten year study of a large family," *Medicine*, vol. 58, no. 3, pp. 209–218, 1979.

[21] K. Takeda, N. Hara, M. Kawaguchi, T. Nishiyama, and K. Takahashi, "Parathyroid hormone-related peptide-producing non-familial pheochromocytoma in a child," *International Journal of Urology*, vol. 17, no. 7, pp. 673–676, 2010.

[22] J. Kirkby-Bott, L. Brunaud, M. Mathonet et al., "Ectopic hormone-secreting pheochromocytoma: a francophone observational study," *World Journal of Surgery*, vol. 36, no. 6, pp. 1382–1388, 2012.

[23] L. V. Neto, G. F. Taboada, L. L. Corrêa et al., "Acromegaly secondary to growth hormone-releasing hormone secreted by an incidentally discovered pheochromocytoma," *Endocrine Pathology*, vol. 18, no. 1, pp. 46–52, 2007.

26

Genotyping of *ABCC8*, *KCNJ11* and *HADH* in Iranian Infants with Congenital Hyperinsulinism

Somayyeh Hashemian,[1] Reza Jafarzadeh Esfehani,[2] Siroos Karimdadi,[1] Nosrat Ghaemi,[1] Peyman Eshraghi,[1] Najmeh Malekzadeh Gonabadi,[3] Amirhossein Sahebkar,[4,5,6] Rahim Vakili,[1] and Mohammad Reza Abbaszadegan[7]

[1]*Department of Pediatric Diseases, Akbar Hospital, Faculty of Medicine, Mashhad University of Medical Sciences, Mashhad, Iran*
[2]*Department of Medical Genetics, Faculty of Medicine, Mashhad University of Medical Sciences, Mashhad, Iran*
[3]*Faculty of Sciences, Sistan and Baluchestan University, Zahedan, Iran*
[4]*Biotechnology Research Center, Pharmaceutical Technology Institute, Mashhad University of Medical Sciences, Mashhad, Iran*
[5]*Applied Biomedical Research Center, Mashhad University of Medical Sciences, Mashhad, Iran*
[6]*School of Pharmacy, Mashhad University of Medical Sciences, Mashhad, Iran*
[7]*Medical Genetic Research Center, Medical School, Mashhad University of Medical Sciences, Mashhad, Iran*

Correspondence should be addressed to Amirhossein Sahebkar; amir_saheb2000@yahoo.com, Rahim Vakili; vakilir@mums.ac.ir, and Mohammad Reza Abbaszadegan; abbaszadeganmr@mums.ac.ir

Academic Editor: Suat Simsek

Background. Congenital hyperinsulinism (CHI) is a heterogeneous disease with various underlying genetic causes. Among different genes considered effective in the development of CHI, *ABCC8, KCNJ11,* and *HADH* genes are among the important genes, especially in a population with a considerable rate of consanguineous marriage. Mutational analysis of these genes guides clinicians to better treatment and prediction of prognosis for this rare disease. The present study aimed to evaluate genetic variants in *ABCC8, KCNJ11,* and *HADH* genes as causative genes for CHI in the Iranian population. *Methods.* The present case series took place in Mashhad, Iran, within 11 years. Every child who had a clinical phenotype and confirmatory biochemical tests of CHI enrolled in this study. Variants in *ABCC8, KCNJ11,* and *HADH* genes were analyzed by the polymerase chain reaction and sequencing in our patients. *Results.* Among 20 pediatric patients, 16 of them had variants in *ABCC8, KCNJ11,* and *HADH* genes. The mean age of genetic diagnosis was 18.6 days. A homozygous missense (c.2041-21G > *A*) mutation in the *ABCC8* gene was seen in three infants. Other common variants were frameshift variants (c.3438dup) in the *ABCC8* gene and a missense variant (c.287-288delinsTG) in the *KCNJ11* gene. Most of the variants in our population were still categorized as variants of unknown significance and only 7 pathogenic variants were present. *Conclusion.* Most variants were located in the *ABCC8* gene in our population. Because most of the variants in our population are not previously reported, performing further functional studies is warranted.

1. Introduction

Congenital hyperinsulinism (CHI) is an important cause of hypoglycemia during the neonatal period and infancy. While transient hypoglycemia could be considered as a common metabolic abnormality among neonates, only 1% of these infants develop repetitive or persistent episodes of hypoglycemia [1]. During CHI, an increased level of insulin within the infant's blood decreases free glucose and results in neurological dysfunction. Repeated episodes of hypoglycemia can also result in neurological damage including mental retardation and developmental delay [2, 3]. Considering the heterogeneous nature of CHI, not all affected infants will have the same clinical presentation and histological findings.

CHI diagnostic algorithms start from the metabolic evaluation followed by molecular investigation and genotyping. Although genetic analysis is the most useful test in hyperinsulinism diagnostic approach, specific radiological modalities such as 18-F-DOPA positron emission tomography (PET) scan are also used to specify lesions [4]. Variants in some specific genes that regulate insulin secretion are considered to be responsible for the development of CHI. *ABCC8* and *KCNJ11* are among the most common genes involved in CHI [5, 6]. These genes encode subunits of ATP sensitive K^+ (KATP) channels in beta cells. *ABCC8* and *KCNJ11* gene variants impair the function of these channels resulting in disrupted membrane depolarization and dysregulated entry of calcium ion ending up in insulin release into plasma [2, 7]. Both of these genes are located on the chromosome 11p15.1 and separated by a few kilobases. *HADH* is the other well-known causative gene for CHI and variants in this gene cause enzymatic defects. *HADH* gene-inactivating variants have been described in CHI patients, resulting in decreased enzymatic activity of L-3-hydroxyacyl-CoA-dehydrogenase [8, 9]. Different types of variants including missense, nonsense, frameshift, and insertions or deletions inactivate these three genes. Determination of such variants in candidate genes is useful in various ways including choosing the best treatment approach [5]. Diazoxide is a KATP channel agonist and the first line of therapy in most of the CHI patients. Those patients who are not responsive to diazoxide may use octreotide as an alternative treatment. Surgical therapy might be used for those CHI patients who are not responsive to pharmacological therapies. Recessive variants in *ABCC8* and *KCNJ11* genes are usually considered to be less responsive to some therapies including diazoxide while compound heterozygotes may have better treatment responses [5, 10]. In contrast to recessive variants, dominant mutations will have a better treatment response [5]. Many case reports and case series have reported new variants in *ABCC8* and *KCNJ11* genes in different populations. We have previously demonstrated rare genetic variants in these two genes in an Iranian population and also demonstrated the clinical efficacy of sirolimus therapy in CHI patients [11]. The prevalence of specific variants in each population seems to be unique and genotyping for CHI has not been widely reported in the Iranian population. Other alternative diagnostic options for CHI include PET scan that helps identifying localization of focal lesions. In the present report, we explored the variants in *ABCC8* and *KCNJ11* genes as the most common genes involved in CHI. Hence, we aimed to evaluate value of genotyping in the diagnostic process, which is a crucial step in CHI treatment.

2. Material and Methods

2.1. Subjects. The present case series was approved by the Mashhad University of Medical Sciences Ethics Committee and included pediatric patients who were referred to the pediatric ward of the Imam Reza Hospital (Mashhad, Iran) from 2008 to 2017. Every neonate/child who had clinical and laboratory features of persistent hypoglycemia underwent assessment of "critical" sample in hypoglycemic state (with hypoglycemia defined as plasma glucose less than 50 mg/dL). Cases who had (1) hyperinsulinemia (defined as plasma insulin greater than 2 μU/mL), or (2) hypofatty acidemia (plasma free fatty acids less than 1.5 mmol/L), or (3) hypoketonemia (defined as plasma beta-hydroxybutyrate less than 2 mmol/L), or (4) inappropriate glycemic response to 1 mg intravenous glucagon (changes in plasma glucose greater than 40 mg/dL) were defined to have hyperinsulinism, and treatment with dextrose fluid therapy, diazoxide, and then octreotide were administered if needed [10]. All patients who had confirmed diagnosis of hyperinsulinism underwent genetic evaluation and were enrolled in the present study if their parents filled an informed consent form. Patients underwent molecular diagnosis for hyperinsulinemic hypoglycemia after genetic counseling. Because of the limitations, genetic testing was limited to the most common genes involved in CHI. Moreover, PET-CT data and surgical specimens of all patients were not available. Among the study population, only six patients were previously reported in the literature and their genotypes and clinical data are considered in the present study as well. Some of them had closed follow-up with PET scan study or surgery, which has been reported previousely (Table 1) [11].

2.2. Sampling and DNA Extraction. To perform molecular tests, venous blood (3 mL) was taken from all subjects and their parents in EDTA tubes. Genomic DNA was extracted using the salting-out method. DNA samples' quality and quantity were examined using nano-drop and gel-electrophoresis and stored in the freezer at −70°C.

2.3. PCR Sequencing. Mutational analysis of coding and flanking intronic regions of the *KCNJ11, HADH,* and *ABCC8* genes was performed using Sanger sequencing following PCR fragment amplification. Interpretation of the pathogenicity of the genetic variants in these genes was checked by VarSome software based on the American College of Medical Genetics (ACMG) instructions [12, 13]. Molecular genetic analysis was performed in the genetic lab of the Mashad University of Medical Sciences and/or genetic lab of the Exeter University in UK.

3. Results

Twenty patients were enrolled in the present study. Among this population, four infants did not have genetic variants in *ABCC8, KCNJ11,* or *HADH* gene. Among the other 16 infants, 11 patients were female and five were male. The mean age of genetic diagnosis was 18.6 days in those who had *ABCC8* or *KCNJ11* variants (except one case who had delay in the diagnosis of CHI). Most of the infants had their genetic tests few weeks after birth. The patient with the most delayed genetic diagnosis was the one who was diagnosed at the age of 3.5 years. Most of the patients had variants in the *ABCC8* gene (Table 1). A missense and aberrant splicing variants in the *ABCC8* gene (c.2041-21G > *A*) were seen in three infants. Other common variants were frameshift variants (c.3438dup) in the *ABCC8* gene and a missense variant (c.287-288delinsTG) in the *KCNJ11* gene. According

TABLE 1: Genotypes and pathogenicity prediction by using online prediction tools and the clinical significance according to Varsome.

Gene	Gender	Birth weight (gr)	Symptom onset	BS-INS at diagnosis	molecular diagnosis	Variant	Zygosity	GnomAD allele frequency	Iranome allele frequency	Clinical significance (varsome.com)	Family history	Surgery	Response to Diazoxide	Clinical Comments (patients did not response to diazoxide underwent surgery or other drugs)
ABCC8	F	4200	4D	27–47	1M	c.331G>A p.Gly111Arg	Hom^	0.000008	—	Pathogenic	—	50D	—	Received diazoxide and octreotide before surgery and sirolimus for 3 months after surgery #
	F	2600	1D	34–63	2.5M	c.2809C>T p.Leu937=	Hom^	—	—	Pathogenic	—	30D	—	Received diazoxide and sirolimus after surgery # histologic features: diffused islet hyperplasia
	F	4350	3D	22–53	1M	c.1671+1G>A	Hom^	—	—	Pathogenic	—	57D	—	—
	F	3400	3D	20–57	3M,6D						+~	—	+	Received octreotide plus diazoxide in some weeks infancy,continued with diazoxide
	M	4000	2D	25–33	1M,4D	c.2041-21G>A	Hom^	0.00002	—	Likely Pathogenic	+~	2M	—	PET scan: no uptake in pancreas He died because of sepsis following the surgery
	M	4200	1D	18–27	1M						+~~	—	—	Received diazoxide plus octreotide but lost follow up
	F	3100	2D	28–69	4M	c.3438dup p.Thr1147HisfsTer48	Het (pat)*	—	—	Pathogenic	—	2M	—	—
	F	3000	4D	40–12	5M,22D	c.1109G>C p.Arg370Thr	Het (de novo)	—	—	Uncertain Significance	—	—	+	—
	F	2800	3D	25–38	6Y,9M	c.3438dup p.Thr1147HisfsTer48	Het (pat)*	—	—	Pathogenic	—	55D	—	Received insulin after surgery because of hyperglycemia
	F	4200	1D	12–28	1M,2D	c.3151dup p.Cys1051LeufsTer64	Hom^	—	—	Pathogenic	—	—	—	Received diazoxide plus octreotide but lost follow up
	M	3150	4D	32–54	1M	c.96C>G p.Asn32Lys c.2041-21G>A	Comp-Het	— 0.00002	—	Uncertain Significance Uncertain Significance	—	—	—	Received sirolimus and responded to sirolimus therapy #
	M	2300	5D	44–34.6	3.5Y	c.3446G>A p.Cys1149Ty	Hom^	—	—	Likely Pathogenic	—	3.5Y	—	Received sirolimus plus diazoxide after surgery PET scan: avid lesion in the head of pancreas histologic features: islet cell hyperplasia

Table 1: Continued.

Gene	Gender	Birth weight (gr)	Symptom onset	BS-INS at diagnosis	molecular diagnosis	Variant	Zygosity	GnomAD allele frequency	Iranome allele frequency	Clinical significance (varsome.com)	Family history	Surgery	Response to Diazoxide	Clinical Comments (patients did not response to diazoxide underwent surgery or other drugs)
KCNJ11	F	3800	3D	28–44	1M,19D	c.287-288delinsTG p.Ala96Val	Hom^	—	—	Uncertain Significance	—	2M	—	—
	F	3500	2D	36–65	2M	c.370T>A p.Ser124Thr	Hom^	—	—	Uncertain Significance	—	2M	—	Received sirulimus ,octreotide and diazoxide before surgery. Continued with low doses of diazoxide after surgery #
	F	4100	1D	28–28	22D	c.362T>G p.Phe121Cys	Hom^	—	—	Uncertain Significance	+~~	—	—	Pet Scan :a mild uptake in the head of pancreas Did not responded to diazoxide alone , continued with octreotide and sirolimus #
HADH	M	3100	15D	38–14	1M	c.706C>T p.Arg236Ter	Hom^	0.00001	—	Pathogenic	—	—	+	PET scan: Uptake in the head of pancreas .Followed by pancreatectomy with no attacks of hypoglycemia

BS: Blood sugar (mg/dl); INS: insulin (IU/ml); D: day; M: Month; Y: year; Pat: paternal; Comp-Het: Compound heterozygote. # The patient previously reported from our center. ^The mother and father are heterozygote for the variant. * The mother did not have any variant in the three genes and the father was asymptomatic and carrying the variant. ~ The patients are first cousins. ~~ The family had child with similar clinical manifestations but without genetic workups.

to the ACMG guideline, most of the genetic variants in our population were reported as variants with uncertain significance.

4. Discussion

According to the results of this study, more than half of the study population with a clinical diagnosis of CHI had variants in the *ABCC8* gene. Additionally, most of these patients had variants with uncertain significance in *ABCC8* or *KCNJ11* genes.

Recurrent or persistent hypoglycemia is the first clue for the diagnosis of CHI. The presentation of CHI usually begins during the neonatal period and some types of CHI including focal CHI can present later in life. Less than half of the children with CHI have the genetic form of this disease [7]. At least variants in nine genes have been reported to be related to CHI. Among these genes, *ABCC8* and *KCNJ11* carry most of the mutations that cause CHI and other mutations are common in specific populations. HADH gene is among the other genes that have been reported to be common in countries with considerable consanguinity including Iran [14]. Variants in both *KCNJ11* and *ABCC8* genes, which are located on chromosome 11p15.1, are characterized by defective Kir6.2 and SUR1 subunits of ATP-dependent K channels in B-cells [6]. KATP channel variants result in various degrees of dysfunction ranging from partial to complete loss of channel function in B-cells [15]. Recessive and dominant variants in both of these genes can cause CHI [7].

Many studies from around the world have evaluated the heterogeneous genotypes of CHI patients. It is noteworthy to mention that even in the same country, a wide range of variants in *ABCC8* and *KCNJ11* genes are present. As summarized in Table 1, only a small number of variants have been previously reported in the literature. Only a few studies from Iran evaluated the genotype of CHI patients. Recently, a study from Iran evaluated six patients with CHI and the only similar variants to our study were the c.96 C *G* variants in the *ABCC8* gene [14]. Alaei et al. [14] reported that one of their patients had this variant in homozygous form while our patient had this variant in compound heterozygous form. Another study from Iran evaluated 23 patients with hyperinsulinemic hypoglycemia [16]. The authors demonstrated that after screening for *ABCC8, HADH, HNF4A, KCNJ11, GLUD1*, and *GCK*, only 4 patients did not show any variant in these genes. Most of their patients had variants in the *HADH* gene and the *ABCC8* gene was the next gene with frequent variants. The only similar variants between this study and the present one are the splicing variants in the *ABCC8* gene (c.2041-21G > *A*) [16]. They reported that their female heterozygous patient had died at the age of 3 months. In our population, we reported a compound heterozygous male with this variant and three homozygous infants. The c.2041-21G > *A* variants were the most common variants in our population.

Other genetic variants were slightly similar to studies from other countries. Kapoor et al. demonstrated that among a CHI population who were referred to a children hospital in England, c.331 G > *A* variant in the *ABCC8* gene was one of the most common variants [2]. Another study from England provided the same results. Among their 53 CHI patients in a 13-year period, only the c.331 G > *A* variant was similar to our study [17]. The c.331 G > *A* variants in *ABCC8* gene were also the only similar variants between our study and a retrospective Chinese study [18].

In our studied population, only one compound heterozygous variant was found. Compound heterozygous status has been reported in other studies while Senniappan et al. have previously reported the same heterozygous variants in the Iranian population [16, 19]. Their patient was a female child who died at 3 months of age [16]. Similar to the Senniappan et al.'s study, Mohnike et al. also demonstrated a case of paternally heterozygous child with c.2041-21G > *A* variant in the *ABCC8* gene and focal CHI [20]. Their patient has undergone surgery but the outcome was not mentioned [20]. Sousa-Santos et al. reported that even patients with the same compound heterozygous variants in the *ABCC8* gene (c.3576delG and c.742 C *T*) can have different phenotypes [21]. Moreover, a combination of heterozygous variants in *ABCC8* and *KCNJ11* genes has been reported to be responsible for CHI [22].

Although genetic analysis can be applied as an important tool for diagnostic and management purposes in some patients, genotyping in our population showed that most of the variants were still categorized as variants of unknown significance (VUS) in *ABCC8* or *KCNJ11* genes. However, further genetic studies are needed to unravel molecular basis of CHI.

4.1. Limitations. In the present study, we used Sanger sequencing for the genotyping of all patients, and therefore, some other possible genetic variants including copy number variations might have been undetectable by using this technique. Moreover, all of our patients did not undergo other diagnostic workups including PET scan. Only six patients with closed follow-up have been reported previously [11]. The high cost of these imaging and other molecular techniques including using multiplex ligation-dependent probe amplification or gene panel analysis by next generation sequencing might have limited the interpretation of the results of our research in its present form. Furthermore, we did not have histological specimens of our patients. Finally, we evaluated a particular gene panel as causative genes for CHI in the Iranian population and we were not able to investigate other genes.

5. Conclusion

The present study evaluated genetic variants in *ABCC8, KCNJ11*, and *HADH* genes in 20 children. Approximately, 75% of children with CHI phenotype had variants in *ABCC8* and *KCNJ11* genes. According to the present results, c.2041-21G > *A* missense variant in the *ABCC8* gene was the most common variant in our Iranian population. Most of the variants in our population were variants with unknown significance and only seven patients had pathogenic variants.

Authors' Contributions

Somayyeh Hashemian and Reza Jafarzadeh Esfehani equally contributed as co-first authors.

Acknowledgments

The authors would like to thank Dr. Mehri Tafazoli in Sadra Lab, Mashhad, Iran, and Dr. Hanieh Yaghootkar in the University of Exeter, UK, for collecting and performing molecular genetic assessments for some of their patients. This study was financially supported by the Mashhad University of Medical Sciences, Mashhad, Iran.

References

[1] P. Goel and S. R. Choudhury, "Persistent hyperinsulinemic hypoglycemia of infancy: an overview of current concepts," *Journal of Indian Association of Pediatric Surgeons*, vol. 17, no. 3, pp. 99–103, 2012.

[2] R. R. Kapoor, S. E. Flanagan, V. B. Arya, J. P. Shield, S. Ellard, and K. Hussain, "Clinical and molecular characterisation of 300 patients with congenital hyperinsulinism," *European Journal of Endocrinology*, vol. 168, no. 4, pp. 557–564, 2013.

[3] E. C. McNay and V. E. Cotero, "Mini-review: impact of recurrent hypoglycemia on cognitive and brain function," *Physiology & Behavior*, vol. 100, no. 3, pp. 234–238, 2010.

[4] A. Casertano, A. De Matteis, E. Mozzillo et al., "Diagnosis of congenital Hyperinsulinism can occur not only in infancy but also in later age: a new flow chart from a single center experience," *Italian Journal of Pediatrics*, vol. 46, no. 1, pp. 1–7, 2020.

[5] C. James, R. R. Kapoor, D. Ismail, and K. Hussain, "The genetic basis of congenital hyperinsulinism," *Journal of Medical Genetics*, vol. 46, no. 5, pp. 289–299, 2008.

[6] S. Galcheva, H. Demirbilek, S. Al-Khawaga, and K. Hussain, "The genetic and molecular mechanisms of congenital hyperinsulinism," *Frontiers in Endocrinology*, vol. 10, p. 111, 2019.

[7] I. Banerjee, M. Salomon-Estebanez, P. Shah, J. Nicholson, K. E. Cosgrove, and M. J. Dunne, "Therapies and outcomes of congenital hyperinsulinism-induced hypoglycaemia," *Diabetic Medicine*, vol. 36, no. 1, pp. 9–21, 2019.

[8] S. Galcheva, H. Demirbilek, S. Al-Khawaga, and K. Hussain, *The Genetic and Molecular Mechanisms of Congenital Hyperinsulinism*, vol. 10, no. 111, 2019.

[9] P. T. Clayton, S. Eaton, A. Aynsley-Green et al., "Hyperinsulinism in short-chain L-3-hydroxyacyl-CoA dehydrogenase deficiency reveals the importance of β-oxidation in insulin secretion," *Journal of Clinical Investigation*, vol. 108, no. 3, pp. 457–465, 2001.

[10] B. Dekel, D. Lubin, D. Modan-Moses, J. Quint, B. Glaser, and J. Meyerovitch, "Compound heterozygosity for the common sulfonylurea receptor mutations can cause mild diazoxide-sensitive hyperinsulinism," *Clinical Pediatrics*, vol. 41, no. 3, pp. 183–186, 2002.

[11] S. Hashemian, R. Jafarzadeh Esfehani, S. Karimdadi, R. Vakili, D. Zamanfar, and A. Sahebkar, "Clinical efficacy evaluation of sirolimus in congenital hyperinsulinism," *International Journal of Endocrinology*, vol. 2020, Article ID 7250406, 6 pages, 2020.

[12] C. Kopanos, V. Tsiolkas, A. Kouris et al., "VarSome: the human genomic variant search engine," *Bioinformatics*, vol. 35, no. 11, pp. 1978–1980, 2019.

[13] S. Richards, N. Aziz, N. Aziz et al., "Standards and guidelines for the interpretation of sequence variants: a joint consensus recommendation of the American College of medical genetics and genomics and the association for molecular pathology," *Genetics in Medicine*, vol. 17, no. 5, pp. 405–423, 2015.

[14] M. R. Alaei, S. Akbaroghli, M. Keramatipour, and A. Alaei, "A case series: congenital hyperinsulinism," *International Journal of Endocrinology and Metabolism*, vol. 14, no. 4, Article ID e37311, 2016.

[15] F.-F. Yan, Y.-W. Lin, C. MacMullen, A. Ganguly, C. A. Stanley, and S.-L. Shyng, "Congenital hyperinsulinism associated ABCC8 mutations that cause defective trafficking of ATP-sensitive K+ channels: identification and rescue," *Diabetes*, vol. 56, no. 9, pp. 2339–2348, 2007.

[16] S. Senniappan, A. Sadeghizadeh, S. E. Flanagan et al., "Genotype and phenotype correlations in Iranian patients with hyperinsulinaemic hypoglycaemia," *BMC Research Notes*, vol. 8, p. 350, 2015.

[17] V. B. Arya, M. Guemes, A. Nessa et al., "Clinical and histological heterogeneity of congenital hyperinsulinism due to paternally inherited heterozygous ABCC8/KCNJ11 mutations," *European Journal of Endocrinology*, vol. 171, no. 6, pp. 685–695, 2014.

[18] W.-Y. Wang, Y. Sun, W.-T. Zhao et al., "Congenital hyperinsulinism in China: a review of Chinese literature over the past 15 years," *Journal of Clinical Research in Pediatric Endocrinology*, vol. 9, no. 3, pp. 194–201, 2017.

[19] B. H. Lee, J. Lee, J.-M. Kim et al., "Three novel pathogenic mutations in KATP channel genes and somatic imprinting alterations of the 11p15 region in pancreatic tissue in patients with congenital hyperinsulinism," *Hormone Research in Paediatrics*, vol. 83, no. 3, pp. 204–210, 2015.

[20] K. Mohnike, I. Wieland, W. Barthlen et al., "Clinical and genetic evaluation of patients with KATPChannel mutations from the German registry for congenital hyperinsulinism," *Hormone Research in Paediatrics*, vol. 81, no. 3, pp. 156–168, 2014.

[21] F. Sousa-Santos, H. Simões, L. Castro-Feijóo et al., "Congenital hyperinsulinism in two siblings with ABCC8 mutation: same genotype, different phenotypes," *Archives of Endocrinology and Metabolism*, vol. 62, no. 5, pp. 560–565, 2018.

[22] K. Rozenkova, A. Nessa, B. Obermannova et al., "Could a combination of heterozygous ABCC8 and KCNJ11 mutations cause congenital hyperinsulinism?" *Journal of Pediatric Endocrinology & Metabolism: JPEM*, vol. 30, no. 12, pp. 1311–1315, 2017.

27

Unstimulated Serum Thyroglobulin Levels after Thyroidectomy and Radioiodine Therapy for Intermediate-Risk Thyroid Cancer are not Always a Reliable Marker of Lymph Node Recurrence: Case Report and a Lesson for Clinicians

Luca Foppiani ,[1] Simona Sola,[2] Manlio Cabria,[3] Gianluca Bottoni,[3] and Arnoldo Piccardo[3]

[1]*Internal Medicine, Galliera Hospital, Genoa, Italy*
[2]*Department of Pathology, Galliera Hospital, Genoa, Italy*
[3]*Nuclear Medicine, Galliera Hospital, Genoa, Italy*

Correspondence should be addressed to Luca Foppiani; luca.foppiani@galliera.it

Academic Editor: Lucy Mastrandrea

Over 50% of patients with papillary thyroid carcinoma (PTC) have cervical lymph-node metastasis on diagnosis, and up to 30% show nodal recurrence after surgery plus radioactive iodine (131I) (RAI) therapy. The combination of ultrasonography (US) and fine-needle aspiration cytology (FNAC) and the measurement of thyroglobulin (Tg) in washout fluid are cornerstones in the diagnosis of nodal metastasis. In the absence of anti-Tg antibodies, unstimulated serum thyroglobulin (Tg) levels are generally a reliable marker of recurrent disease, and 18F-FDG positron emission tomography (PET)/computed tomography (CT) plays an important role in the imaging work-up. We report the case of a 65-year-old man evaluated for a large multinodular goitre which caused compressive symptoms; the dominant nodule in the left lobe presented suspicious features on US. Thyroid function showed subclinical hypothyroidism, calcitonin was normal, serum thyroglobulin levels were low, and anti-thyroid antibodies were absent. The prevalent left nodule showed an intense uptake on 18F-FDG PET/CT but proved benign at FNAC. On the basis of the suspicious clinical and imaging features, total thyroidectomy was performed. Histology revealed a tall-cell variant of PTC with scattered expression of Tg and diffuse high expression of cytokeratin (CK) 19; RAI therapy was performed. Within 6 years of surgery, left laterocervical lymph-node recurrence was twice detected (first at levels II and III, then at levels IV and VI) by US and 18F-FDG-PET/CT and was confirmed by FNAC. Tg levels in the washout fluid proved clearly diagnostic of metastasis only in the second, larger, recurrence, whereas serum Tg levels (in the absence of anti-Tg antibodies) always remained undetectable on L-thyroxine therapy. Surgery was performed on both recurrences, and histology confirmed lymph-node metastasis of PTC. Immunohistochemical expression of Tg and CK 19 was similar to that of the primary tumour. No further relapses have occurred to date. Posttherapy (surgery and RAI) unstimulated serum Tg levels may not be a reliable marker of nodal recurrence in patients with differentiated thyroid cancer (DTC) that produces low amounts of Tg.

1. Introduction

DTC is the most common endocrine malignancy and generally has an excellent prognosis. Despite the hugely increased number of diagnoses over the last 20 years, mostly due to the detection of micro-PTC by the widespread use of neck US, cancer-related mortality has not risen accordingly. Cervical lymph node metastases are present in a significant percentage of patients with PTC (up to 50–60% or even 90% in the case of occult metastases) at the time of diagnosis [1].

The treatment paradigm for DTC consists of total thyroidectomy, followed by remnant ablation with RAI, and L-thyroxine therapy; the amount of TSH-suppression must be tailored according to the patient's category of risk [2].

Cornerstones of follow-up are neck US and the measurement of serum Tg levels, anti-Tg antibodies, and TSH levels.

During follow-up, US detects locoregional disease (i.e., thyroid bed or lymph nodes) in 7%–28% of PTC patients. The progression of cancer recurrence in these anatomical sites is generally slow, and the impact on clinical outcome is not well ascertained. 18F-FDG PET/CT is a reliable tool for the restaging of DTC patients who have undergone surgery and display increased (generally >10 ng/ml) Tg levels and negative neck US or whole-body scan (WBS) [3, 4]. Surgery is the reference treatment for locoregional disease [2].

We report the case of a man with a large multinodular goitre and low Tg levels, in whom the prevalent left thyroid nodule, which was negative on FNAC, proved to be a tall-cell variant of PTC on histopathology. Posttherapy (surgery and RAI) unstimulated serum Tg levels (in the absence of anti-Tg antibodies) always remained undetectable and therefore were not a reliable marker of the lymph-node recurrences that were detected over the years.

2. Case Report

Eight years ago, a 65-year-old man with hypertension on therapy with candesartan 16 mg/hydrochlorothiazide 12.5 mg and benign prostatic hyperplasia treated with alfuzosin started complaining discomfort in the left part of the neck where he noticed a lump. He was evaluated by his general practitioner who palpated a large, hard left thyroid nodule and referred the patient to the thyroid out-patient clinic of our hospital. The patient reported no family history of thyroid disease or cancer. US revealed a multinodular goitre with a prevalent 4 cm hypoechoic nodule with taller-than-wide shape in the mid-lower part of left thyroid lobe which was deemed at high risk for malignancy (European Thyroid Imaging and Reporting Data System (EU-TIRADS) 5) (Figure 1(a)); no pathological lymph nodes were detected. FT4 levels were in the lower normal range: 1 ng/dl (n.v. 1.1–1.7), whereas TSH levels were slightly increased: 4.9 μU/ml (n.v. 0.3–4.2), and L-thyroxine therapy (up to 75 μg/day) was started. Further examinations showed normal calcitonin levels, absence of thyroid autoantibodies, and very low serum Tg levels: 1.4 ng/ml (n.v. 1.4–78). Because of the suspicious features of the left thyroid nodule, 18F-FDG PET/CT was performed, which showed intense uptake (standardized uptake value (SUV) max: 14; SUV ratio: 7.3; this latter defined as the ratio between the SUV of the nodule and that of the contralateral normal thyroid parenchyma) (Figure 1(b)). US-guided FNAC results revealed normal thyrocytes, fibrin, and histiocytes, and the nodule was classified as benign (Thyroid (Thy) 2). However, due to the clinical features, total thyroidectomy was performed. On histology, the large left thyroid nodule proved to be a tall-cell variant of PTC (pT3 pNx) which infiltrated the capsule, reached the fatty tissue, and invaded the vessels (Figure 2(a)). The tumour was deemed multifocal on the basis of the finding of another 6 mm neoplastic nodule in the right lobe. Immunohistochemistry showed scattered cytoplasmatic positivity for Tg (Figure 2(b)) and diffuse strong cytoplasmatic and membrane positivity for cytokeratin 19 (Figure 2(c)), an integral protein of the cytoskeleton of the epithelial cells which is highly expressed in PTC [5]. The thyroid tumour was classified as stage II, and the patient as being at intermediate risk of recurrence. L-thyroxine (up to 150/175 μg on alternate days) was started in order to maintain TSH levels between 0.1 and 0.5 μU/ml. Nearly two months after surgery, L-throxine was withdrawn until TSH levels >30 μU/ml, and he was treated with ablative dose of 131I therapy (3.7 GBq). The preablative Tg level was 0.3 ng/ml, and anti-Tg antibodies were negative. Posttherapy whole-body scan (WBS) was performed 2 days after the administration of 131I and did not show any uptake. Over the first three years following surgery/RAI while on suppressive L-thyroxine therapy, Tg levels were undetectable (ultrasensitive immunoassay, analytical sensitivity: 0.04 ng/ml), and anti-Tg antibodies were absent. During the fourth year of follow-up, neck US revealed a few (diameter 1.0–1.5 cm) oval laterocervical lymph nodes, with no visible hilum and focal hyperechogenicity at levels III and IV (Figures 3(a) and 3(b)), which aroused the suspicion of recurrence; serum Tg levels on L-thyroxine therapy and anti-Tg antibodies remained undetectable. An rh-TSH stimulation test (0.9 mg intramuscularly on two consecutive days) did not result in increase in Tg levels (baseline <0.04 ng/ml, +72 h: 0.3 ng/ml). FNAC was performed on the prevalent lymph node, together with the assay of Tg levels in 1 ml of normal saline washout fluid. Washout Tg levels proved "negative" (0.24 ng/ml); by contrast, FNAC showed epithelial cells with irregular nuclei and nuclear pseudoinclusions suggestive of PTC metastasis (Figure 4). Left laterocervical lymphadenectomy (levels II, III, and IV) was performed, and 21 lymph nodes (8 of levels II and 13 of levels III and IV) were removed; on histopathology, one of the level III nodes and one of the level IV nodes showed PTC metastasis (maximum diameter 1.5 cm) (Figure 5(a)) and had scattered positivity for Tg (Figure 5(b)) and diffuse strong positivity for CK 19 (Figure 5(c)). The next year following lymphadenectomy, neck US was unremarkable, and serum Tg levels remained undetectable. Nevertheless, two years after the first recurrence, a left supraclavicular lymph node was palpated. US confirmed a 20 mm pathological (hypoechoic, with irregular shape, no visible hilum, and focal hyperechogenicity) lymph node in the left supraclavicular region (level IV) (Figure 6(a)) and a smaller one (10 mm) with the same features in the paratracheal region (level VI). 18F-FDG PET/CT showed significant tracer uptake (SUV max: 20.7) by left supraclavicular lymph node and, to a lesser extent (SUV max: 11), by left paratracheal lymph node (Figure 6(b)). FNAC of the left larger supraclavicular lymph node showed epithelial cells with enlarged and hyperchromatic nuclei that were diagnostic of metastatic PTC; this diagnosis was strengthened by the finding of increased Tg levels: 220 ng/ml in the washout fluid, in the presence of undetectable serum Tg levels. Lymphadenectomy (level IV and level VI) was performed, and histology confirmed the cytological findings. Imaging procedures six months (neck US and 18F-FDG PET/CT) and one year later (neck US) were negative, and unstimulated serum Tg was undetectable. The patient is healthy, and imaging and hormonal follow-up have been scheduled.

3. Discussion

More than half of patients with PTC have cervical lymphatic spread at the time of diagnosis [1, 6]. In the follow-up after surgery and RAI (when performed), US is the cornerstone technique for evaluating locoregional recurrence (thyroid

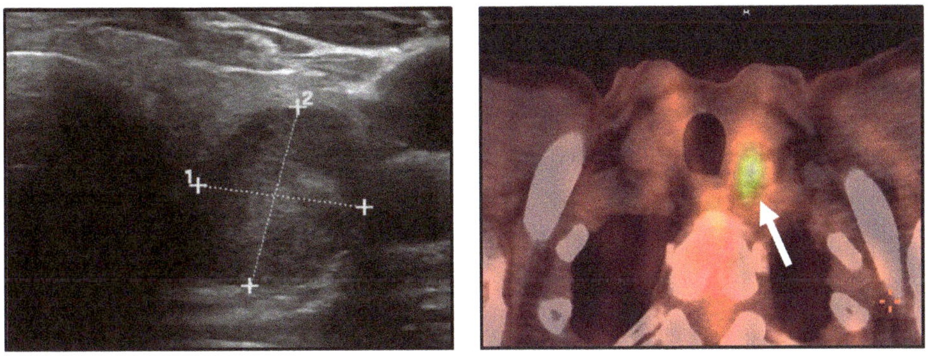

(a) (b)

Figure 1: Ultrasonographic suspicious features of the large solid hypoechoic and taller-than-wide shape thyroid nodule located in the mid-inferior part of the left lobe (a), which showed significant tracer uptake at 18F-FDG PET/CT (arrow, (b)).

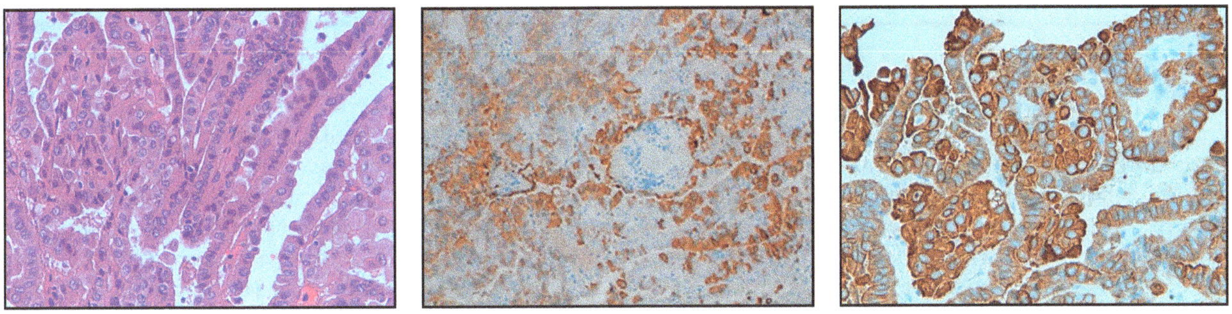

(a) (b) (c)

Figure 2: Histology after thyroidectomy showing a tall-cell variant of papillary thyroid carcinoma: papillary architecture neoplasm consisting of proliferation of elongated cells with a large eosinophilic cytoplasm, "ground glass" nuclei, and evident nuclear grooves and pseudoinclusions (haematoxylin-eosin stain, 40X, (a)). The tumour showed scattered thyroglobulin cytoplasmatic staining of different intensity (20X, (b)) and strong and diffuse CK19 cytoplasmatic staining (40X, (c)). Immunohistochemical staining was performed using specific antibodies by indirect biotin streptavidin 3, 3′-diaminobenzidine (DAB) system.

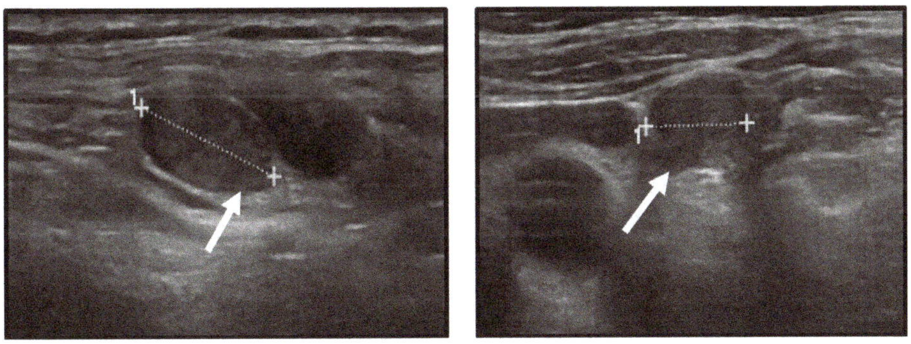

(a) (b)

Figure 3: During the fourth year of follow-up after surgery and radioactive 131I therapy, ultrasonography showed small (maximum 1.5 cm) suspicious laterocervical lymph nodes with oval shape and no visible hilum (a, b, arrows).

bed and lymph nodes), which occurs in up to 30% of patients [7]. Two-thirds of patients show tumour recurrence within 5 years after surgery [8]. The evaluation of Tg levels in the washout fluid from FNA, the values of which correlate

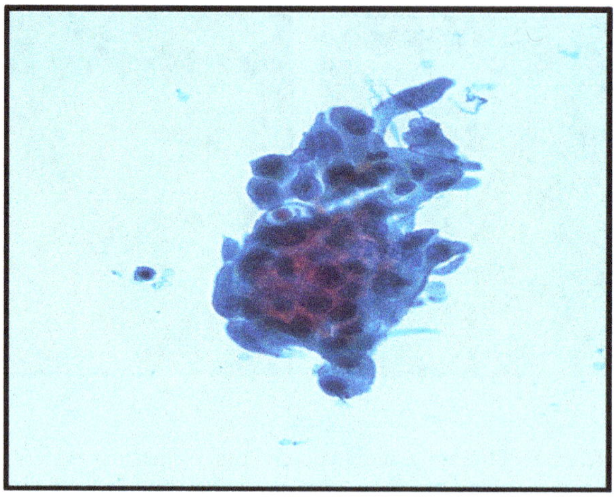

Figure 4: Fine needle aspiration cytology of the left laterocervical lymph-node recurrence detected during the fourth year of follow-up after surgery and radioactive 131I therapy, which showed three-dimensional papillary flaps of medium size cells with pseudoinclusions and grooves which proved compatible with metastasis of papillary thyroid carcinoma (ThinPrep method, Papanicolaou stain, 40X).

positively with TSH levels and serum Tg levels, improves the accuracy of the diagnosis of nodal metastasis from PTC when used in combination with FNAC [9].

The ATA [3] staging system enables the initial risk of recurrence to be restratified as a function of response to therapies (surgery and RAI if performed). The rate of recurrence may be downgraded to as low as 2% in intermediate-risk PTC patients, when the initial treatments yield an excellent response to therapy (i.e., no evidence of structural disease, unstimulated Tg < 0.2 ng/ml, or stimulated Tg < 1 ng/ml) [10]. Using these criteria, our patient, who had been categorized as being at intermediate risk of recurrence at the time of diagnosis, was subsequently downgraded to a low risk of recurrence.

US displays good sensitivity but has some limitations, such as suboptimal specificity and operator dependency [1]. In our patient, the combination of clinical examination and suspicious ultrasound features prompted us to perform 18F-FDG PET/CT in order to stratify cancer risk, which is about 35% in the case of 18F-FDG-avid nodules, while a nodule with absent/low uptake is deemed at low risk for malignancy [4].

A recent study evaluated the predictivity tests of dedicated 18F-FDG PET/CT in ninety-three patients having a thyroid nodule larger than 1 cm with US assessment of intermediate risk (EUTIRADS 4, $n = 48$) or high risk (EUTIRADS 5, $n = 45$). All patients underwent thyroidectomy, and histology was the gold standard. Overall, 18F-FDG PET/CT sensitivity and specificity were 94% and 53%, respectively. With regards to EUTIRADS 5 thyroid nodules, sensitivity, specificity, positive predictive value, and negative predictive value of 18F-FDG PET/TC were 96%, 61%, 79%, and 92%, respectively [11].

The risk of nodal recurrence is related to the presence of nodal disease at the time of initial surgery and to the number and ratio (number of positive nodes/number of nodes removed) of lymph nodes [12].

As no lymph node dissection was performed during the initial surgery, we do not know the status of nodal disease at the time of thyroidectomy.

In our patient, US detected lymph nodes suspicious for recurrences in the lateral compartment (levels III, IV, and VI) during follow-up. These locations are the most common sites of nodal spread in PTC [1]. In addition to general criteria for the detection of suspicious/tumourous lymph node, peculiar US features of lymph node metastasis from DTC include focal/diffuse hyperechogenicity, as was ascertained in our patient [13].

The two nodal recurrences, which occurred over the years, were confirmed by FNAC, which showed metastasis from PTC. US-guided FNAC of the cervical lymph nodes has high specificity; however, it yields 5–20% of inadequate results and up to 50% of false-negative results in the presence of small lymph nodes and cystic metastases [6, 14].

Serum Tg levels reflect the tumour burden or the capacity of the tumour to synthesize and secrete Tg and are used to detect recurrence of thyroid cancer after primary treatment (surgery and RAI when performed). The greatest accuracy on the basal ultrasensitive Tg assay is achieved by setting a cut-off of 0.2–0.3 ng/ml [2].

In our patient, presurgical serum Tg levels (in the absence of anti-Tg antibodies) were low and remained persistently undetectable, irrespective of two lymph node recurrences of different sizes over the years. We hypothesize that these findings were not related to reduced Tg synthesis, since no evidence of poor differentiation of the primary thyroid tumour or dedifferentiation of lymph node recurrences was reported by the pathologist. The production by the tumour of a Tg variant which was not recognized by the immunoassay cannot be excluded but seems unlikely [15].

While serum Tg is often able to indicate recurrent PTC even before the disease becomes structurally detectable on US levels, Rosario and colleagues demonstrated that serum Tg may not increase in patients with small (<1 cm) lymph node recurrence

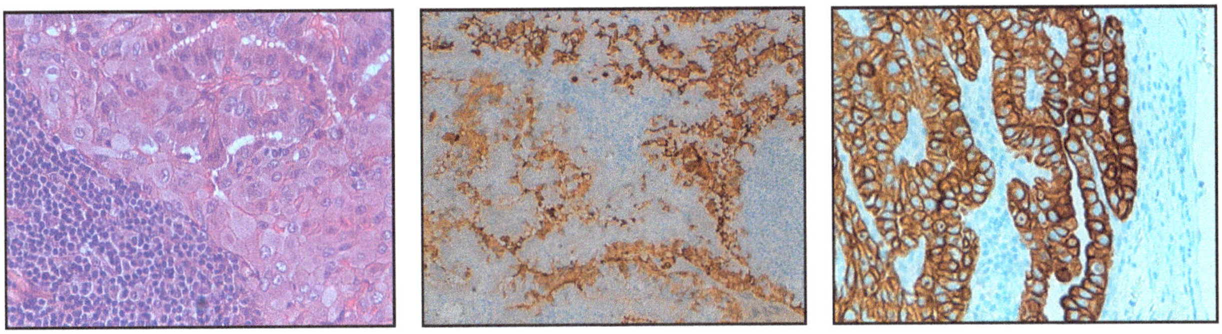

(a) (b) (c)

FIGURE 5: Histology of lymph node metastasis (first recurrence detected during the fourth year of follow-up after surgery and radioactive 131I therapy) of tall-cell variant of papillary thyroid carcinoma: proliferation of cells with a large eosinophilic cytoplasm, "ground glass" nuclei, and evident nuclear grooves and pseudoinclusions (left side) and residual patrimonial lymphoid tissue (right side) (haematoxylin-eosin stain, 40X, (a)). The neoplastic thyroid cells showed scattered thyroglobulin cytoplasmatic staining of different intensity (40X, (b)) and diffuse strong cytoplasmatic CK19 staining (40X, (c)). Immunohistochemical staining was performed using specific antibodies by indirect biotin streptavidin 3, 3′-diaminobenzidine (DAB) system.

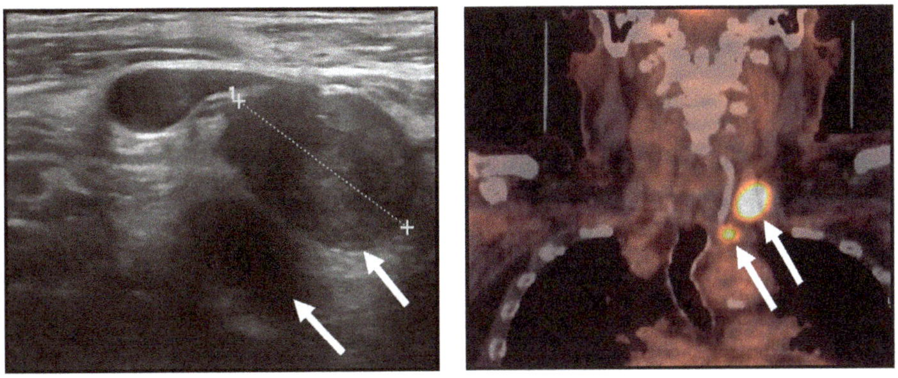

(a) (b)

FIGURE 6: Ultrasonographic features of second nodal recurrences (6 years after surgery and radioactive iodine 131I therapy) of papillary thyroid carcinoma (two laterocervical metastatic hypoechoic lymph nodes, 2.2 cm and 1 cm, respectively) with irregular shape, no visible hilum and focal hyperechogenicity ((a), arrows). At 18F-FDG PET/CT, both lymph nodes showed significant tracer uptake (arrows) (the larger one: SUV max: 20.7; the smaller one: SUV max: 11) (b).

[16]. This fits well with our patient's first small nodal recurrence, but less so with the second, larger, one, in which an increase in serum Tg levels might be expected.

Overall, our findings may imply that the thyroid tumour was able to produce Tg (as shown by immunohistochemistry both in the primary tumour and in the lymph node recurrence) but had lost its functional ability to secrete it. With regards to nodal recurrences, Tg therefore remained confined within the tumoural intranodal space, and its levels in the systemic circulation subsequently remained undetectable [17]. On the rh-TSH stimulation test performed at the time of the first small recurrence, Tg showed only a minimal response vs baseline (peak <0.5 ng/ml).

In addition, patients with PTC of different histopathologic variants (included tall-cell variant) who have normal or low serum Tg (as found in our patient) before surgery may not show rising serum Tg on disease recurrence [18]. Hence, undetectable serum Tg should not be considered a reliable criterion for excluding a relatively small tumour burden in patients who have already been treated with RAI [18].

In our patient, the first laterocervical lymph-node recurrence was small (diameter 1–1.5 cm) and the very low level of Tg found in the FNA washout fluid may have been due to several factors: a procedural error, an increased clearance of Tg from plasma, loss of the immunological activity of Tg or, more likely, small amounts of Tg produced by the tumour [17]. Interference by anti-Tg antibodies in the Tg assay seems unlikely, given their absence in the serum; however, they were not measured in the FNA fluid.

A large retrospective cohort study, which evaluated Tg in the washout fluid from FNAC in 428 PTC patients by means of an ultrasensitive assay, validated 1.0 ng/ml as a cut-off value for diagnosing PTC lymph-node metastases [9], and this cut-off has been supported by a recent meta-analysis

[19]. However, a universal cut-off has not yet been established, owing to the high variability among the Tg assays used [19, 20].

In this regard, Yap et al. [14] claimed that all FNA-Tg levels ≥ functional sensitivity of the assay (0.1 ng/ml in our case) were suggestive of nodal recurrence, with a high (95%) positive predictive value; if this criterion were applied, to our patient, his washout Tg levels in the first nodal recurrence would not be strictly defined as "negative." In this setting, the marked expression of CK-19 in metastatic lymph nodes, albeit alone nonspecific for PTC [5], might strengthen the FNAC findings of recurrence and overcome the non-diagnostic result of washout Tg.

In conclusion, in the absence of anti-Tg antibodies, posttherapy unstimulated serum Tg levels may remain undetectable and hence not be a reliable marker of lymph node recurrences in DTC. This may be particularly true in DTC patients with low presurgical serum Tg levels, in whom the tumour either produces little Tg or, alternatively, has lost the capacity to secrete Tg. In these patients, US and, when appropriate, 18F-FDG PET/CT are fundamental tools for the identification of tumour recurrence.

Consent

Written informed consent was obtained from the patient for this research.

References

[1] G. H. Sakorafas, A. Koureas, I. Mpampali, D. Balalis, D. Nasikas, and S. Ganztzoulas, "Patterns of lymph node metastasis in differentiated thyroid cancer; clinical implications with particular emphasis on the emerging role of compartment-oriented lymph node dissection," *Oncology Research and Treatment*, vol. 42, no. 3, pp. 143–147, 2019.

[2] L. Lamartina, S. Leboulleux, M. Terroir, D. Hartl, and M. Schlumberger, "An update on the management of low-risk differentiated thyroid cancer," *Endocrine-Related Cancer*, vol. 26, no. 11, pp. R597–R610, 2019.

[3] B. R. Haugen, E. K. Alexander, K. C. Bible et al., "2015 American Thyroid Association management guidelines for adult patients with thyroid nodules and differentiated thyroid cancer: the American Thyroid Association Guidelines Task Force on thyroid nodules and differentiated thyroid cancer," *Thyroid*, vol. 26, no. 1, pp. 1–133, 2016.

[4] L. Giovanella, A. M. Avram, I. Iakovou et al., "EANM practice guideline/SNMMI procedure standard for RAIU and thyroid scintigraphy," *European Journal of Nuclear Medicine and Molecular Imaging*, vol. 46, no. 12, pp. 2514–2525, 2019.

[5] N. S. Abouhashem and S. M. Talaat, "Diagnostic utility of CK19 and CD56 in the differentiation of thyroid papillary carcinoma from its mimics," *Pathology - Research and Practice*, vol. 213, no. 5, pp. 509–517, 2017.

[6] J. H. Lim, D. W. Kim, J. Y. Park et al., "Ultrasonography, cytology, and thyroglobulin measurement results of cervical nodal metastasis in patients with unclear papillary thyroid carcinoma," *Frontiers in Endocrinology (Lausanne)*, vol. 10, no. 395, 2019.

[7] L. Lamartina, G. Grani, M. Biffoni et al., "Risk stratification of neck lesions detected sonographically during the follow-up of differentiated thyroid cancer," *The Journal of Clinical Endocrinology & Metabolism*, vol. 101, no. 8, pp. 3036–3044, 2016.

[8] C. Durante, T. Montesano, M. Torlontano et al., "Papillary thyroid cancer: time course of recurrences during postsurgery surveillance," *The Journal of Clinical Endocrinology & Metabolism*, vol. 98, no. 2, pp. 636–642, 2013.

[9] J. H. Moon, Y. I. Kim, J. A. Lim et al., "Thyroglobulin in washout fluid from lymph node fine-needle aspiration biopsy in papillary thyroid cancer: large-scale validation of the cutoff value to determine malignancy and evaluation of discrepant results," *The Journal of Clinical Endocrinology & Metabolism*, vol. 98, no. 3, pp. 1061–1068, 2013.

[10] R. M. Tuttle, H. Tala, J. Shah et al., "Estimating risk of recurrence in differentiated thyroid cancer after total thyroidectomy and radioactive iodine remnant ablation: using response to therapy variables to modify the initial risk estimates predicted by the new American Thyroid Association staging system," *Thyroid*, vol. 20, no. 12, pp. 1341–1349, 2010.

[11] P. Trimboli, A. Piccardo, M. Alevizaki et al., "Dedicated neck 18 F-FDG PET/CT: an additional tool for risk assessment in thyroid nodules at ultrasound intermediate risk," *Clinical Endocrinology*, vol. 90, no. 5, pp. 737–743, 2019.

[12] M. F. Bates, M. R. Lamas, R. W. Randle et al., "Back so soon? Is early recurrence of papillary thyroid cancer really just persistent disease?" *Surgery*, vol. 163, no. 1, pp. 118–123, 2018.

[13] D. W. Kim, H. J. Choo, Y. J. Lee, S. J. Jung, J. W. Eom, and T. K. Ha, "Sonographic features of cervical lymph nodes after thyroidectomy for papillary thyroid carcinoma," *Journal of Ultrasound in Medicine*, vol. 32, no. 7, pp. 1173–1180, 2013.

[14] N. S.-J. Yap, R. Maher, and D. L. Learoyd, "Any detectable thyroglobulin in lymph node biopsy washouts suggests local recurrence in differentiated thyroid cancer," *Endocrine Connections*, vol. 3, no. 4, pp. 150–155, 2014.

[15] W. Li, D. Sun, H. Ming, G. Zhang, and J. Tan, "A rare case report of very low thyroglobulin and a negative whole-body scan in a patient with a solid variant of papillary thyroid carcinoma with distant metastases," *Medicine (Baltimore)*, vol. 96, no. 7, Article ID e6086, 2017.

[16] P. W. Rosario, G. F. Mourão, and M. R. Calsolari, "Can the follow-up of patients with papillary thyroid carcinoma of low and intermediate risk and excellent response to initial therapy be simplified using second-generation thyroglobulin assays?" *Clinical Endocrinology*, vol. 85, no. 4, pp. 596–601, 2016.

[17] J. M. Han, W. B. Kim, J. H. Yim et al., "Long-term clinical outcome of differentiated thyroid cancer patients with undetectable stimulated thyroglobulin level one year after initial treatment," *Thyroid*, vol. 22, no. 8, pp. 784–790, 2012.

[18] R. T. Kloos, "Thyroid cancer recurrence in patients clinically free of disease with undetectable or very low serum thyroglobulin values," *The Journal of Clinical Endocrinology & Metabolism*, vol. 95, no. 12, pp. 5241–5248, 2010.

[19] L. Giovanella, M. Bongiovanni, and P. Trimboli, "Diagnostic value of thyroglobulin assay in cervical lymph node fine-needle aspirations for metastatic differentiated thyroid cancer," *Current Opinion in Oncology*, vol. 25, no. 1, pp. 6–13, 2013.

[20] G. Grani and A. Fumarola, "Thyroglobulin in lymph node fine-needle aspiration washout: a systematic review and meta-analysis of diagnostic accuracy," *The Journal of Clinical Endocrinology & Metabolism*, vol. 99, no. 6, pp. 1970–1982, 2014.

28

Sheehan Syndrome Presenting with Psychotic Manifestations Mimicking Schizophrenia in a Young Female: A Case Report and Review of the Literature

Nipun Lakshitha de Silva,[1] **Janith Galhenage**,[2] **Madhubhashinee Dayabandara**,[2] **and Noel Somasundaram**[1]

[1]*Diabetes and Endocrine Unit, National Hospital of Sri Lanka, Colombo 10, Sri Lanka*
[2]*University Psychiatry Unit, National Hospital of Sri Lanka, Colombo 10, Sri Lanka*

Correspondence should be addressed to Nipun Lakshitha de Silva; nipunlak@gmail.com

Academic Editor: Osamu Isozaki

Introduction. Sheehan syndrome presents with features of multiple hormone deficiencies including lactation failure and amenorrhoea as well as with features of central hypothyroidism and adrenocorticotropic hormone deficiency. Psychiatric manifestations are mostly limited to cognitive impairment. Psychotic presentations are rare and limited to case reports. *Case Presentation*. A 32-year-old female was evaluated for fearfulness and delusions for one year. She had persecutory and bizarre delusions, delusion of thought possession, and elementary auditory hallucinations. These began four months after the birth of her third child. The delivery had been complicated with postpartum haemorrhage. Her symptoms caused the functional decline and progressively worsened, resulting in suicidal ideation. Cognitive assessment revealed mild impairment in attention. Further inquiry revealed lethargy, constipation, cold intolerance, and lactation failure. She was slow, having dry skin, puffy face, and bradycardia with a blood pressure of 80/60 mmHg (supine) and 70/50 mmHg (standing). She had hyponatraemia, elevated creatine phosphokinase, low thyroxine, prolactin, FSH, LH, and IGF-1. She had poor cortisol and growth hormone response to the insulin tolerance test. MRI-pituitary showed empty sella. A diagnosis of Sheehan syndrome was made. Her symptoms improved completely after the initiation of levothyroxine and hydrocortisone. *Conclusions*. Sheehan syndrome can present with psychotic symptoms mimicking schizophrenia with variable involvement of cognition. Detailed reporting of these patients would enhance better characterization of the clinical presentation and risk profile of these patients.

1. Introduction

Sheehan syndrome is postpartum hypopituitarism caused by necrosis of the pituitary gland. This is thought to be a result of hypotension caused by postpartum haemorrhage. The risk is higher in those with predisposing factors of the enlarged pituitary gland during pregnancy, small sella turcica, vasospasm, and a thrombophilic state [1]. The prevalence of Sheehan syndrome was high in an era of poor obstetric care. There has been a marked reduction due to improved obstetric care especially in the developed world.

The presentation of Sheehan syndrome can vary; some patients are diagnosed soon after childbirth while delayed diagnosis even up to 20 years has been reported [1, 2]. Common manifestations include failure of lactation, amenorrhoea, and asthenia [2–4]. Psychiatric manifestations are less common and are mostly limited to cognitive impairment [2]. Psychotic manifestations with preserved cognitive functions are limited to few case reports. We report a patient who had Sheehan syndrome presenting one year after delivery with psychotic symptoms that were similar to schizophrenia.

2. Case Presentation

A 32-year-old Sri Lankan female presented to the psychiatry services with fearfulness, undue suspicion, and hearing voices. She believed that somebody has implanted a camera inside her head to record her thoughts. She was irritable. In addition, she had begun to neglect her functions as a housewife and a mother. These symptoms were present for one year and had worsened over the previous two weeks.

Over the previous year, she was also experiencing lethargy, constipation, and cold intolerance. Symptom review was negative for postural dizziness, polyuria, polydipsia, headache, and visual disturbances.

She was a mother of three children; the youngest was one year and four months old. Her last pregnancy was complicated with gestational diabetes and pregnancy-induced hypertension. Childbirth by vaginal delivery was complicated with heavy bleeding. She experienced inability to lactate her child. An intrauterine contraceptive device was inserted six weeks postpartum. She did not experience any menstrual bleeding since childbirth.

She had no other comorbidities. Assessment of personality indicated that she was a well-adjusted person prior to the onset of illness without any maladaptive traits. This was her first presentation to a psychiatry service.

She was from a poor socioeconomic setting having poor family support, and her husband was alcohol dependent. This has led to a delay in seeking healthcare advice.

She was average built with a weight of 49 kg and a height of 151 cm. She was slow in response with dry skin of normal complexion and facial puffiness. There was no goitre. She had bradycardia (heart rate of 56/min) with a supine blood pressure of 80/60 mmHg and a standing blood pressure of 70/50 mmHg. The rest of the physical examination was normal.

Her mental state examination revealed an anxious mood with fleeting passive suicidal ideas. She had persecutory delusions involving an unidentified persecutor and a bizarre delusion that an external object has been implanted in her head to monitor her mental activity. She also had delusions of thought possession and elementary auditory hallucinations. Her delusions and hallucinations were observed to be transient. They were changing throughout the hospital stay. Initial persecutory delusions disappeared and the content of bizarre delusions changed in subsequent mental state examinations.

Her orientation with regard to time, day, month, place, and city was normal. Attention and concentration tested with digit span were impaired, and she could repeat only four digits forward (normal is 5 to 9 digits) and three in reverse (normal being 6 or more). Her short-term and long-term memory as well as other aspects of extended cognitive assessment was normal.

Initial laboratory investigations showed hyponatraemia, elevated creatine phosphokinase, and low free T4 with normal thyroid-stimulating hormone (TSH) (Table 1). A provisional diagnosis of organic delusional disorder (schizophrenia-like) was made and risperidone 1 mg daily was started.

Table 1: Summary of laboratory investigations.

Investigation	Result	Reference range
Haemoglobin (g/dL)	11.8	11–16
Serum creatinine (mg/dL)	0.84	0.5–1.1
Sodium (mmol/L)	122	135–145
Potassium (mmol/L)	3.8	3.5–5.1
Aspartate transaminase (U/L)	56	<40
Alanine transaminase (U/L)	22	<40
Creatine phosphokinase (U/L)	1381	26–192
Fasting blood glucose (mg/dL)	96	<100
Thyroid-stimulating hormone (mIU/l)	3.428	0.5–4.7
Free T4 (ng/dl)	<0.1	0.89–1.76
9am cortisol (nmol/l)	221	118–618
Prolactin (mIU/l)	26.94	59–619
Follicle-stimulating hormone (IU/L)	2.88	
Luteinizing hormone (IU/L)	0.94	
Insulin-like growth factor (ng/ml)	8	177–382
Insulin tolerance test		
Lowest random blood glucose (mg/dL)	13.9	<40
Highest growth hormone (μg/L)	<0.1	>7
Highest cortisol (nmol/L)	88.1	>550

She was referred to the endocrinology team for further evaluation and management. With a 9am cortisol of 221 nmol/L, she was started on levothyroxine under the cover of hydrocortisone. After normalizing free T4, she underwent an insulin tolerance test withholding hydrocortisone for 24 hours (Table 1). A diagnosis of panhypopituitarism was made. MRI of the pituitary gland showed a normal-sized sella turcica filled with cerebrospinal fluid (CSF). There was no pituitary gland, suggesting empty sella. The pituitary stalk was slightly deviated to the right extending up to the sellar floor showing normal signal and diameter (Figure 1).

Levothyroxine and hydrocortisone were continued. Symptoms, including psychotic symptoms and hyponatraemia, improved remarkably within two weeks and risperidone was discontinued. Oestrogen and progesterone replacement therapy was initiated later. The patient is currently satisfied with her clinical outcome.

3. Discussion

Our patient presented to a psychiatry service with disturbing delusions and hallucinations with fairly intact cognition. The presentation would usually fit into a schizophrenia-like disorder.

However, detailed history and clinical examination suggested an organic pathology with the presence of hypothyroid features. Early endocrine referral led to the confirmation of diagnosis and initiation of specific treatment leading to marked clinical improvement. The diagnosis of Sheehan syndrome was made based on the temporal relationship of symptoms to childbirth, history suggestive of postpartum haemorrhage, characteristic anterior pituitary

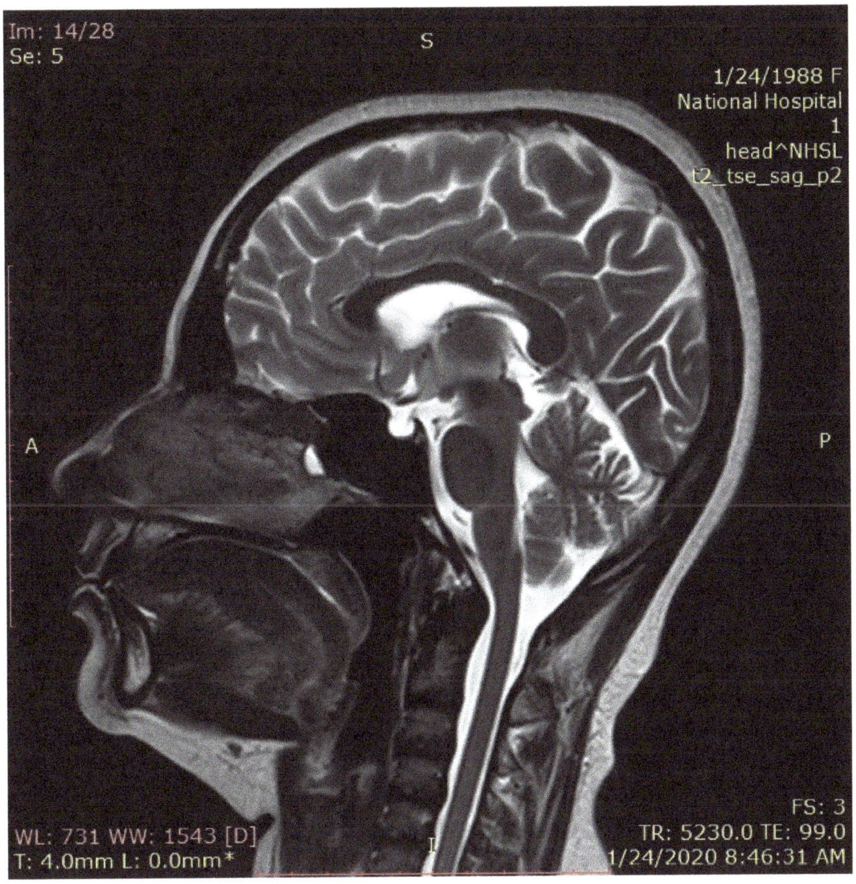

FIGURE 1: MRI-pituitary of the patient showing empty sella. T2 sagittal section of MRI-sellar region shows normal-sized pituitary fossa filled with CSF. The pituitary gland is not seen in the sella.

dysfunction, and imaging evidence of empty sella. Low prolactin leading to lactation failure noted in our patient is characteristically seen in Sheehan syndrome. Most of the other causes of hypopituitarism including lymphocytic hypophysitis cause normal or elevated prolactin [1]. This further strengthened our clinical diagnosis.

The delusions of thought possession and the bizarre delusion initially suggested the possibility of schizophrenia. Organic psychosis can present with persecutory delusions and even first rank symptoms or thought disorder. Patients with intact cognitive function are known to present with complex delusions such as in this case. A strong suspicion of organic psychosis was aroused due to the changing nature of her symptoms coupled with physical signs [5].

Psychotic manifestations in patients with Sheehan syndrome are limited to several case reports. We performed a systematic literature search in PubMed and Google Scholar to identify case reports on psychotic manifestations in Sheehan syndrome. Further reports were recognized using cross-referencing of the initial articles. Articles which did not provide full text in English were excluded. Thirteen full-text articles were reviewed for eligibility. One reported a patient without clear psychotic manifestations [6]. Another report described a patient with delirium precipitated with sepsis and severe hyponatraemia. There were no psychiatric manifestations until the acute insult [7]. Another patient misdiagnosed with depressive disorder did not have any psychotic manifestations [8]. Though one report described protracted delirium as a result of Sheehan syndrome, the original presentation was with seizures and cerebral oedema associated with hyponatraemia and hypoglycaemia [9].

After excluding the above cases, nine reports of women with Sheehan syndrome presenting with psychotic manifestations were reviewed in detail [10–18]. Clinical details of these patients are summarised in Table 2. In one patient, details of lactation were not reported. All the other patients had evidence of lactation failure and secondary amenorrhoea. Secondary hypothyroidism and ACTH deficiency were noted in all the patients. None had diabetes insipidus. Growth hormone deficiency was not tested in any of the patients. All patients except one patient had a clear history of postpartum haemorrhage. Except the first three patients reported before 1980, all the other patients had imaging evidence of empty sella. None of the patients had prior psychiatric comorbidities.

The interval between childbirth and onset of psychiatric manifestations ranged from few days [10, 14, 15] to about three decades. There seems to be a bimodal distribution. Few patients present acutely and others develop psychiatric symptoms more than few years later. In patients who developed psychiatric manifestations later, most had developed lactation failure and amenorrhoea soon after childbirth,

Table 2: Summary of case reports describing patients presenting with psychotic manifestations due to Sheehan syndrome.

Author, year	Age at presentation	Interval between psychiatric manifestations and childbirth	Psychiatric manifestations	Hormone deficiencies*	Notes
Lightenberg and Cader, 1959 [10]	37 years	12 days	Auditory and olfactory hallucinations, delusions. Apathy, disorientation. No details on other cognitive functions.	TSH, ACTH, gonadotropin, and prolactin	Twice improves without replacing deficient hormones, but relapsed. MRI-pituitary not reported.
Hanna, 1970 [11]	55 years	19 years	Delusions and auditory hallucinations Impaired cognition including disorientation and poor memory.	Gonadotropin, TSH, ACTH. Symptoms of hypopituitarism have lasted long before psychiatric manifestations No details about prolactin levels or lactation	One week after presentation developed seizures, coma, and hypotension. MRI pituitary not reported.
Kitis and Johnson, 1976 [12]	48 years	10 years	Auditory hallucinations, paranoid delusions, and aggressive behavior. Depression. No details on cognition, attention, and concentration.	Gonadotropins, prolactin, TSH, ACTH (hormone deficiency persisted at least 4 years before the onset of psychiatric manifestations)	Six years after childbirth, Sheehan syndrome diagnosed, but the patient defaulted. MRI pituitary not reported.
Leo et al., 1998 [13]	57 years	29 years	Paranoid delusions and auditory hallucinations. Apathy and dysphoria. Normal memory and attention	Gonadotropins, prolactin, TSH, ACTH (onset of any of the hormone deficiencies not clear from history)	Initially diagnosed as schizoaffective disorder with poor response.
Kale et al., 1999 [14]	21 years	15–20 days	Hallucinations, persecutory delusions, and delusions of infidelity.Orientation normal. No cognitive assessment.	Gonadotropins, prolactin, TSH, ACTH	No history of postpartum haemorrhage.
Shoib, 2013 [15]	31 years	16–18 days	Persecutory delusions, auditory hallucinations. Intact memory, poor attention, concentration, and verbal fluency.	Gonadotropins, prolactin, TSH, ACTH	
Reddy, 2017 [16]	42 years	11 years	Delusions of persecutions and second person auditory hallucinations. Has forgetfulness, no details on cognition, attention, and concentration.	Gonadotropins, prolactin (onset soon after childbirth) TSH, ACTH (onset not defined)	
Nath et al., 2018 [17]	43 years	13 years	Catatonia, reduced speaking, and reduced emotional reactivity. No details about cognition, attention, and concentration.	Gonadotropins, prolactin (onset soon after childbirth) TSH, ACTH (onset not defined)	
Shiekh et al., 2018 [18]	37 years	2 years	Persecutory delusions, auditory hallucinations. Normal memory. Poor attention and concentration.	Gonadotropins, prolactin (onset soon after childbirth) TSH, ACTH (onset not defined)	

*No diabetes insipidus in any of the patients. Growth hormone was not tested in any of the patients.

suggesting early-onset hypopituitarism. But the time of the onset of hypothyroidism and ACTH deficiency was not clear from the reports in some [16–18]. In two patients, other features of hypopituitarism have lasted long before the onset of psychiatric manifestations [11, 12]. In our patient, symptoms have developed early though they were left unattended.

Our patient had psychotic manifestations with mildly impaired attention and concentration but otherwise intact cognitive functions. Cognitive involvement, attention, and concentration were variable among different patients in the reported cases. Details of these aspects were not reported in five patients. Of the other four, one had normal cognition, attention, and concentration [13]. One had impaired cognition and disorientation [11]. Two patients had intact memory with impaired attention and concentration [15, 18]. This is in contrast to the observation that impaired cognition is one of the commonest manifestations of Sheehan syndrome [2].

The pathophysiology of psychiatric manifestations in Sheehan syndrome is not clear. Psychiatric symptoms are hypothesized to be caused by the complex interaction of hormonal deficiencies with metabolic and electrolyte changes in the central nervous system [19]. All patients have had dramatic improvement with glucocorticoid and thyroxine replacement therapy, suggesting a possible link to these hormonal deficiencies. None of the patients received growth hormone and oestrogen/progesterone replacement therapy. Therefore, growth hormone and gonadotropin deficiencies seem to be of lesser clinical relevance. Hyponatraemia is also known to cause psychiatric manifestations. However, it is usually associated with delirium presenting with subtle cognitive deficits to overt fleeting psychotic symptoms with global impairment of consciousness [20]. Frank, well-formed delusions and hallucinations in the absence of impairment of consciousness and neurological signs have not been reported in hyponatraemia [19, 21, 22]. Hypothyroidism may be more important in pathogenesis as it is consistently associated with neuropsychiatric manifestations [23]. Hypothyroidism is associated with mood symptoms rather than psychosis though overt psychotic presentations without significant mood symptoms have been reported [24].

Psychosis has been noted in male and female patients with hypopituitarism due to other causes [25-29]. Therefore, it could be a rare manifestation of hypopituitarism per se. The postpartum state is known to predispose to psychosis. Lactation failure characteristically seen in Sheehan syndrome might have a psychological impact on the woman. At least in patients developing psychiatric manifestations early, these might be contributory. Postpartum psychosis typically presents within the first 3–10 days after childbirth [30]. It is noted for its delirium-like presentation with rapid mood fluctuations.

There are several unanswered questions regarding psychotic manifestations in patients with Sheehan syndrome. Long interval between symptoms and onset of hormone deficiencies in some patients remains elusive. Whether there are any predisposing factors for psychiatric manifestations in these patients compared to a large number of patients with Sheehan syndrome without any psychotic manifestations is another interesting question. Detailed attention to patients' personality traits and triggering external factors might help to find answers.

4. Conclusions

This rare presentation of Sheehan syndrome with psychosis not only represents the close association of organic pathology to psychiatric manifestations but also illustrates the possible psychiatric adverse effects of panhypopituitarism and its metabolic consequences.

Abbreviations

ACTH: Adrenocorticotropic hormone
FSH: Follicle-stimulating hormone
IGF-1: Insulin-like growth factor-1
LH: Luteinizing hormone
MRI: Magnetic resonance imaging
TSH: Thyroid-stimulating hormone.

Acknowledgments

The authors would like to acknowledge the patient for providing consent for publication of this case report.

References

[1] Z. Karaca, "Sheehan syndrome," *Nature Reviews Disease Primers*, vol. 2, no. 1, pp. 1-15, 2016.
[2] O. Gei-Guardia, E. Soto-Herrera, A. Gei-Brealey, and C. Chen-Ku, "Sheehan syndrome in Costa Rica: clinical experience with 60 cases," *Endocrine Practice*, vol. 17, no. 3, pp. 337–344, 2011.
[3] C. Shivaprasad, "Sheehan's syndrome: newer advances," *Indian Journal of Endocrinology and Metabolism*, vol. 15, no. 3, p. S203, 2011.
[4] R. J. Dash, V. Gupta, and S. Suri, "Sheehan's syndrome: clinical profile, pituitary hormone responses and computed sellar tomography," *Australian and New Zealand Journal of Medicine*, vol. 23, no. 1, pp. 26–31, 1993.
[5] J. L. Cummings, "Organic psychosis," *Psychosomatics*, vol. 29, no. 1, pp. 16–26, 1988.
[6] M. Wawhal, "Postpartem psychosis with sheehan's syndrome: a rare case report and a brief review of literature," *International Journal of Science and Research*, vol. 4, no. 5, pp. 973–977, 2013.
[7] T. Umekawa, T. Yoshida, N. Sakane, and M. Kondo, "A case of Sheehan's syndrome with delirium," *Psychiatry and Clinical Neurosciences*, vol. 50, no. 6, pp. 327–330, 1996.
[8] M. I. Qadri, "Sheehan's syndrome presenting as major depressive disorder," *Iranian Journal of Medical Sciences*, vol. 40, no. 1, pp. 73–76, 2015.
[9] M. Gahr, S. Hügl, and R. Freudenmann, "Protracted delirium with Sheehan's syndrome," *Acta Neuropsychiatrica*, vol. 24, no. 3, pp. 183–185, 2012.
[10] J. D. Lichtenberg and G. Cader, "The interrelationship between physical and psychic stress in a case of sheehan's disease: postpartum necrosis of the anterior pituitary," *Southern Medical Journal*, vol. 52, no. 5, pp. 594–600, 1959.
[11] S. M. Hanna, "Hypopituitarism (sheehan's syndrome presenting with organic psychosis," *Journal of Neurology, Neurosurgery & Psychiatry*, vol. 33, no. 2, p. 192, 1970.
[12] G. Kitis and V. Johnson, *Sheehan's Syndrome with Psychosis*, Sage Publications, New York, NY, USA, 1976.
[13] R. J. Leo, G. J. Burnett, and M. J. Hassett, "Psychosis associated with hypopituitarism," *General Hospital Psychiatry*, vol. 20, no. 4, pp. 248–254, 1998.
[14] K. Kale, N. Nihalani, N. Karnik, and N. Shah, "Postpartum psychosis in a case of sheehan's syndrome," *Indian Journal of Psychiatry*, vol. 41, no. 1, p. 70, 1999.
[15] S. Shoib, "Sheehan's syndrome presenting as psychosis: a rare

clinical presentation," *Medical Journal of the Islamic Republic of Iran*, vol. 27, no. 1, p. 35, 2013.
[16] M. S. S. Reddy, A. Nahar, H. Thippeswamy, and C. S. Kumar, "Psychosis as a late manifestation of sheehan's syndrome," *Asian Journal of Psychiatry*, vol. 25, pp. 228–230, 2017.
[17] S. Nath, R. Ranjan, D. Mohapatra, and B. R. Mishra, "Successful management of patient with sheehan's syndrome presenting with psychosis and catatonia," *Indian Journal of Psychological Medicine*, vol. 40, no. 3, p. 276, 2018.
[18] N. A. Sheikh, S. K. Gakkhar, and S. K. Gakkhar, "Sheehan's syndrome and psychosis," *Indian Journal of Forensic Medicine and Pathology*, vol. 11, no. 3, p. 207, 2018.
[19] S. Kate, "Acute psychosis as a presentation of hypopituitarism," *Case Reports*, vol. 2013, Article ID bcr2012008516, 2013.
[20] S. Sivaraman and M. Rajajeyakumar, "Psychiatric aspects of hyponatremia-a clinical approach," *Journal of Psychology and Psychotherapy*, vol. 6, pp. 1-2, 2016.
[21] M. M. Gehi, R. H. Rosenthal, N. B. Fizette, L. R. Crowe, and W. L. Webb, "Psychiatric manifestations of hyponatremia," *Psychosomatics*, vol. 22, no. 9, pp. 739–743, 1981.
[22] V. John, P. Evans, and A. Kalhan, "Delayed dyskinesia and prolonged psychosis in a patient presenting with profound hyponatraemia," *Endocrinology, Diabetes & Metabolism Case Reports*, vol. 2017, no. 1, 2017.
[23] J. Davis and G. Tremont, "Neuropsychiatric aspects of hypothyroidism and treatment reversibility," *Minerva Endocrinologica*, vol. 32, no. 1, p. 49, 2007.
[24] M. F. Mohamed, "Acute psychosis and concurrent rhabdomyolysis unveiling diagnosis of hypothyroidism," *BMJ Case Reports CP*, vol. 12, no. 10, Article ID e231579, 2019.
[25] S. A. Dissanayake and D. M. Leiberman, "Hypopituitarism with paranoid psychosis: a description of two cases," *Journal of Neurology, Neurosurgery & Psychiatry*, vol. 32, no. 3, p. 233, 1969.
[26] O. Jegede, "Neuropsychiatric manifestations in a patient with panhypopituitarism," *Case Reports in Psychiatry*, vol. 2017, Article ID 5082687, 3 pages, 2017.
[27] B. Ratnakaran, V. P. Punnoose, S. Das, and A. Kartha, "Psychosis in secondary empty sella syndrome following a Russell's viper bite," *Indian Journal of Psychological Medicine*, vol. 38, no. 3, p. 254, 2016.
[28] M. Nwokolo and J. Fletcher, "A rare case of hypopituitarism with psychosis," *Endocrinology, Diabetes & Metabolism Case Reports*, vol. 2013, no. 1, 2013.
[29] J. Alexander, P. Mann Mah, N. Laddipeerla, and T. Mohan, "Panhypopituitarism and psychosis in a male patient," *Australian & New Zealand Journal of Psychiatry*, vol. 44, no. 4, pp. 393-394, 2010.
[30] V. Bergink, N. Rasgon, and K. L. Wisner, "Postpartum psychosis: madness, mania, and melancholia in motherhood," *American Journal of Psychiatry*, vol. 173, no. 12, pp. 1179–1188, 2016.

The Glucose-Lowering Effects of Coconut Oil: A Case Report and Review of the Literature

Samar Malaeb[1] **and Christopher Spoke**[2]

[1]Division of Diabetes, Endocrinology and Metabolism, Department of Medicine, University of Minnesota, Minneapolis, MN 55407, USA
[2]Department of Medical Education, Abbott Northwestern Hospital, Minneapolis, MN 55455, USA

Correspondence should be addressed to Samar Malaeb; malae002@umn.edu

Academic Editor: J. Paul Frindik

Background. Coconut oil, a saturated fat comprised mostly of the medium-chain fatty acid, lauric acid, has become increasingly popular over the past few decades due to its touted anti-inflammatory, metabolic, and lipid-lowering properties. There have been many studies with mixed results evaluating the effects of coconut oil consumption on lipid metabolism and cardiometabolic risk. However, the effects on glucose metabolism are less clear. There are few trials on the effects of coconut oil on glucose homeostasis but no case reports prior to the current one. *Case.* We present a case of a 66-year-old man with a history of type 2 diabetes managed with insulin who developed recurrent hypoglycemia and required reduction in insulin therapy quickly after consuming coconut oil supplementation. *Conclusion.* This is the first known case report of coconut oil supplementation in a diabetic patient on insulin resulting in hypoglycemia. Review of the literature shows that coconut oil supplementation can have a favorable effect on glycemic control, possibly through phenolic compounds mediating anti-inflammatory effects. This effect is inconsistent throughout the studies reviewed, likely due to variations in types of coconut oil supplementation and scarcity of trials. Further research is required both in animal models and in humans before coconut oil intake is widely advised and popularized. This is especially true in patients with diabetes, who are at increased risk of cardiovascular disease, and in whom reduction in saturated fat intake is advised.

1. Background

The use of coconut oil has become increasingly popular over the past few decades due to claims regarding anti-inflammatory, metabolic, and lipid-altering properties. As a result, there has been an increase in demand for research and clinical trials to evaluate the cardiometabolic and energy metabolism effects of coconut oil. The usual coconut oil commercial product is obtained from the fresh mature kernel of the coconut plant as either refined, bleached, and deodorized coconut oil or, more recently, virgin (i.e., unrefined) coconut oil [1, 2]. The predominant type of fat in coconut oil is lauric acid (comprising about 50%), with smaller amounts of myristic and palmitic acid. Lauric acid is a saturated fatty acid (SFA) with a structure that is C12 : 0, classifying it as a medium-chain fatty acid (MCFA) [1]. While recent dietary guidelines have recommended a diet low in SFA, specifically aiming for less than 10% of daily total caloric intake and replacing SFA with unsaturated fats [3, 4], coconut oil's medium-chain fatty acid property, as well as its high content of polyphenolic compounds, which have been implicated in its anti-inflammatory and enhanced metabolism qualities [5], has been thought to be the basis to its possible health benefits. For this reason, it has been proposed that coconut oil not be considered in the same context as other saturated fats and has been termed by some proponents as a "healthy fat" [6, 7].

There have been few case reports or research into the effects of coconut oil on energy metabolism, specifically glycemic changes. We present a case of a 66-year-old man with a history of type 2 diabetes mellitus managed with insulin who developed recurrent hypoglycemia and required reduction in insulin therapy quickly after consuming coconut oil supplementation. We review the current literature on coconut oil's effect on energy metabolism and glucose homeostasis and propose future areas of research into these properties of coconut oil.

2. Case

A 66-year-old male presented to the endocrine clinic for consultation regarding new onset hypoglycemia. He was diagnosed with type 2 diabetes mellitus at age 42 and was initially managed with metformin. Subsequently, insulin was added due to worsening glycemic control. His insulin regimen, until recently, consisted of NPH insulin 20 units subcutaneously twice daily and regular insulin 15 units before each meal. A few weeks prior to presentation to the endocrine clinic, he started taking coconut oil supplements because he heard about some health benefits. Specifically, he started taking a dose of 1000 mg daily. Within 1-2 days of starting the supplement, he began experiencing hypoglycemia. He denied any changes in his appetite or caloric intake. There were no other factors that would have explained his onset of hypoglycemia. Specifically, his weight, which was 253 lbs at baseline (for a body mass index of 33.5), had not changed. He did not start taking any other new medications or supplements. Based on advice from his primary care provider, he reduced his insulin doses: initially, NPH down to 15 units twice daily and then to 10 units twice daily. He then started avoiding some of the regular insulin doses. When he took regular insulin, he would have hypoglycemia at bedtime.

During his visit to the endocrine clinic, he reported a stable weight. He was experiencing hypoglycemia (defined as blood glucose below 70 mg/dL [8]) about once weekly. These episodes tended to occur after he had supper, close to bedtime. His lowest glucose reading was 50 mg/dL in the past 2 weeks. His hemoglobin A1c, a long-term measure of glycemic control, was 6.2%. This was lower than his previous level of 6.4% checked 3 months prior to starting coconut oil, despite cutting the dose of his long-acting insulin in half and occasionally skipping his meal-time insulin. His lipid levels prior to coconut oil intake were as follows: total cholesterol of 116 mg/dL, LDL of 36 mg/dL, HDL of 34 mg/dL, and triglycerides of 232 mg/dL. He was taking a statin medication before and continued to take it after initiating coconut oil. By the time he was seen in the endocrine clinic, a lipid panel was not repeated, due to short-time duration since being on the new supplement. The patient was intending to raise his coconut oil dose to 2000 mg per day and had questions regarding the effects of coconut oil on his blood glucose and implications of taking coconut oil supplementation on his diabetes management. This prompted a review of the literature as detailed in the remainder of this report.

3. Discussion

Research into the effects of coconut oil has increased over the past few decades. It has been proposed to have anti-inflammatory, antioxidant, enhanced metabolism, as well as antidiabetic properties. Coconut oil has been implicated in improving the quality of life in cancer treatments, reducing inflammation markers, reducing toxic side effects of chemotherapy, and even improving bone mineral density in animal studies [9–14]. The metabolism of coconut oil has been heavily researched. Coconut oil is high in saturated fatty acids, with more than 60% consisting of medium-chain fatty acids (MCFAs), a large percentage of which is lauric acid (C 12 : 0). Its medium-chain fatty acid property has been thought to be the source of its health benefits as MCFA have been shown to improve metabolism and positively affect cardiometabolic risk factors [5]. The metabolism of MCFA differs from other fatty acids as they are hydrolyzed and absorbed faster than other fats. They do not undergo degradation and re-esterification processes and can be directly used in the body to produce energy. This is thought to result in faster gastric emptying, thus leading to less stimulation of gut hormones [6, 15]. After their absorption, MFCAs are transported directly into the liver and undergo β-oxidation. Compared with long-chain fatty acids (LCFAs), MCFAs do not require chylomicron transport via the lymphatic system to reach their target tissues, thereby favoring hepatic metabolism and mitochondrial oxidation [2, 16]. This results in preferential metabolism of MCFAs over LCFAs, and different animal and human trials have proposed this property to positively effect satiety, weight loss, energy expenditure, and glucose homeostasis [5, 17].

One of the most heavily researched aspects of coconut oil is its effect on lipid metabolism and cardiovascular risk reduction. Epidemiologic studies have found that population groups that consume coconut as part of their traditional diets had higher HDL and lower rates of cardiovascular disease [2]. It is important to note that the type of coconut these populations consume is not the same as what is in a typical Western diet and in processed coconut products. Results of studies on effects of coconut oil on cholesterol metabolism have been mixed, with most studies favoring an increase in HDL, LDL cholesterol and triglyceride levels [18–20]. The proposed mechanisms are thought to be due to effects of lauric acid, which acts as a substrate in the liver for the production of ApoA-I and ApoB production. A second mechanism is through a decrease in HDL cholesterol and ApoA-I catabolism and increased reverse cholesterol transport due to increased size of the HDL cholesterol molecule [9]. One randomized control trial found that HDL cholesterol levels increased on average by 3.1 mg/dL with coconut oil supplementation [19]. Some evidence (though inconsistent) points to butter raising LDL cholesterol more than coconut oil. When coconut oil replaces carbohydrates, a slight reduction in LDL-to-HDL cholesterol ratio has been reported. However, when coconut oil replaces monounsaturated or polyunsaturated oils, LDL is raised. Since cardiovascular risk is more correlated with raising LDL than raising HDL and because coconut oil increases LDL cholesterol, a cause of CVD, the American Heart Association Presidential advisory panel in 2017 recommended against the use of coconut oil [4]. This recommendation is further supported by 2 recent systematic reviews and meta-analyses on the effects of coconut oil on cardiovascular risk factors. One review included 16 trials and showed that compared with nontropical vegetable oils, coconut oil consumption increased total cholesterol, LDL cholesterol, and HDL cholesterol and did not significantly change C-reactive protein, fasting glucose concentrations, or measures of body adiposity. The findings prompted the authors to express concern about increased consumption of the saturated fat, coconut oil, in the population [21]. Another review, which included 12 trials, showed similar findings on cholesterol profile when compared with other plant oils. However, in this review, a comparison with animal oils found that coconut oil reduced LDL cholesterol. Despite the HDL cholesterol-raising effect, the authors were cautious to not recommend replacing a significant amount of unsaturated plant oil with coconut oil [22]. The latter review did not evaluate effects on glycemia.

The patient in this case report developed recurrent hypoglycemia and had decreased insulin requirements after the addition of coconut oil supplementation to his diet. We hypothesize that the metabolic and anti-inflammatory properties of coconut oil contributed to the patient's decreased insulin requirements. This is the first known case report of coconut oil supplementation in a diabetic patient on insulin resulting in hypoglycemia. There have been multiple studies into the effects of coconut oil on glucose homeostasis in animal models. In a study on streptozocin-induced diabetic rats fed various types of fats, the coconut oil-fed rats exhibited the best (lowest rise in glucose) response to an oral glucose tolerance test (compared with palm oil and groundnut oil). These same rats also exhibited lower levels of total cholesterol and non-HDL cholesterol. It was hypothesized that the mechanism of improved insulin sensitivity was related to the triglyceride levels, which were reduced in the coconut oil-fed rats [23]. This may or may not be generalizable to human populations where triglyceride levels have been found to rise after coconut oil supplementation. A more recent study on alloxan-induced diabetic rats showed that virgin coconut oil intake resulted in reduction in food intake and body weight gain, as well as improvement in microbiota profile (increase in certain probiotic bacteria) in diabetic rats [24]. A study on C57/BL6 male mice fed a diet moderately high in fat from coconut oil + soybean oil vs. coconut oil only or fructose only showed that addition of soybean oil was most detrimental to metabolic outcomes such as diabetes, insulin resistance, and fatty liver [25]. Another study on a similar mouse model was mainly conducted to evaluate the effect of coconut oil on cardiomyopathy (vs. standard chow diet). Though it did show an aggravation of cardiomyopathy from coconut oil consumption, specific effects on insulin resistance were evaluated and found to be neutral [26]. In an attempt to better mimic a human diet-induced obesity model, one study in female Ossabaw minipigs fed a high fat diet rich in hydrogenated fats, fructose, and coconut oil surprisingly showed that despite developing obesity, those pigs manifested similar glucose concentrations and lower systemic inflammatory cytokine levels compared with controls, as well as a shift of their urogenital microbiota towards a more anti-inflammatory phenotype. It was hypothesized that coconut oil in their diet conferred those benefits [27]. Finally, it is worth noting that the various chemical forms of coconut oil may not behave similarly. A study on the effect of thermally oxidized coconut oil (the kind that would naturally occur from cooking at high temperatures and not what is present in virgin coconut oil supplements) on glucose metabolism in rats showed negative effects. Specifically, those rats were fed a high-fructose diet and developed insulin resistance, hyperglycemia, and systemic inflammation. Those effects were all exacerbated, or made worse, in the group supplemented with thermally oxidized coconut oil [28]. All of these studies combined show that the data on the effect of coconut oil on glucose homeostasis in animals have shown some favorable, but overall mixed results.

As far as human studies on effects of coconut oil intake on glucose homeostasis, an older study conducted in 1992 by Eckel et al. showed improved insulin mediated glucose metabolism after medium-chain triglyceride (MCT) supplementation for four days (vs. isocaloric long-chain triglyceride supplementation). This effect was seen in subjects with and without type 2 diabetes, and in diabetics, it was independent of severity of diabetes or intake of sulfonylureas. Using the euglycemic clamp technique following an MCT supplemented diet, the amount of glucose needed to maintain euglycemia during an intravenous insulin infusion was increased in diabetic subjects by 30%, in nondiabetic subjects with hypertriglyceridemia by 30%, and in normotriglyceridemic subjects by 17%, all indicating higher insulin sensitivity [29]. More recently, a randomized trial on 75 adult obese women all following a hypocaloric lifestyle modification program divided the women into 4 groups of vegetable oil supplementation: coconut, safflower, chia, and soybean. Compared to baseline, all groups saw a significant ($p < 0.001$) reduction in weight, LDL cholesterol, triglycerides, blood glucose, and hemoglobin A1c and an increase in HDL cholesterol. Addition of 6 grams of coconut oil supplementation to the diet resulted in the largest decrease amongst the 4 groups in average blood glucose (−25 mg/dL vs. baseline) and in glycated hemoglobin A1c (−0.86% vs baseline). The coconut oil group also saw the greatest reduction in weight (about 8% reduction vs. baseline), with a concomitant reduction in body mass index, waist-to-height ratio, and increase in % lean mass. The coconut oil consumed about 613 less Kcal/day at the end of the study compared to baseline, which was significantly lower than the calorie reduction in the other three groups. The authors hypothesized that this preferential weight loss effect may have been related to increased satiety effects of coconut oil. Most of the calorie reduction was from reduced carbohydrate intake. The glycemic effects were also hypothesized to be related to phenolic compounds in coconut oil, discussed in the next paragraph of this report, although these compounds were not directly measured. The chia seed oil saw the greatest improvement in lipid parameters [17]. Finally, a randomized crossover controlled study on 15 adult women with excess body fat (defined as far comprising >32% of body composition) evaluated acute effects of virgin coconut oil (VCO) administration on energy metabolism, cardiometabolic risk markers, and appetitive responses. Subjects were fed a breakfast supplemented with 25 mL of MCFA in the form of VCO (vs. control: olive oil), and postprandial data were obtained for up to 240 minutes. The VCP group did not exhibit any significant differences in postprandial glucose response compared to placebo. Also, notable was that the VCO group has less satiety response than placebo. There were no differential effects on lipid levels. It was hypothesized by the authors that differences in fatty acid composition, and hence structure, of VCO (compared to other synthetic forms of coconut oil) may explain some of these negative findings. This prompted the authors to caution against prescribing this form of coconut oil as a supplement, given no clear benefit in this acute study [15]. The above human studies show that data remain mixed on effects of coconut oil supplementation on glucose homeostasis in humans. This may be related to varying forms of coconut oil supplementation, as well as confounding of weight loss from calorie restriction. One important observation in the case report presented in this current paper is that the hypoglycemic effects were seen after 2 days of ingestion of 1 g of coconut oil supplements. The human studies cited above had durations that varied from 240 minutes postprandial (which showed a negative result) to 4 days (using 40 grams of MCT oil/1000 calories per day) to 8 weeks (using 6 grams/day of coconut oil supplementation). This shows that it is difficult at this point, based on the data reported in the literature, to predict or validate whether ingestion of 1 g per day for 2 days is sufficient enough to show a response. More studies are needed before a consensus is reached on the glycemic effects.

When it comes to the proposed mechanisms to any likely benefit on glycemia, coconut oil's high concentration of polyphenolic compounds has been proposed to increase the efficiency of glucose metabolism [1]. Coconut oil is known to contain phenolic antioxidants such as caffeic acid, ferulic acid, syringic acid, catechin, and epigallocatechin. Phenolic compounds have been shown to have antidiabetic and insulin-sensitizing effects, as well and anti-inflammatory and immune modulatory priorities [17, 30]. Phenolic compounds have been implicated in inhibiting the COX pathway, downregulating TNF alpha and cytokine production, and inactivating peroxisome proliferator-activated receptor gamma (PPARγ) [30]. Given these properties, it has been proposed that coconut oil ingestion results in less demand for enzyme production of the pancreas, thus improving insulin secretion and utilization of blood glucose [31]. One specific example is ferulic acid, which has been shown to contain high levels of phenolic acids, and when added to the diet in type 2 diabetes mice models, resulted in reduction in serum glucose, increase in serum insulin, and increased hepatic glycogen production and glucokinase activity [32]. Coconut kernel protein has also been shown to have antidiabetic properties, hypothesized to improve pancreatic beta-cell regeneration by means of arginine [16, 33]. One challenge remains and that is to determine the correlation between coconut oil doses, phenolic content, and clinically meaningful antioxidant activity. Rigorous studies using various extraction methods have shown that the antioxidant properties of coconut oil correlate with phenolic compound content, and that both of those vary with the method of extraction used. Virgin coconut oil (VCO), especially when produced by the chilling method, tends to have the highest phenolic acid content (as measured by gallic acid equivalents) and antioxidant activity (as measured by scavenging activity of the stable 1,1-diphenyl-2-picrylhydrazyl (DPPH) free radical, b-carotene-linoleate bleaching activity, and reducing power) [34, 35]. In one study, the total phenolic content and DPPH radical-scavenging activity of VCO was found to be in the range of 1.16–12.54 mg gallic acid equivalents (GAE)/g and 7.49–104.52 mg/ml [35]. However, the correlation of this data with the amounts usually present in supplements (1000 mg per supplement) or in diets rich in coconut oil, and their clinical relevance, i.e., the dose needed to give a clinical effect, has not been published. More controlled experiments need to be done to answer these questions.

4. Back to the Patient

The patient presented in this case report was advised to stop the prandial insulin due to evidence of postprandial hypoglycemia. He was started on a GLP-1 agonist medication to help maintain good glycemic control as the prandial insulin was withdrawn. He was given dietary advice specific to diabetes management and weight loss. He was advised to continue taking the statin medication for cardiovascular prevention given his age and history of diabetes. He wished to continue the coconut oil supplements knowing that the evidence for their use is not consistent. The next steps in his management will include attempting to reduce his long-acting insulin (NPH) if enough weight is lost. At the time of completion of this case report, the patient had not returned for a follow-up visit to the endocrine clinic.

5. Conclusion

This is the first known case report of coconut oil supplementation in a diabetic patient on insulin resulting in hypoglycemia. Summary of the literature shows that coconut oil supplementation may have an effect on glycemic control, possibly through phenolic compounds mediating anti-inflammatory effects. This effect is inconsistent throughout the studies reviewed, likely due to variations in types of coconut oil supplementation and scarcity of animal mechanistic studies and human clinical trials. One of the limitations of this case report is that it was not a controlled experimental trial, and patient report was the primary source of data; thus, we cannot conclude with certainty that it was coconut oil ingestion that resulted in the reported hypoglycemia. This case report is clinically relevant because it highlights the importance of checking supplement history in patients in general and specifically in patients with diabetes. Patients with diabetes are at increased risk of cardiovascular complications, and this is especially important since coconut oil is a saturated fat that has been shown to increase LDL cholesterol. Therefore, even if the evidence points to some improvement in glycemic control, further outcomes research is required in humans before coconut oil intake is advised and popularized, to the general population as well as to patients with diabetes in particular.

Abbreviations

BG: Blood glucose
MCFA: Medium-chain fatty acids
SFA: Saturated fatty acids
VCO: Virgin coconut oil.

References

[1] A. S. Babu, S. K. Veluswamy, R. Arena, M. Guazzi, and C. J. Lavie, "Virgin coconut oil and its potential cardioprotective effects," *Postgraduate Medicine*, vol. 126, no. 7, pp. 76–83, 2014.

[2] L. Eyres, M. F. Eyres, A. Chisholm, and R. C. Brown, "Coconut oil consumption and cardiovascular risk factors in humans," *Nutrition Reviews*, vol. 74, no. 4, pp. 267–280, 2016.

[3] K. B. DeSalvo, R. Olson, and K. O. Casavale, "Dietary guidelines for Americans," *The Journal of the American Medical Association*, vol. 315, no. 5, pp. 457-458, 2016.

[4] F. M. Sacks, A. H. Lichtenstein, J. H. Y. Wu et al., "Dietary fats and cardiovascular disease: a presidential advisory from the American heart association," *Circulation*, vol. 136, no. 3, pp. e1–e23, 2017.

[5] K. C. Maki, W. Hasse, M. R. Dicklin et al., "Corn oil lowers plasma cholesterol compared with coconut oil in adults with above-desirable levels of cholesterol in a randomized crossover trial," *The Journal of Nutrition*, vol. 148, no. 10, pp. 1556–1563, 2018.

[6] W. Amarasiri, "Coconut fats," *Ceylon Medical Journal*, vol. 51, no. 2, p. 47, 2009.

[7] T. Tholstrup, C. Ehnholm, M. Jauhiainen et al., "Effects of medium-chain fatty acids and oleic acid on blood lipids, lipoproteins, glucose, insulin, and lipid transfer protein activities," *The American Journal of Clinical Nutrition*, vol. 79, no. 4, pp. 564–569, 2004.

[8] P. E. Cryer, L. Axelrod, A. B. Grossman et al., "Evaluation and management of adult hypoglycemic disorders: an endocrine society clinical practice guideline," *The Journal of Clinical Endocrinology & Metabolism*, vol. 94, no. 3, pp. 709–728, 2009.

[9] H. O. Santos, S. Howell, C. P. Earnest, and F. J. Teixeira, "Coconut oil intake and its effects on the cardiometabolic profile-a structured literature review," *Progress in Cardiovascular Diseases*, vol. 62, no. 5, pp. 436–443, 2019.

[10] K.-T. Khaw, S. J. Sharp, L. Finikarides et al., "Randomised trial of coconut oil, olive oil or butter on blood lipids and other cardiovascular risk factors in healthy men and women," *BMJ Open*, vol. 8, no. 3, p. e020167, 2018.

[11] A. C. Famurewa, A. M. Folawiyo, E. B. Enohnyaket et al., "Beneficial role of virgin coconut oil supplementation against acute methotrexate chemotherapy-induced oxidative toxicity and inflammation in rats," *Integrative Medicine Research*, vol. 7, no. 3, pp. 257–263, 2018.

[12] K. S. Law, N. Azman, E. A. Omar et al., "The effects of virgin coconut oil (VCO) as supplementation on quality of life (QOL) among breast cancer patients," *Lipids in Health and Disease*, vol. 13, no. 1, p. 139, 2014.

[13] Z. Hayatullina, N. Muhammad, N. Mohamed, and I.-N. Soelaiman, "Virgin coconut oil supplementation prevents bone loss in osteoporosis rat model," *Evidence-based Complementary and Alternative Medicine*, vol. 2012, pp. 1–8, 2012.

[14] K. A. Page, A. Williamson, N. Yu et al., "Medium-chain fatty acids improve cognitive function in intensively treated type 1 diabetic patients and support in vitro synaptic transmission during acute hypoglycemia," *Diabetes*, vol. 58, no. 5, pp. 1237–1244, 2009.

[15] F. X. Valente, F. G. Cândido, L. L. Lopes et al., "Effects of coconut oil consumption on energy metabolism, cardiometabolic risk markers, and appetitive responses in women with excess body fat," *European Journal of Nutrition*, vol. 57, no. 4, pp. 1627–1637, 2018.

[16] M. Debmandal and S. Mandal, "Coconut (Cocos nucifera L.: arecaceae): in health promotion and disease prevention," *Asian Pacific Journal of Tropical Medicine*, vol. 4, no. 3, pp. 241–247, 2011.

[17] L. Oliveira-de-Lira, E. M. C. Santos, R. F. de Souza et al., "Supplementation-dependent effects of vegetable oils with varying fatty acid compositions on anthropometric and biochemical parameters in obese women," *Nutrients*, vol. 10, no. 7, 2018.

[18] M. Vijayakumar, D. M. Vasudevan, K. R. Sundaram et al., "A randomized study of coconut oil versus sunflower oil on cardiovascular risk factors in patients with stable coronary heart disease," *Indian Heart Journal*, vol. 68, no. 4, pp. 498–506, 2016.

[19] D. A. Cardoso, A. S. Moreira, G. M. de Oliveira, R. Raggio Luiz, and G. Rosa, "A coconut extra virgin oil-rich diet increases hdl cholesterol and decreases waist circumference and body mass in coronary artery disease patients," *Nutricion Hospitalaria*, vol. 32, no. 5, pp. 2144–2152, 2015.

[20] C. M. Sciarrillo, N. A. Koemel, P. M. Tomko, K. B. Bode, and S. R. Emerson, "Postprandial lipemic responses to various sources of saturated and monounsaturated fat in adults," *Nutrients*, vol. 11, no. 5, p. 1089, 2019.

[21] N. Neelakantan, J. Y. H. Seah, and R. M. van Dam, "The effect of coconut oil consumption on cardiovascular risk factors," *Circulation*, vol. 141, no. 10, pp. 803–814, 2020.

[22] M. Teng, Y. J. Zhao, A. L. Khoo, T. C. Yeo, Q. W. Yong, and B. P. Lim, "Impact of coconut oil consumption on cardiovascular health: a systematic review and meta-analysis," *Nutrition Reviews*, vol. 78, no. 3, pp. 249–259, 2020.

[23] B. M. Kochikuzhyil, K. Devi, and S. R. Fattepur, "Effect of saturated fatty acid-rich dietary vegetable oils on lipid profile, antioxidant enzymes and glucose tolerance in diabetic rats," *Indian Journal of Pharmacology*, vol. 42, no. 3, pp. 142–145, 2010.

[24] S. Djurasevic, S. Bojic, B. Nikolic et al., "Beneficial effect of virgin coconut oil on alloxan-induced diabetes and microbiota composition in rats," *Plant Foods for Human Nutrition*, vol. 73, no. 4, pp. 295–301, 2018.

[25] P. Deol, J. R. Evans, J. Dhahbi et al., "Soybean oil is more obesogenic and diabetogenic than coconut oil and fructose in mouse: potential role for the liver," *PLoS One*, vol. 10, no. 7, p. e0132672, 2015.

[26] I. Muthuramu, R. Amin, A. Postnov et al., "Coconut oil aggravates pressure overload-induced cardiomyopathy without inducing obesity, systemic insulin resistance, or cardiac steatosis," *International Journal of Molecular Sciences*, vol. 18, no. 7, 2017.

[27] A. E. Newell-Fugate, K. Lenz, C. Skenandore et al., "Effects of coconut oil on glycemia, inflammation, and urogenital microbial parameters in female Ossabaw mini-pigs," *PLoS ONE*, vol. 12, no. 7, p. e0179542, 2017.

[28] A. Narayanankutty, B. T. Kuzhivelil, and A. C. Raghavamenon, "A high-fructose diet formulated with thermally oxidized monounsaturated fat aggravates metabolic dysregulation in colon epithelial tissues of rats," *Journal of the American College of Nutrition*, pp. 1–12, 2020.

[29] R. H. Eckel, A. S. Hanson, A. Y. Chen, J. N. Berman, T. J. Yost, and E. P. Brass, "Dietary substitution of medium-chain triglycerides improves insulin-mediated glucose metabolism in NIDDM subjects," *Diabetes*, vol. 41, no. 5, pp. 641–647, 1992.

[30] N. Yahfoufi, N. Alsadi, M. Jambi, and C. Matar, "The immunomodulatory and anti-inflammatory role of polyphenols," *Nutrients*, vol. 10, no. 11, p. 1618, 2018.

[31] A. Saat, R. Rosli, and N. Syakroni, "Potential hypoglycemic property of Albizia myriophylla and virgin coconut oil in streptozotocin induced diabetic rats," *International Journal of Pharmacy and Pharmaceutical Sciences*, vol. 5, no. 4, pp. 199–202, 2013.

[32] E. H. Jung, S. Ran Kim, I. K. Hwang, and T. Youl Ha, "Hypoglycemic effects of a phenolic acid fraction of rice bran and ferulic acid in C57BL/KsJ-db/dbMice," *Journal of Agricultural and Food Chemistry*, vol. 55, no. 24, pp. 9800–9804, 2007.

[33] G. Salil, K. G. Nevin, and T. Rajamohan, "Arginine rich coconut kernel protein modulates diabetes in alloxan treated rats," *Chemico-biological Interactions*, vol. 189, no. 1-2, pp. 107–111, 2011.

[34] A. M. Marina, Y. B. Che man, S. A. H. Nazimah, and I. Amin, "Antioxidant capacity and phenolic acids of virgin coconut oil," *International Journal of Food Sciences and Nutrition*, vol. 60, no. sup2, pp. 114–123, 2009.

[35] N. A. A. Ghani, A.-A. Channip, P. Chok Hwee Hwa, F. Ja'afar, H. M. Yasin, and A. Usman, "Physicochemical properties, antioxidant capacities, and metal contents of virgin coconut oil produced by wet and dry processes," *Food Science & Nutrition*, vol. 6, no. 5, pp. 1298–1306, 2018.

30

Asymptomatic and Biochemically Silent Pheochromocytoma with Characteristic Findings on Imaging

Andrew Spiro, Aqueel Usman, Asif Ajmal, Thanh D. Hoang, and Mohamed K. M. Shakir

Division of Endocrinology, Walter Reed National Military Medical Center, 8901 Wisconsin Ave., Bethesda, MD 20889, USA

Correspondence should be addressed to Mohamed K. M. Shakir; mohamed_shakir@hotmail.com

Academic Editor: Osamu Isozaki

Pheochromocytomas are tumors that originate from the chromaffin tissue of the adrenal medulla and commonly produce catecholamines. The diagnosis is typically established by the measurement of catecholamines or their metabolites in urine or plasma, and tumors are localized with the use of radiographic and scintigraphic studies. Pheochromocytomas can occur in asymptomatic patients, and the preferred treatment is surgical removal of the tumor. We report a 48-year-old male with a left adrenal incidentaloma, which progressively increased in size from 1.1 cm to 2.6 cm over a 4-year period, as measured by an adrenal computed tomography (CT) scan. Throughout his entire course of treatment, he was asymptomatic with normal blood pressure readings. His biochemical screening was unremarkable for the first three years of tumor surveillance. Follow-up imaging, including CT and MRI, showed findings suspicious for pheochromocytoma, and the diagnosis was ultimately made with the combination of imaging and laboratory studies. He underwent laparoscopic resection of the adrenal mass with confirmation of pheochromocytoma on histology. This case illustrates how CT and MRI findings can alert providers to the presence of a pheochromocytoma, even in an asymptomatic, biochemically negative patient.

1. Introduction

Catecholamine-producing tumors arise from chromaffin cells in the sympathoadrenal system. Approximately 80 to 85% of catecholamine-producing tumors originate from the adrenal medulla, and these are called pheochromocytomas. About 15 to 20% derive from the sympathetic paravertebral ganglia and are known as catecholamine-secreting paragangliomas. It is worth noting, that non-catecholamine-secreting paragangliomas usually arise from the parasympathetic ganglia in the neck and base of the skull. Among patients with hypertension in the outpatient setting, the prevalence of catecholamine-producing tumors is estimated to be 0.2% to 0.6% [1]. The adrenal medulla normally secretes about 80% epinephrine, but the tumors of the adrenal medulla predominantly secrete more norepinephrine than epinephrine [2]. The elevated catecholamines can give rise to symptoms including sustained or paroxysmal hypertension, headaches, palpitations, tremors, diaphoresis, dyspnea, anxiety, chest pain, nausea, vomiting, and paresthesia. Catecholamines also have anti-insulinemic actions, which can cause elevated blood glucose levels and may result it polydipsia and polyuria. In severe cases, patients may experience myocardial infarction, heart failure, pulmonary edema, arrhythmias, or intracranial hemorrhage. A diagnosis is usually established by measuring the levels of metanephrines in the urine or blood [3]. Computed tomography (CT) or magnetic resonance imaging (MRI) are used for tumor localization. The tumor can also present as an asymptomatic adrenal incidentaloma, identified radiographically. Here, we report one such interesting case.

2. Case Presentation

A 48-year-old male with a left adrenal incidentaloma was evaluated in the endocrine clinic in 2013. CT showed a 1.1 cm left adrenal mass, with attenuation of 55 Hounsfield Units (HU). He was completely asymptomatic, with blood pressure readings in the normal range. A biochemical evaluation was unremarkable, including urine and plasma metanephrine levels, 1 mg dexamethasone suppression test, and plasma aldosterone-to-renin ratio. Repeat biochemical evaluations in 2014 and 2015 were also unremarkable; however, the size of the adrenal mass increased to 1.5 cm in 2014 and to 1.8 cm in 2015.

In 2016, adrenal CT (Figure 1) showed the mass had increased to 2.6 cm, with an attenuation of 40 HU. An MRI scan confirmed a 2.4 × 2.4 × 2.5 cm left adrenal mass with hyperintense T2 signal, isotense T1 signal without drop of signal on out-of-phase images, and homogenous enhancement postcontrast. The patient denied any symptoms consistent with pheochromocytoma. Physical examination was normal, including heart rate and blood pressure measurement. Plasma metanephrines and chromogranin A were unremarkable. A 24-hour urine metanephrine level was normal at 160 mcg (ref 45–290), while a 24-hour urine normetanephrine level was elevated at 1415 mcg (ref 82–500). An ^{123}I-metaiodobenzylguanidine (MIBG) scintigraphy scan revealed abnormal focal intense radiotracer accumulation in the left adrenal lesion (Figures 2(a) and 2(b)). With the presumptive diagnosis of pheochromocytoma, the patient was treated with phenoxybenzamine and underwent laparoscopic resection of the left adrenal mass. A 3.0 × 2.6 × 2.5 cm left adrenal pheochromocytoma was confirmed on histology (Figure 3). Postoperatively, the patient continued to be asymptomatic and normotensive, with normal levels of serum and urine metanephrine levels.

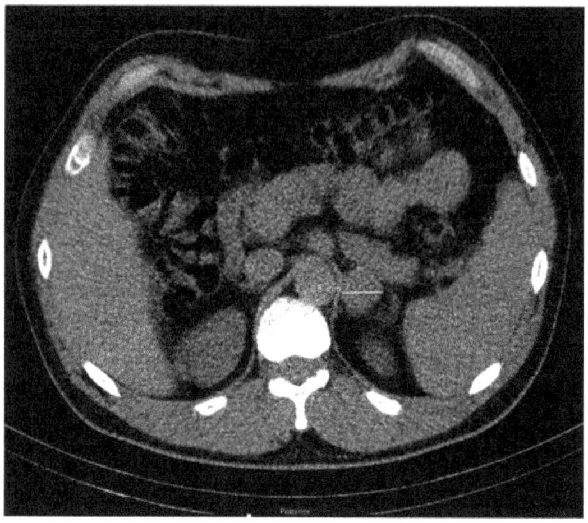

Figure 1: CT scan showing a 2.6 cm left adrenal mass.

3. Discussion

Our patient demonstrated an asymptomatic incidentaloma that was biochemically negative for the first three years after it was identified. The diagnosis of pheochromocytoma was ultimately made with the combination of follow-up imaging and lab work. In addition to curing hypertension, the early diagnosis of pheochromocytoma is important because if unrecognized, it can be a lethal condition. Medications, anesthetic agents, pregnancy, and surgery can precipitate hypertensive crisis or shock, even in asymptomatic patients [4]. The widespread use of radiological imaging has increased the detection of adrenal incidentalomas in individuals over 30 years of age. The clinical parameters of the tumor that need to be considered include functionality and aggressiveness. Assessing functionality involves identifying the secretion of cortisol, aldosterone, catecholamines, and androgens [5]. A retrospective study evaluated 42 patients with adrenal incidentalomas who were treated between 1995 and 2005, to determine the diagnostic significance of borderline-elevated urine or plasma metanephrines, defined as 1-2 times the upper limit of normal. The study found that 30% of the patients with adrenal incidentalomas and borderline-elevated urine or plasma metanephrines had a pheochromocytoma [6]. In another study of 27 patients with pheochromocytomas, 19 patients (70%) had an incidentally discovered tumor, six patients (22%) were normotensive, and two patients had near-normal urinary metanephrine levels [7]. For three years after the adrenal incidentaloma was identified, our patient's biochemical parameters, including urine and plasma metanephrine levels, were normal. Four years after the identification of the incidentaloma, it had significantly increased in size, and the 24-hour urine normetanephrine level was elevated; however, 24-hour urine metanephrine values remained normal, and serum metanephrine levels were never elevated.

In general, a CT scan with contrast-enhancement and MRI are used to localize pheochromocytomas [8]. The Endocrine Society Guidelines recommend CT rather than MRI as the initial imaging modality for most patients, due to excellent spacial resolution in the thorax, abdomen, and pelvis [1]. A retrospective study of 41 patients, who had undergone surgery for pheochromocytoma between 1990 and 2002, found that the classic association of headaches, palpitations, and sweating was only present in 24% of the cases. In roughly half of the cases, the tumor was discovered incidentally by imaging that was not part of a diagnostic workup for abnormal blood pressure readings [9]. Several imaging findings can be indicative of pheochromocytoma, adrenocortical carcinoma, or metastasis, including heterogeneity, cystic or hemorrhagic changes, high Hounsfield density (>10 HU) on CT, marked enhancement with intravenous contrast, delayed contrast washout (less than 60% at 10 minutes), or a high signal intensity on a T2-weighted MRI. It should be noted that a pheochromocytoma with lipid degeneration can result in low attenuation scores (<10 HU) and more than 60% washout in delayed CT scanning, which can appear similar to adrenal adenomas [10]. Characteristic features of benign adrenal adenomas include a size less than 5 cm, sharp margins, lack of significant growth on serial imaging, low attenuation scores, and more than 60% washout by delayed CT [8, 11]. Our patient's initial imaging was not concerning for pheochromocytoma, largely because of the small size of the mass. Serial CT imaging showed a progressive increase in size, and the most recent scan showed a Hounsfield density of 40 HU. Additionally, MRI showed a hyperintense T2 signal, isotense T1 signal without drop of signal on out-of-phase images, and homogenous enhancement postcontrast.

In our patient, ^{123}I-MIBG scintigraphy showed abnormal focal radiotracer accumulation in the left adrenal lesion with no other foci. MIBG is a compound that resembles norepinephrine and is actively concentrated within the

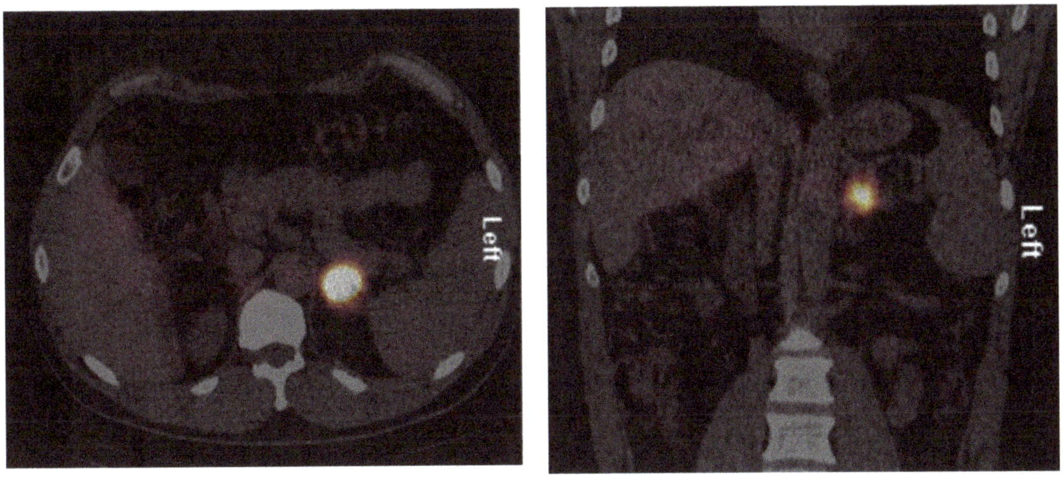

(a) (b)

FIGURE 2: ^{123}I-metaiodobenzylguanidine (MIBG) scintigraphy scan showed abnormal focalintense radiotracer accumulation in the left adrenal lesion

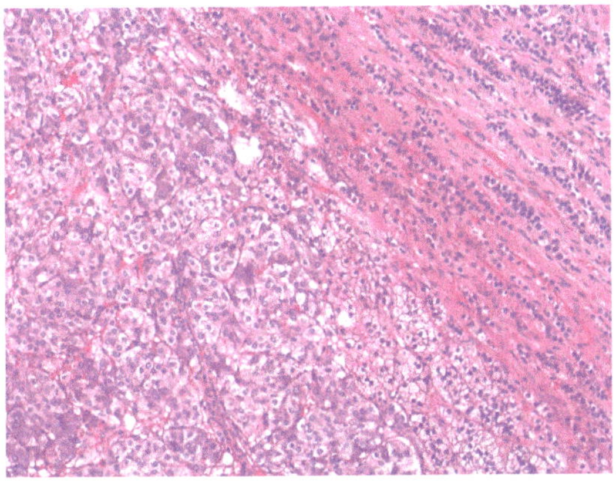

FIGURE 3: Histology demonstrates the well-circumscribed nature of the typical pheochromocytoma. There is an abrupt and distinct border between the pheochromocytoma on the left and the surrounding normal adrenal gland on the right. The tumor has the typical low-power architecture with cells arranged in nests and cords.

sympathomedullary tissue. ^{123}I-MIBG scintigraphy may be useful for identification of tumors missed by MRI or CT. It can also be used for identifying catecholamine-secreting paragangliomas, multifocality, or multiple smaller masses throughout the body, such as metastasis [12, 13].

One contributing factor for our patient's initial negative biochemical profile could be the relatively small tumor size. The average size of pheochromocytomas at the time of diagnosis is 4.9 cm, and there is evidence that tumor size correlates with the hormone level [14]. Even with relatively large pheochromocytomas though, there are reasons why a patient may be asymptomatic. A large tumor can have only a small amount of functional tissue, or rapid turnover in the tumor may result in the release of predominantly metabolized catecholamines. A tumor may be stress-activated or only secrete catecholamines episodically. There can also be false-negative laboratory results because of handling the sample at a high room temperature or due to caffeine ingestion within 24 hours prior to testing [15].

4. Conclusions

The early diagnosis of pheochromocytoma is important because if unrecognized, it can lead to high morbidity and mortality. Our patient demonstrated an asymptomatic incidentaloma that was biochemically negative for the first few years after identification. Follow-up imaging, including CT and MRI, showed findings suspicious for pheochromocytoma, and the diagnosis was ultimately made with the combination of imaging and laboratory studies. This case shows how CT and MRI findings can alert providers to the presence of a pheochromocytoma, even in an asymptomatic, biochemically negative patient.

Disclosure

This abstract was presented as a poster at the 2018 Endocrine Society meeting in Chicago.

References

[1] J. W. M. Lenders, Q.-Y. Duh, G. Eisenhofer et al., "Pheochromocytoma and paraganglioma: an endocrine society clinical practice guideline," *The Journal of Clinical Endocrinology & Metabolism*, vol. 99, no. 6, pp. 1915–1942, 2014.

[2] G. H. Anderson Jr., N. Blakeman, and D. H. P. Streeten, "The effect of age on prevalence of secondary forms of hypertension in 4429 consecutively referred patients," *Journal of Hypertension*, vol. 12, no. 5, pp. 609–615, 1994.

[3] J. W. Lenders, K. Pacak, M. M. Walther et al., "Biochemical diagnosis of pheochromocytoma: which test is best?" *JAMA*, vol. 287, no. 11, pp. 1427–1434, 2002.

[4] E. L. Bravo and R. W. Gifford Jr., "Pheochromocytoma: di-

agnosis, localization and management," *New England Journal of Medicine*, vol. 311, no. 20, pp. 1298-1303, 1984.
[5] Y. Y. Chen, "Pheochromocytoma presenting with normal urinary catecholamines and metabolites: a case report," *Formosan Journal of Endocrinology and Metabolism*, vol. 1, pp. 33–37, 2009.
[6] J. A. Lee, R. Zarnegar, W. T. Shen, E. Kebebew, O. H. Clark, and Q. Y. Duh, "Adrenal incidentaloma, borderline elevations of urine or plasma metanephrine levels, and the "subclinical" pheochromocytoma," *Archives of Surgery*, vol. 142, no. 9, pp. 870–874, 2007.
[7] C. R. McHenry, "Pheochromocytoma: a clinical enigma," *AACE Clinical Case Reports*, vol. 3, no. 2, pp. e180–e181, 2017.
[8] D. H. Szolar, M. Korobkin, P. Reittner et al., "Adrenocortical carcinomas and adrenal pheochromocytomas: mass and enhancement loss evaluation at delayed contrast-enhanced CT," *Radiology*, vol. 234, no. 2, pp. 479–485, 2005.
[9] J. Baguet, L. Hammer, T. Mazzuco et al., "Circumstances of discovery of phaeochromocytoma: a retrospective study of 41 consecutive patients," *European Journal of Endocrinology*, vol. 150, no. 5, pp. 681–686, 2004.
[10] M. A. Blake, S. K. Krishnamoorthy, G. W. Boland et al., "Low-density pheochromocytoma on CT: a mimicker of adrenal adenoma," *American Journal of Roentgenology*, vol. 181, no. 6, pp. 1663–1668, 2003.
[11] P. Boraschi, G. Braccini, L. Grassi et al., "Incidentally discovered adrenal masses: evaluation with gadolinium enhancement and fat-suppressed MR imaging at 0.5 T," *European Journal of Radiology*, vol. 24, no. 3, pp. 245–252, 1997.
[12] E. L. Bravo, "Pheochromocytoma: new concepts and future trends," *Kidney International*, vol. 40, no. 3, pp. 544–556, 1991 Sep.
[13] B. Bennett, D. Johnson, A. Panakos, and A. Rozenberg, "Unsuspected pheochromocytoma incidentally found on chest CT," *Radiology Case Reports*, vol. 13, no. 1, pp. 191–196, 2017.
[14] M. A. Guerrero, J. M. J. Schreinemakers, M. R. Vriens et al., "Clinical spectrum of pheochromocytoma," *Journal of the American College of Surgeons*, vol. 209, no. 6, pp. 727–732, 2009.
[15] S. K. Kota, S. K. Kota, S. Panda, and K. D. Modi, "Pheochromocytoma: an uncommon presentation of an asymptomatic and biochemically silent adrenal incidentaloma," *Malaysian Journal of Medical Sciences*, vol. 19, no. 2, pp. 86–89, 2012 Apr.

31

Coincidence of Large Adrenal Cyst and Prominent Hyporeninemic Hyperaldosteronism

Takaaki Sakaue,[1] Yosuke Okuno,[1] Kosuke Mukai,[1] Shingo Fujita,[1] Junji Kozawa,[1] Hitoshi Nishizawa,[1] Taka-Aki Matsuoka,[1] Hiromi Iwahashi,[1,2] Maeda Norikazu,[1,3] Yuto Yamazaki,[4] Hironobu Sasano,[4] Michio Otsuki,[1] and Iichiro Shimomura[1]

[1]*Department of Metabolic Medicine, Osaka University Graduate School of Medicine, Osaka 565-0871, Japan*
[2]*Department of Diabetes Care Medicine, Osaka University Graduate School of Medicine, Osaka 565-0871, Japan*
[3]*Department of Metabolism and Atherosclerosis, Osaka University Graduate School of Medicine, Osaka 565-0871, Japan*
[4]*Department of Pathology, Tohoku University Graduate School of Medicine, Sendai 980-8574, Japan*

Correspondence should be addressed to Yosuke Okuno; wokuno@endmet.med.osaka-u.ac.jp and Michio Otsuki; otsuki@endmet.med.osaka-u.ac.jp

Academic Editor: Mihail A. Boyanov

A 67-year-old Japanese woman who had end-stage renal disease was referred to our hospital for kidney transplantation. Abdominal CT revealed a large adrenal mass with inhomogeneity. She had a history of hospitalization for stroke and heart failure and exhibited prominent hyporeninemic hyperaldosteronism. Histological examination of the resected tumor with anti-CYP11B2 antibody indicated that she had a vascular endothelial cyst with primary aldosteronism (PA) due to multiple adrenocortical micronodules. This report implicates the pathological interaction between adrenal vascular cysts and PA-mediated vascular damage of the adrenal vein.

1. Introduction

Adrenal cysts are rare and form a heterogeneous group of lesions. Their incidence in autopsy has been reported to be 0.064–0.18% [1]. However, the frequency with which they are disclosed appears to be increasing because of improved radiological imaging techniques such as computed tomography (CT) and magnetic resonance imaging (MRI) [2]. Adrenal vascular endothelial cysts are one of the subtypes of adrenal cysts and associated with vascular damage [3]. Although aldosterone is directly involved in such vascular damage, coincidence of these two disorders was scarcely reported.

Etiologically, hypertension induced by excess aldosterone secretion features more prominent renal damage than essential hypertension [4]. When not treated appropriately, it eventually leads to end-stage renal disease (ESRD). Under these circumstances, endocrinological examinations are less valuable because of aberrant hormone metabolism and the risk of confirmation tests.

We herein present a case of combination of large adrenal endothelial cyst and prominent hyporeninemic hyperaldosteronism with ESRD where immunohistological examination was useful.

2. Case Presentation

A 67-year-old Japanese woman was referred to our hospital for renal replacement therapy and kidney transplantation. She had been diagnosed as hypertension at her late 20s, but blood pressure was poorly controlled despite treatment with antihypertensive drugs without an aldosterone antagonist. She had a history of hospitalization for stroke at 48 years old and heart failure at 53 years old. She was administrated with warfarin for atrial fibrillation. She was diagnosed as diabetes at 62 years old, but her glycemia was well-controlled with linagliptin. Her renal function had gradually impaired, most likely due to nephrosclerosis. In April 2018, her estimated glomerular filtration rate (eGFR) was 7 ml/min/1.73 m^2.

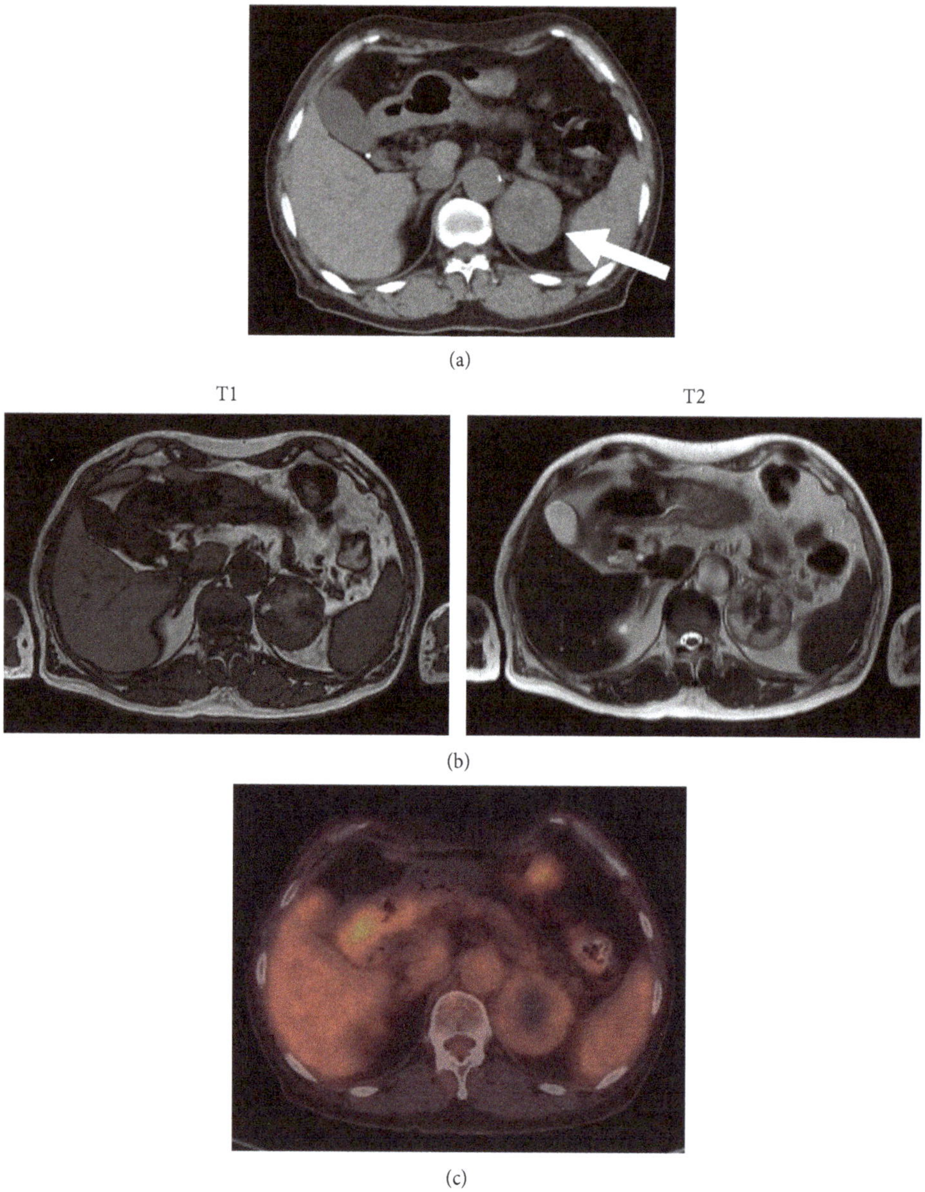

FIGURE 1: (a) Abdominal plain CT. Arrow: left adrenal mass (52 mm × 50 mm). (b) T1-weighed (left) and T2-weighed (right) images of plain MRI. (c) PET-CT.

During the checkup for kidney transplantation, abdominal CT revealed a left adrenal mass, which was 5 cm in diameter with inhomogeneity of density and smooth borders (Figure 1(a)). She was admitted in August 2018 for endocrinological examination.

On admission, her blood pressure was 133/89 mmHg with 5 mg amlodipine, 60 mg azosemide, and 0.625 mg bisoprolol fumarate. She had no Cushingoid appearances. The plasma parameters are shown in Table 1. Her serum potassium level was at the lower limit of normal despite ESRD. She exhibited prominent hyporeninemic hyperaldosteronism. The plasma aldosterone concentration (PAC) was 514.9 pg/ml, and plasma renin activity (PRA) was <0.2 ng/ml/hr, but we could not perform saline infusion test nor captopril challenge test in afraid of deteriorating renal function and heart failure. The plasma ACTH level and serum cortisol level were within normal limits. The serum dehydroepiandrosterone-sulfate (DHEA-S) level was below the lower limit of normal. The midnight serum cortisol level was above 5 μg/dl. Overnight 1 mg dexamethasone suppression test could not suppress the serum cortisol level below 3 μg/dl. Twenty-four-hour urinary excretion of cortisol was below the detection limit. Twenty-four-hour urinary excretion of catecholamines and their metabolites did not exceed normal limits. The serum testosterone and estradiol levels were within normal limits.

High-intensity in T1-weighted images (T1WI) and low-intensity in T2WI of abdominal MRI suggested bleeding in the adrenal mass (Figure 1(b)). ^{123}I-metaiodobenzylguanidine (MIBG) was not uptaken into the adrenal mass (data not shown). On the positron emission tomography with fluorodeoxyglucose (FDG-PET), the mass

Table 1: Plasma parameters.

Blood sample: on admission					
WBC	4.52×10^3	/μL	RBC	4.41×10^6	/μL
Hb	11.9	g/dL	Plt	187×10^3	/μL
Creatinine	6.61	mg/dL	eGFR	5.4	ml/min/1.73 m^2
Na	144	mEq/L	K	3.7	mEq/L
PRA	≦0.2	ng/mL/hr	PAC	514.9	pg/mL
ACTH	25	pg/mL	Cortisol	14.5	μg/dL
DHEA-S	25	μg/dL	Estradiol	<14.0	ng/mL
Testosterone	0.24	ng/mL	HbA1c	5.6	%
Urine sample					
U-adrenaline	1.08	μg/day	U-VMA	2.16	mg/day
U-noradrenaline	55.26	μg/day	U-metanephrine	0.036	mg/day
U-dopamine	100.8	μg/day	U-normetanephrine	0.126	mg/day
U-cortisol	Below the detection limit				
Diurnal profile of ACTH and cortisol					
Time	6:00	23:00			
ACTH (pg/mL)	23	7			
Cortisol (μg/dL)	16.4	6.9			
Low-dose dexamethasone suppression test					
	After 1 mg				
ACTH (pg/mL)	2				
Cortisol (μg/dL)	4.5				
Blood sample: one month after surgery					
K	4.4	mEq/L	eGFR	5.1	ml/min/1.73 m^2
PRA	≦0.2	ng/mL/hr	PAC	533.6	pg/mL
ACTH	31	pg/mL	Cortisol	13.5	μg/dL
DHEA-S	3.8	μg/dL			

had activity less than that of the liver (Figure 1(c)). Considering the size above 4 cm and bleeding inside, the tumor was laparoscopically resected for suspected malignancy. After surgery, PAC, PRA, plasma ACTH, and serum cortisol remained almost unchanged, while blood pressure was decreased to 108/70 mmHg and serum potassium level was increased to 4.4 mEq/L (Table 1).

On gross inspection, the tumor exhibited multiple nodular solid lesions with prominent bleeding (Figure 2). The blood tumor was an adrenal vascular endothelial cyst surrounded by CD31-positive/PDPN-negative endothelial lining and papillary hyperplasia (Figure 3(a)). There was no arteriovenous malformation. As a possible source of hyperaldosteronism, CYP11B2-positive multiple adrenocortical micronodules (MN) surrounded by hyperplastic zona glomerulosa without diffuse overexpression of CYP11B2 were identified (Figure 3(b)). The expression of dehydroepiandrosterone sulfotransferase (DHEA-ST) in zona reticularis was normal (Figure 3(c)).

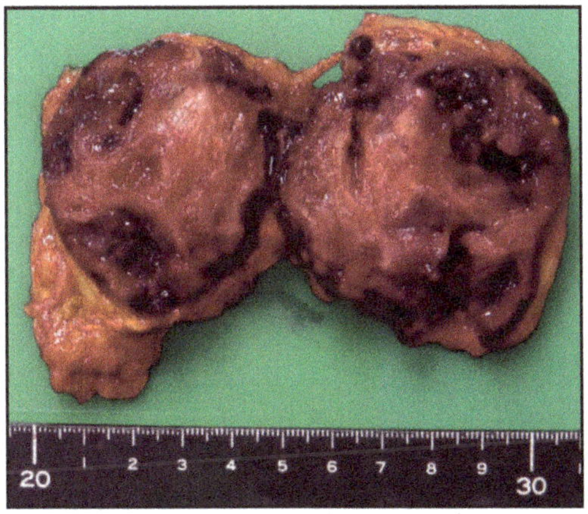

Figure 2: Gross inspection of the resected tumor.

3. Discussion

In this paper, we report the unique case of prominent hyporeninemic hyperaldosteronism with a large vascular endothelial cyst. The coincidence of hyporeninemic hyperaldosteronism and adrenal cyst was reported only in one case report, where primary aldosteronism (PA) by adrenal adenoma was combined with ipsilateral pseudocyst [5].

The cause of adrenal vascular endothelial cysts and pseudocysts is not clear, but they are considered to originate from prior hemorrhage from pre-existing vascular hamartoma or adrenal vein [3, 6]. As aldosterone is known to be directly involved in vascular damage [7] and hemodynamics within the tissue [8], it might attribute to such adrenal hemorrhages. For example, intra-adrenal veins are considered to be uniquely fragile in patients with PA, from the fact that extremely high rate of intra-adrenal hemorrhage was experienced specifically in adrenal venography of PA [9]. As a possible mechanism, mineralocorticoid receptor was expressed in vascular smooth muscle cells (VSMC) [10] and direct mineralocorticoid effect on vascular tone and contractility has been suggested [11-13]. Aldosterone also stimulates fibroblast-mediated fibrosis in a vascular matrix

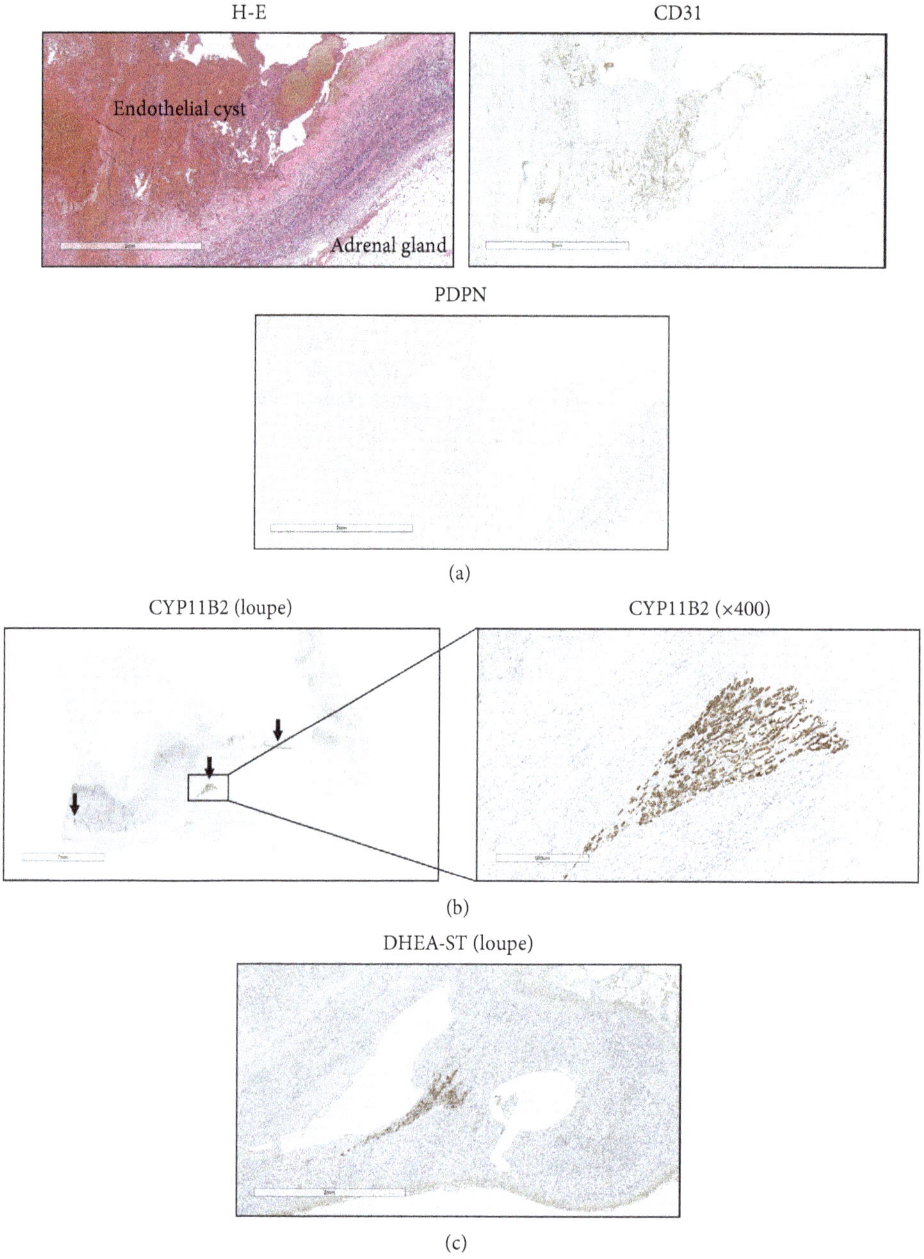

FIGURE 3: (a) H-E staining (H-E) immunostaining with anti-CD31 antibody (CD31) or anti-PDPN (D2-40) antibody (PDPN) of the resected tumor (magnification: x200). (b) Immunostaining of the resected tumor with anti-CD11B2 antibody. Left: loupe, right: x400 magnification. Arrow: CYP11B2-positive regions. (c) Immunostaining with anti-DHEA-ST antibody of the adjacent adrenal gland (magnification: x20).

[14–16]. PA not only increases intravascular volume in the whole body [17] but also decreases local vascular resistance, at least in the kidney [8], which may increase the flow volume in the tissue. Analogically, PA might also increase the flow volume of the adrenal vein and make it prone to hemorrhage. In this case, hemorrhagic diathesis by warfarin would be attributed to adrenal hemorrhages. ESRD may also be attributed to vascular cysts, as congestion or hemorrhage was frequently observed in the adrenal of patients with ESRD in an autopsy analysis [18].

In patients with ESRD, it is difficult to evaluate autonomous aldosterone secretion. The aldosterone-to-renin ratio (ARR) is elevated in chronic renal disease [19], and saline infusion test or captopril challenge test need caution as they might exaggerate the renal impairment. In this case, we could not endocrinologically diagnose but strongly suspected PA from poorly controlled hypertension, multiple PA-related complications, and low serum potassium despite ESRD, together with prominent hyporeninemic hyperaldosteronism. Identification of CYP11B2-positive lesions surrounded by hyperplastic zona glomerulosa further supported this speculation [20]. In this case, as serum potassium level and blood pressure were improved after surgery, significant amount of aldosterone may be produced by the same side of adrenal. Although hyporeninemic hyperaldosteronism still existed after removal of the left adrenal containing CYP11B-positive lesions, it was not surprising as the majority of MN is bilateral [21]. If this case was PA, aldosterone concentration would be much higher in the adrenal vein than in the blood, which further accelerated the formation of adrenal endothelial cyst.

It is also challenging to evaluate autonomous cortisol secretion in ESRD. The morning plasma cortisol is higher, and 1 mg dexamethasone fails to suppress plasma total cortisol in patients with chronic renal failure [22]. The serum DHEA-S level is decreased in hemodialysis patients [23]. In this case, the possibility of coexisting subclinical Cushing syndrome could not be ruled out by dexamethasone suppression test or midnight serum cortisol, but was unlikely from the normal expression of DHEA-ST in zona reticularis. We assumed that the patient was in the pseudo-Cushing state caused by ESRD.

This case implicated the pathological interaction between adrenal vascular cyst and aldosterone-mediated vascular damage or hemodynamics of adrenal vein and showed the usefulness of immunohistochemistry to understand the endocrinological state in ESRD.

LH: luteinizing hormone, FSH: follicle-stimulating hormone, PRL: prolactin, ACTH: adrenocorticotropic hormone, DHEA-S: dehydroepiandrosterone-sulfate, TSH: thyroid stimulating hormone, FT3: free triiodothyronine, FT4: free thyroxine, PRA: plasma renin activity, PAC: plasma aldosterone concentration, and U-VMA: urinary vanillyl mandelic acid.

Disclosure

This research was performed as part of the employment of the authors by Iichiro Shimomura.

Authors' Contributions

Iichiro Shimomura was involved in manuscript editing.

References

[1] L. M. Neri and F. C. Nance, "Management of adrenal cysts," *The American Surgeon*, vol. 65, no. 2, pp. 151–163, 1999.

[2] J. Fan, J. Tang, J. Fang et al., "Ultrasound imaging in the diagnosis of benign and suspicious adrenal lesions," *Medical Science Monitor : International Medical Journal of Experimental and Clinical Research*, vol. 20, pp. 2132–2141, 2014.

[3] E. Carvounis, A. Marinis, N. Arkadopoulos, T. Theodosopoulos, and V. Smyrniotis, "Vascular adrenal cysts: a brief review of the literature," *Archives of Pathology & Laboratory Medicine*, vol. 130, no. 11, pp. 1722–1724, 2006.

[4] G. P. Rossi, G. Bernini, G. Desideri et al., "Renal damage in primary aldosteronism," *Hypertension*, vol. 48, no. 2, pp. 232–238, 2006.

[5] M. Watanabe, H. Matsuura, T. Oshima et al., "Primary aldosteronism with ipsilateral adrenal cyst: report of a case," *Endocrine Journal*, vol. 40, no. 5, pp. 619–624, 1993.

[6] A. Kawashima, C. M. Sandler, R. D. Ernst et al., "Imaging of nontraumatic hemorrhage of the adrenal gland," *Radiographics*, vol. 19, no. 4, pp. 949–963, 1999.

[7] D. Duprez, M. De Buyzere, E. R. Rietzschel, and D. L. Clement, "Aldosterone and vascular damage," *Current Hypertension Reports*, vol. 2, no. 3, pp. 327–334, 2000.

[8] L. A. Sechi, A. Di Fabio, M. Bazzocchi, A. Uzzau, and C. Catena, "Intrarenal hemodynamics in primary aldosteronism before and after treatment," *The Journal of Clinical Endocrinology & Metabolism*, vol. 94, no. 4, pp. 1191–1197, 2009.

[9] J. J. Bookstein, J. Conn, and S. R. Reuter, "Intra-adrenal hemorrhage as a complication of adrenal venography in primary aldosteronism," *Radiology*, vol. 90, no. 4, pp. 778-779, 1968.

[10] Y. Takeda, I. Miyamori, S. Inaba et al., "Vascular aldosterone in genetically hypertensive rats," *Hypertension*, vol. 29, no. 1, pp. 45–48, 1997.

[11] L. Tobian and P. D. Redleaf, "Effect of hypertension on arterial wall electrolytes during desoxycorticosterone administration," *American Journal of Physiology-Legacy Content*, vol. 189, no. 3, pp. 451–454, 1957.

[12] T. R. Hansen and D. F. Bohr, "Hypertension, transmural pressure, and vascular smooth muscle response in rats," *Circulation Research*, vol. 36, no. 5, pp. 590–598, 1975.

[13] L. Kornel, "The role of vascular steroid receptors in the control of vascular contractility and peripheral vascular resistance," *The Journal of Steroid Biochemistry and Molecular Biology*, vol. 45, no. 1-3, pp. 195–203, 1993.

[14] A. Benetos, P. Lacolley, and M. E. Safar, "Prevention of aortic fibrosis by spironolactone in spontaneously hypertensive rats," *Arteriosclerosis, Thrombosis, and Vascular Biology*, vol. 17, no. 6, pp. 1152–1156, 1997.

[15] R. MacFadyen, C. S. Barr, and A. D. Struthers, "Aldosterone blockade reduces vascular collagen turnover, improves heart rate variability and reduces early morning rise in heart rate in heart failure patients," *Cardiovascular Research*, vol. 35, no. 1, pp. 30–34, 1997.

[16] Y. Sun, F. J. Ramires, and K. T. Weber, "Fibrosis of atria and great vessels in response to angiotensin II or aldosterone infusion," *Cardiovascular Research*, vol. 35, no. 1, pp. 138–147, 1997.

[17] R. C. Tarazi, M. M. Ibrahim, E. L. Bravo, and H. P. Dustan, "Hemodynamic characteristics of primary aldosteronism," *New England Journal of Medicine*, vol. 289, no. 25, pp. 1330–1335, 1973.

[18] A. N. Elias, N. D. Vaziri, S. Farooqui, D. C. Martin, and M. K. Mirahmadi, "Pathology of endocrine organs in chronic renal failure-an autopsy analysis of 66 patients," *The International Journal of Artificial Organs*, vol. 7, no. 5, pp. 251–256, 1984.

[19] R. J. Hené, P. Boer, H. A. Koomans, and E. J. Dorhout Mees, "Plasma aldosterone concentrations in chronic renal disease," *Kidney International*, vol. 21, no. 1, pp. 98–101, 1982.

[20] S. Boulkroun, B. Samson-Couterie, J.-F. G. Dzib et al., "Adrenal cortex remodeling and functional zona glomerulosa hyperplasia in primary aldosteronism," *Hypertension*, vol. 56, no. 5, pp. 885–892, 2010.

[21] Y. Yamazaki, Y. Nakamura, K Omata et al., "Histopathological classification of cross-sectional image-negative hyperaldosteronism," *The Journal of Clinical Endocrinology and Metabolism*, vol. 102, no. 4, pp. 1182–1192, 2017.

[22] E. Z. Wallace, P. Rosman, N. Toshav, A. Sacerdote, and A. Balthazar, "Pituitary-adrenocortical function in chronic

renal failure: studies of episodic secretion of cortisol and dexamethasone suppressibility," *The Journal of Clinical Endocrinology & Metabolism*, vol. 50, no. 1, pp. 46–51, 1980.

[23] R. Kakiya, T. Shoji, T. Hayashi et al., "Decreased serum adrenal androgen dehydroepiandrosterone sulfate and mortality in hemodialysis patients," *Nephrology Dialysis Transplantation*, vol. 27, no. 10, pp. 3915–3922, 2012.

32

Falsely Elevated 25-Hydroxy-Vitamin D Levels in Patients with Hypercalcemia

Moon Kyung Choi,[1] **Prapaipan Putthapiban**,[1] **and Patamaporn Lekprasert**[2]

[1]*Department of Internal Medicine, Einstein Medical Center Philadelphia, 5501 Old York Road, Philadelphia, PA 19141, USA*
[2]*Department of Endocrinology, Einstein Endocrine Associates, 50 East Township Line Road Medical Arts Building, Suite G01, Elkins Park, PA 19027, USA*

Correspondence should be addressed to Moon Kyung Choi; moonkyungchoi7@gmail.com

Academic Editor: Osamu Isozaki

Symptomatic hypercalcemia is a commonly encountered clinical scenario. Though it is important to collect detailed history to find clinical clues connecting to the etiology of hypercalcemia, the diagnostic workup of hypercalcemia depends heavily on laboratory analysis. Accurate measurement of the parathyroid hormone and vitamin D levels is essential. However, commercial laboratory measurement of vitamin D levels can be erroneous in the setting of abundant paraprotein in the serum. One of the most common conditions that can cause an increased amount of paraproteins is multiple myeloma. We report 2 cases of falsely elevated 25-hydroxy-vitamin D levels in patients presenting with hypercalcemia and an underlying diagnosis of MM.

1. Introduction

Hypercalcemia is a well-established complication in patients with multiple myeloma (MM). Hypercalcemia due to MM is mediated by increased production of osteoclast-activating paracrine molecules by the tumor cells. Even in patients with underlying MM who present with hypercalcemia, measurement of the parathyroid hormone (PTH) and 25-hydroxy-vitamin D (25 (OH)-vit D) levels is integral for complete diagnostic investigation. Unfortunately, commercial laboratory analysis of the 25-hydroxy-vitamin D level carries limitations. This possibility of laboratory error is often overlooked by clinicians which may lead to invalid interpretation of laboratory results. Here, we describe 2 cases of erroneously elevated 25-hydroxy-vitamin D levels in MM patients presenting with symptomatic hypercalcemia.

2. Case Presentation

2.1. Case 1. A 65-year-old woman with a past medical history of hypertension and MM presented with fatigue. She was not started on treatment for MM except for recent radiation therapy to a metastatic lesion in the thoracic spine. Laboratory analysis was notable for chronic anemia (hemoglobin 7.0 g/dL, normal 12–16 g/dL), acute kidney injury (creatinine 3.1 mg/dL, normal 0.6–1.0 mg/dL), and serum calcium level of 16.6 mg/dL (corrected calcium 18.0 mg/dL, normal 8.4–10.3 mg/dL). Total protein level was elevated to 11.1 g/dL (normal 6–8.3 g/dL), and gamma globulin level was 6.0 g/dL (normal 0.6–1.6 g/dL). As there was no worsening of patient's anemia from her personal baseline, her fatigue was attributed to hypercalcemia. Further blood work revealed a PTH level of 8.0 pg/mL (normal 9–73 pg/mL). 25 (OH)-vit D level was >96.0 ng/mL via immunoassay with a reference normal range of 30 to 50 ng/mL. 1,25-Dihyroxy-vitamin D level was 12 pg/mL (normal 18–72 pg/mL). PTH-related protein (PTHrP) level was 12 pg/mL (normal 14–27 pg/mL). These laboratory findings indicated that the patient had PTH and PTHrP-independent hypercalcemia. The elevated 25 (OH)-vit D level suggested vitamin D toxicity. However, the patient was not on any vitamin D supplements, and the clinical suspicion for vitamin D intoxication was very low. To evaluate for laboratory error, 25 (OH)-vit D level was measured via liquid chromatography-tandem mass spectrometry (LC-MS/MS) which revealed a normal value of 46 ng/mL (normal 30–100 ng/mL). Based on low PTH level, normal 25 (OH)-vit D level, low 1,25-dihydroxy-vitamin D level, and low PTHrP level, the patient was diagnosed with hypercalcemia secondary to multiple myeloma. Her hypercalcemia was treated with intravenous fluids, calcitonin, and zoledronic acid. The patient's hypercalcemia showed a good response to treatment in the following days.

2.2. Case 2. A 72-year-old man with MM receiving melphalan and dexamethasone for palliation presented with confusion. His other comorbidities were hypertension, paroxysmal atrial fibrillation, chronic systolic heart failure, and a history of ischemic stroke. The family provided medical history on the patient's behalf. The patient had complained of thirst few hours ago and then became disoriented. Family members have not observed any focal weakness or dysarthria. The patient had not mentioned chest pain or shortness of breath. Initial blood work showed chronic anemia (hemoglobin 7.7 g/dL), acute kidney injury (creatinine 1.3 mg/dL), and hypercalcemia 14.9 mg/dL (corrected calcium 16.1 mg/dL). Total protein level was increased to 12.3 g/dL. A CT head scan did not reveal any acute disease process. Further investigation revealed a PTH level of 16.2 pg/mL and 25 (OH)-vit D level >96.0 ng/mL via immunoassay. 1,25-Dihyroxy-vitamin D and PTHrP levels were not measured. Similar to the previous case, the patient was not on any vitamin D supplements, and this raised concerns of an erroneous measurement of the 25 (OH)-vit D level. 25 (OH)-vit D level was measured again by LC-MS/MS and was found to be in the normal range (68 ng/mL). Normal PTH and 25 (OH)-vit D levels supported the high clinical suspicion for hypercalcemia secondary to MM. The patient's hypercalcemia improved when treated with intravenous fluid, calcitonin, and zoledronic acid. He was also continued on a palliative regimen for MM including dexamethasone. The patient's hypercalcemia and disorientation improved, and he was safely discharged to a nursing facility.

3. Discussion

25 (OH)-vit D level is widely accepted as a standard value representing the vitamin D status of a patient. Various methods are utilized to measure 25 (OH)-vit D levels such as automated immunoassay, competitive protein-binding assay, and LC-MS/MS [1]. Among these different methods, automated immunoassay is the most commonly used technique in commercial laboratories [2].

The initial measurements of the 25 (OH)-vit D level for the above 2 cases were carried out by Abbott Architect i2000 automated immunoassay. In the Architect i2000 immunoassay method, sheep polyclonal anti-vitamin D IgG is incubated with patient's serum. After sheep polyclonal anti-vitamin D IgG binds to 25 (OH)-vit D in the sample, chemiluminescence-labeled 25-hydroxy-vitamin D is added. Excess sheep polyclonal anti-vitamin D IgG that was not bound to 25 (OH)-vit D in the sample will bind to this exogenous vitamin D. After washing, only sheep anti-vitamin D IgG that is bound to exogenous vitamin D will emit chemiluminescence. Thus, the amount of chemiluminescence will be inversely associated with the quantity of 25 (OH)-vit D in the sample.

The repeat measurements of 25 (OH)-vit D levels were carried out by the AB SCIEX 6500 LC-MS/MS system. LC-MS/MS is largely accepted as the most accurate method of measuring 25 (OH)-vit D levels [1]. During LC-MS/MS, 25 (OH)-vit D is separated from other potential interfering molecules via chromatography. We hypothesize that the abundant paraprotein from MM may have interfered with the binding of sheep polyclonal anti-vitamin D IgG in the immunoassay. The abundant paraprotein may have had cross-reactivity to sheep polyclonal anti-vitamin D IgG, thus decreasing the amount of chemiluminescence. Total protein level was elevated in both cases, pointing to the abundance of the paraprotein from underlying MM. Cross-reactivity is a well-described interference in all immunoassays regardless of the measured molecule [3]. Further studies are required to investigate whether the concentration and cross-reactivity of paraproteins both affect the likelihood of laboratory error in 25 (OH)-vit D quantification.

We found 2 previous case reports of laboratory interference in the immunoassay measurement of 25 (OH)-vit D levels [2, 4]. Similar to our cases presented here, Ong et al. suspected that the falsely elevated measure of 25 (OH)-vit D was caused by an increased number of immunoglobulins from MM. In the second case report, immunoglobulins due to MM and rheumatoid factor were both considered as possible interfering molecules. Other serum molecules known to interfere with the 25 (OH)-vit D immunoassay include bilirubin, triglyceride, and anti-animal antibodies [2]. Our 2 patients did not have rheumatologic disease or hypertriglyceridemia. Total bilirubin levels were also normal in both patients.

In conclusion, it is important for clinicians to be aware of the limitations of the immunoassay measurement of the 25 (OH)-vit D level in the setting of MM. Careful interpretation of laboratory data in correlation with clinical manifestation is important. When there is discordance between laboratory data and clinical clues, close collaboration with the laboratory is crucial to perform analysis with alternative methods and evaluate for laboratory interference.

Disclosure

An earlier version of this case series was presented at the ENDO 2019 Conference, New Orleans, LA, 2019.

References

[1] C.-J. Farrell and M. Herrmann, "Determination of vitamin D and its metabolites," *Best Practice & Research Clinical Endocrinology & Metabolism*, vol. 27, no. 5, pp. 675–688, 2013.

[2] M. W. Ong, R. Salota, T. Reeman, M. Lapsley, and L. Jones, "Artefactual 25-OH vitamin D concentration in multiple

myeloma," *Annals of Clinical Biochemistry*, vol. 54, no. 6, pp. 716–720, 2017.
[3] Y. Ismail, A. A. Ismail, and A. A. Ismail, "Erroneous laboratory results: what clinicians need to know," *Clinical Medicine*, vol. 7, no. 4, pp. 357–361, 2007.
[4] N. Belaidi, A. Georges, I. Lacroix et al., "Hypercalcemia and elevated concentration of vitamin D: a case report too easy to be true," *Clinica Chimica Acta*, vol. 457, pp. 123-124, 2016.

33

Case Report and Literature Review of Insulinoma in the Geriatric Population: An 86-Year-Old Female with Syncope of Unknown Origin

Gerry Samantha Eichelberger[1] **Jordan Carbono,**[2] **Zachary Field,**[2] **KanwarAnoop Kainaur,**[3] **and Federico Montalvo**[1,2]

[1]*Florida State University College of Medicine, 1115 W. Call Street, Tallahassee, FL, USA 32304*
[2]*Department of Internal Medicine, Orlando Regional Healthcare, 21 W. Columbia St., Orlando, FL, USA 32806*
[3]*Department of Pathology, Orlando Regional Healthcare, 52 W. Underwood St., Orlando, FL, USA 32806*

Correspondence should be addressed to Gerry Samantha Eichelberger; gse12@my.fsu.edu

Academic Editor: Suat Simsek

Insulinomas are extremely rare pancreatic endocrine tumors. The tumor is characterized by endogenous hypersecretion of insulin and ensuing development of symptoms of neuroglycopenia and the catecholaminergic response. Symptoms may not always be present, particularly in patients compensating appropriately with increased appetites and caloric intake due to low glucose levels. Early localization of the disease is essential to prevent lethal hypoglycemia and timely treatment. This case report and literature review depict the case of a pancreatic insulinoma in an 86-year-old female, an exceptionally rare presentation based on age and absence of clinical symptoms for one or more years prior to hospitalization. Despite its rarity, similar presentations have been reported in the literature and are further outlined with characteristics and treatment plans. This case highlights a unique presentation of insulinoma and suggests the need for clinical vigilance and further study. It also discusses diagnosis, localization, and management of this uncommon disease in patients above the age of seventy-five.

1. Introduction

Pancreatic endocrine tumors are unusual findings. Among pancreatic endocrine tumors, the most common type is an insulinoma. Insulinomas are in fact quite rare with an annual incidence of four cases per million people in the general population [1]. Insulinomas occur more frequently in women than in men, with a 3 : 2 female-to-male ratio [2]. No racial predilection appears to exist. These tumors typically present in the fifth decade of life with a median age of diagnosis of 47 years of age, except in patients with a history of multiple endocrine neoplasia (MEN) type one syndrome, in whom the median age is typical during the second decade of life [3]. Insulinomas are typically sporadic, benign tumors, with a solitary small (<2 cm in diameter) mass [4]. However, 10% of insulinomas are multiple and occur as a part of MEN type one syndrome. The diagnosis is often delayed or missed due to the rarity of insulinomas and nonspecific symptoms.

Most symptomatic patients present with hypoglycemic episodes resulting from inappropriate intermittent insulin secretion by the tumor. Symptoms can include diaphoresis, tremor, palpitations, tachycardia, and neuroglycopenic symptoms such as personality changes, visual disturbances, weakness, confusion, syncope, seizures, and even coma. Diagnosis is achieved by satisfying the criteria of Whipple's triad—hypoglycemia (plasma glucose <50 mg/dL), neuroglycopenic symptoms, and prompt relief of symptoms following the administration of glucose. The gold standard for biochemical diagnosis includes measuring plasma glucose, insulin, C-peptide, and proinsulin during a 72-hour fast. This prolonged fasting test can detect up to 99% of insulinomas. Approximately 65% of patients will experience hypoglycemic episodes within the first 24 hours of fast [5].

Additionally, more than one imaging modality may be necessary for the localization of the tumor. Localization is performed using computed tomography (CT), magnetic resonance imaging (MRI), endoscopic ultrasonography (EUS), intra-arterial calcium stimulation test with hepatic venous sampling or angiography, and arterial stimulation venous sampling (ARVS). Because of their small size, localization is often difficult. Diagnosis of this pathology relies on a high index of suspicion based on clinical findings and symptomatology along with laboratory testing and imaging to aid in localization. Although medical therapy can be used in the initial treatment, surgical removal is often curative and is the standard of care to prevent permanent neurological deficits associated with prolonged hypoglycemia [6]. Nonetheless, surgery in the elderly population, particularly above the age of 75, can present with a greater risk of complications.

2. Case Presentation

An 86-year-old Caucasian female presents to the emergency room after a syncopal episode. She gives a history of multiple syncopal episodes in the past. Her most recent episode was three months ago and resulted in a fracture of her right femur, which was subsequently treated surgically. Detailed cardiac and neurological evaluations at that time were unable to establish a clear etiology for her syncope. The rest of her pertinent past medical history includes essential hypertension, hyperlipidemia, and breast cancer for which she underwent a bilateral mastectomy. Emergency responders found the patient unresponsive with a blood glucose of 38 mg/dL (70–99 mg/dL fasting). The patient received 50 mL of 50% dextrose in water and became responsive. Repeat glucose was 260 mg/dL. Upon further questioning, the patient admitted to skipping lunch to explain her low blood sugar. She also admitted to having multiple falls of unclear etiology during the past year.

At the time of her current admission, vital signs were notable for an elevated blood pressure of 151/70 mmHg. Physical examination, including complete neurological examination, was normal. Postural blood pressure readings did not show any orthostatic hypotension. Basic laboratory studies including a complete metabolic panel and complete blood count were normal except for the glucose level. Glucose was noted to be 125 mg/dL (70–99 mg/dL fasting). Her hemoglobin A_1C was noted to be 4.7% (4–5.6%); C-peptide was noted to be 2.16 ng/mL (0.78–5.19 ng/mL). Additional workup including TSH, electrocardiogram, troponins, and computerized tomography of the head were within normal limits.

Throughout the hospital course, the patient experienced recurrent hypoglycemic episodes. Fasting blood sugar was as low as 56 mg/dL on day three of her hospitalization requiring frequent doses of intravenous dextrose. Eventually, a continuous dextrose infusion was needed to maintain adequate blood glucose levels. The patient was tested for adrenal insufficiency with a morning cortisol level, which was found to be normal. Additionally, she was screened for exogenous hypoglycemic agents including sulfonylurea levels, which were negative.

Finally, the patient underwent a 72-hour fasting trial to assess for an insulinoma. The patient experienced symptomatic hypoglycemia within 48 hours, with a blood glucose of 32 mg/dL. Fasting trial was discontinued and insulin and C-peptide levels were 22.05 uIU/mL (1.90–23.00 uIU/mL) and 3.61 ng/mL (0.78–5.19 ng/mL), respectively, during the time of the hypoglycemic episode. High normal insulin and normal C-peptide levels in conjunction with very low plasma glucose levels strongly indicated the presence of an insulinoma.

Shown in Figure 1, the computerized tomography scans of the chest, abdomen, and pelvis demonstrated a well-defined enhancing pancreatic tail mass highly suggestive of insulinoma. The computerized tomography scans ruled out metastatic disease. The patient underwent elective laparoscopic-assisted pancreatic mass enucleation on day twelve of her hospitalization. Pathology results showed a low-grade well-differentiated noninvasive pancreatic neuroendocrine tumor, 1.5 cm diameter in size with no invasion present and negative margins as depicted in Figure 2.

Postoperatively, blood glucose levels normalized, without requiring any additional dextrose. The patient was discharged three days later. Two months after her hospitalization, the patient continued to show improvement in her clinical symptoms. She did not report any additional syncopal episodes or falls. Follow-up laboratory work demonstrated euglycemia. Repeat insulin and C-peptide levels were not obtained because of symptomatic improvement.

3. Discussion

Insulinomas have variable and nonspecific presentations particularly in the elderly population usually related to the hypoglycemic episodes. This can be attributable to the episodic and intermittent nature of the secretion of insulin from the tumor. Moreover, the pathogenesis of insulinomas remains unclear. In patients with insulinomas, there is continued secretion of insulin despite a low glucose level. Catecholaminergic and neuroglucopenic symptoms aid in reaching the diagnosis. However, due to the wide range of symptoms and severity, insulinomas can go undiagnosed for a substantial length of time. A broad differential diagnosis of syncope in the geriatric population further prevents prompt diagnosis of insulinoma. In fact, the median duration of symptoms before diagnosis remains variable and can be 12–18 months on average or even years in rarer circumstances from the onset of symptoms [7]. Delayed diagnosis and treatment of insulinomas represents a potentially dangerous condition. Early diagnosis prevents cognitive impairment as well as falls and improves the quality of life of elderly patients.

Insulinomas are defined by meeting Whipple's triad including hypoglycemia (plasma glucose <50 mg/dL),

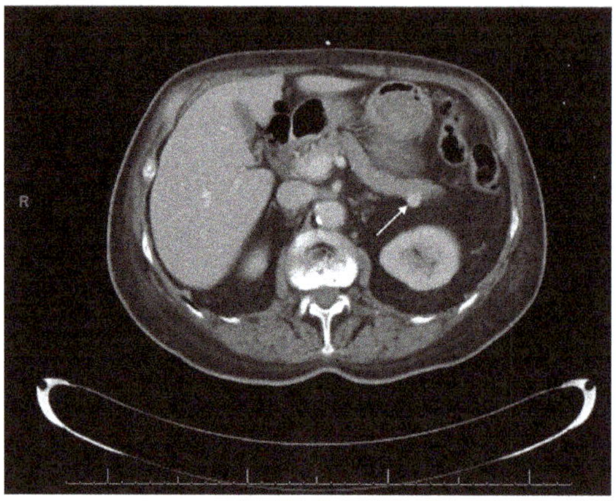

Figure 1: Computerized tomography of the abdomen and pelvis demonstrating enhanced pancreatic tail mass (1.5 cm) suggestive of insulinoma in the setting of unexplained hypoglycemia.

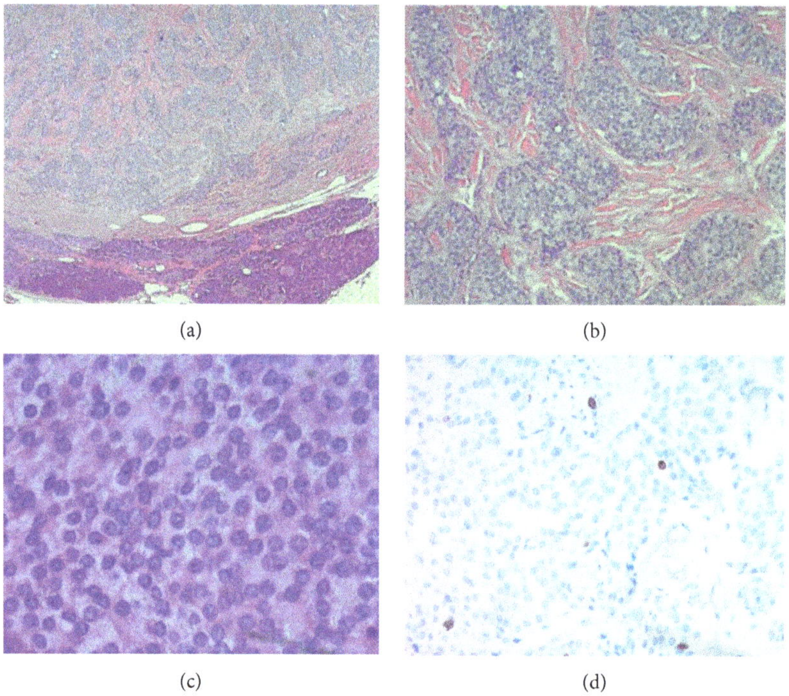

Figure 2: Low-grade pancreatic neuroendocrine tumor. (a) Low-power (20x) view shows a well-circumscribed nested pattern of the tumor cells within the eosinophilic stromal background with adjacent pancreatic parenchyma and (b) 100x view. (c) 400x exhibits uniform nuclei with "salt and pepper" chromatin. (d) 200x shows an immunohistochemical stain for Ki67, which demonstrated 1% reactivity, supporting a low-grade designation.

neuroglycopenic symptoms, and relief of symptoms following the administration of glucose. The 72-hour fasting test remains the gold standard for biochemical diagnosis with measurements of plasma glucose, insulin, C-peptide, and proinsulin levels during the onset of the hypoglycemic episodes. Various imaging modalities may be used to localize the tumor. Imaging type may be limited to what is available at each institution. However, studies have shown a higher sensitivity and preference for helical computerized tomography and endoscopic ultrasound, both of which have up to 94% sensitivity [8]. For most insulinomas, surgery can be curative. Alternatively, medical treatment with octreotide or streptozotocin may be used especially in those with contraindications to surgery or metastatic disease. In cases of malignant insulinomas, an aggressive medical approach is used for enhancing the quality of life by preventing hypoglycemic episodes and improving survival.

Exposure and recognition of an insulinoma case may be limited due to lack of clinical experience amongst healthcare providers. This is especially true in the event of an atypical presentation such as diagnosing insulinomas in the geriatric population. The importance of this case outlines the

TABLE 1: Outline of the literature with insulinoma cases including characteristics of patients, image modality of choice for diagnosis, location of tumor, and treatment plan.

Literature review of insulinomas in elderly patients (above 75 years of age)											
Name of study	Year	Age of presentation	Male vs. fatale	History of multiple endocrine neoplasia	Initial glucose level (mg/dL)	Glucose level within 72-hour fast trial	Imaging modality for diagnosis	Tumor size and location	Metastasis	Surgical management	Medical management
An elderly patient with an insulinoma who had prolonged dementia-like symptoms [12]	1998	77	Female	—	34 mg/dL	—	Abdominal ultrasound; mass not seen on CT or MRI; tumor localized via abdominal arteriography	1 cm tumor localized at the pancreatic tail	—	Pancreatectomy	—
Malignant insulinoma: spectrum of unusual clinical features [13]	2005	82	Female	No	26 mg/dL	—	Abdominal MRI	8.0 cm tumor localized at the dome of the liver	Yes	Percutaneous radiofrequency ablation	—
Successful treatment of insulinoma by a single daily dose of octreotide in two elderly female patients [14]	2006	76	Female	No	—	39 mg/dL after 6 hours	Abdominal angiography	1.5 cm tumor localized at the dome of the liver	No	Refused surgical management	Octreotide 50 μg subcutaneous once daily
Successful treatment of insulinoma by a single daily dose of octreotide in two elderly female patients [14]	2006	85	Female	No	61 mg/dL	37 mg/dL	Abdominal CT	1.5 cm tumor localized at the pancreatic uncus	No	Unsuitable for surgery due to obesity	Initial management was octreotide 100 μg subcutaneous once daily and subsequently reduced to octreotide 50 μg subcutaneous once daily
Pancreatic insulinoma coexisting with gastric GIST in the absence of neurofibromatosis 1 [15]	2009	76	Female	No	—	—	Abdominal CT	1.3 cm localized at the pancreatic tail	No	Pancreatectomy	Initial management with diazoxide

Table 1: Continued.

Literature review of insulinomas in elderly patients (above 75 years of age)											
Insulinoma in the elderly: a report of 3 cases and review literature [11]	2014	82	Female	Yes	—	—	Abdominal MRI	Unknown size; location initially pancreas with metastasis to liver	Yes	Pancreatectomy w/ partial hepatectomy (1993); radiofrequency (2004 and 2006); selective angiographic embolization (2010)	Metastasis in 2011: initial management with subcutaneous injection of octreotide 0.1 mg twice a day and switched to long-acting lanreotide 120 mg every four weeks upon discharge; further progression of metastasis in 2012; lanreotide was switched to diazoxide 100 mg three times a day w/ symptomatic improvement
Insulinoma in the elderly: a report of 3 cases and review literature [11]	2014	84	Male	No	—	—	Abdominal MRI	1 cm tumor localized at pancreatic tail that progressed to 2.2 cm in size	No	Refused surgery (2006); received unsuccessful selective embolization (2012)	Octreotide 0.2 mg three times a day
Insulinoma in the elderly: a report of 3 cases and review literature [11]	2014	85	Male	No	—	—	Abdominal MRI	4 cm tumor localized at the pancreatic head	No	Refused surgical management	Initial management with subcutaneous injection of octreotide 0.1 mg twice a day and switched to long-acting lanreotide 120 mg every four weeks upon discharge
Octreotide LAR was useful for avoiding hypoglycemia in an elderly patient with insulinoma [16]	2017	80	Female	No	—	—	—	—	No	Refused surgical management	Initial management with octreotide 50 mg subcutaneous injection every day; subsequently switched to lanreotide 120 mg every 4 weeks

Table 1: Continued.

Literature review of insulinomas in elderly patients (above 75 years of age)											
Insulinoma case report and literature review of insulinoma in 86-year-old female with late onset hypoglycemia of unknown origin	2020	86	Female	No	38 mg/dL	32 mg/dL	Abdominal CT	1.6 cm tumor localized at pancreatic tail	No	Pancreatectomy with enucleation	—

difficulty in diagnosing insulinomas in patients above the age of seventy-five. Syncopal episodes increase during aging with a prevalence of more than 20% in patients above the age of 75 [9]. Multiple etiologies of syncope exist including cardiovascular disease, arrhythmias, orthostatic hypotension, and neurological causes [10]. Risk factors for hypoglycemia in geriatric patients can include baseline dementia, polypharmacy, and inadequate diet, all of which are common characteristics of patients within this age group, making a diagnosis of an insulinoma more challenging [11]. Nonetheless, it is critical for healthcare providers to maintain insulinoma as a potential diagnosis in this patient population. Missing the diagnosis can lead to morbidity and mortality.

Despite the rarity of this disease, clinicians should be aware of the occurrence of insulinomas in the geriatric population, and how the clinical manifestations can widely vary. Table 1 depicts insulinoma cases in the geriatric population reported in the literature. Insulinomas are not restricted to a particular demographic or age group, as demonstrated by this case. While the classic demographic for insulinomas presents between 40 and 60 years of age, this patient presented at 86 years old, illustrating the wide demographic variance. Creating a proper differential diagnosis and having a high clinical index of suspicion will aid in making a diagnosis earlier. Healthcare providers that encounter syncope in the setting of hypoglycemic episodes should still consider the diagnosis of insulinoma in a geriatric patient. Ultimately, the best treatment is surgical removal or enucleation [11].Laparoscopic surgery can be performed; however, in approximately 44% of cases, open exploration was needed presenting greater possibility of complications [17]. Thus, in the geriatric population, particularly in those above the age of 75, the treatment plan can be medical or surgical. Due to the higher risks of surgical and postsurgical complications in this population, patients and physicians should engage in shared medical decision-making. However, with advancements in surgical techniques, more data are necessary to assess the relative risk and mortality from surgical management.

4. Conclusion

Insulinomas are a rare pancreatic endocrine tumor and disease, but can cause severe neurologic damage and complications resulting from repeated hypoglycemia in geriatric patients. Insulinomas are a difficult diagnosis to make and require a high index of clinical suspicion focusing on the significant recurrent hypoglycemic episodes. It is imperative for physicians to keep in mind insulinomas as a rare cause of syncope in patients above the age of 75 with hypoglycemic episodes, as missing the diagnosis can ultimately lead to morbidity and mortality. Patients and physicians should engage in shared medical decision-making of whether to opt for surgical or medical management, especially in the geriatric population who may be particularly vulnerable to complications.

Acknowledgments

The authors thank Dr. Vinayak Purandare, MD, from Florida State University College of Medicine for peer editing the case report.

References

[1] F. J. Service, M. M. McMahon, P. C. O'Brien, and D. J. Ballard, "Functioning insulinoma—incidence, recurrence, and long-term survival of patients: a 60-year study," *Mayo Clinic Proceedings*, vol. 66, no. 7, pp. 771–779, 1991.

[2] D. Andronesi, A. Andronesi, S. Andrei, A. Tonea, and I. Popescu, "Etiopathogeny of the insulinoma," *Annals of Fundeni Hospital*, vol. 13, no. 1-2, pp. 51–57, 2008.

[3] Z. A. Ali, "Insulinoma," 2013, https://emedicine.medscape.com/article/283039-overview.

[4] R. Sotoudehmanesh, A. Hedayat, N. Shirazian et al., "Endoscopic ultrasonography (EUS) in the localization of insulinoma," *Endocrine*, vol. 31, no. 3, pp. 238–241, 2007.

[5] F. J. Service and N. Natt, "The prolonged fast," *The Journal of Clinical Endocrinology & Metabolism*, vol. 85, no. 11, pp. 3973-3974, 2000.

[6] G. J. Abood, A. Go, D. Malhotra, and M. Shoup, "The surgical and systemic management of neuroendocrine tumors of the pancreas," *Surgical Clinics*, vol. 89, no. 1, pp. 249–266, 2016.

[7] K. Bouslama, H. Maghrebi, H. Bedioui, and K. Bouslama, "Pancreatic insulinoma: diagnostic approach and therapeutic modalities," *Journal Africain d'Hépato-Gastroentérologie*, vol. 8, no. 1, pp. 11–15, 2014.

[8] G. McAuley, H. Delaney, J. Colville et al., "Multimodality preoperative imaging of pancreastic insulinomas," *Clinical Radiology*, vol. 60, no. 10, pp. 1039–1050, 2005.

[9] E. S. Soteriades, J. C. Evans, M. G. Larson et al., "Incidence and prognosis of syncope," *New England Journal of Medicine*, vol. 347, no. 12, pp. 878–885, 2002.

[10] P. Goyal and M. S. Maurer, "Syncope in older adults," *Journal of Geriatric Cardiology*, vol. 13, no. 5, pp. 380–386, 2016.

[11] K. Bernaerts, L. Gers, A. Verhaegen, C. D. Block, and L. V. Gaal, "Insulinoma in the elderly: a report of three cases and review literature," *JSM Clinical Case Reports*, vol. 2, no. 1, p. 1020, 2014.

[12] H. Hattori, M. Matsumoto, H. Tsuchiya et al., "An elderly patient with an insulinoma who had prolonged dementia-like symptoms," *Nippon Ronen Igakkai Zasshi. Japanese Journal of Geriatrics*, vol. 35, no. 7, pp. 566–570, 1998.

[13] B. Hirshberg, C. Cochran, M. C. Skarulis et al., "Malignant insulinoma: spectrum of unusual clinical features," *Cancer*, vol. 104, no. 2, pp. 264–272, 2005.

[14] H. Kishikawa, Y. Okada, A. Hirose, T. Tanikawa, K. Kanda, and Y. Tanaka, "Successful treatment o finsulinoma by a single daily dose of octreotide in two elderly female patients," *Endocrine Journal*, vol. 53, no. 1, pp. 79–85, 2006.

[15] E. Alabraba, S. Bramhall, B. O'Sullivan, B. Mahon, and P. Taniere, "Pancreatic insulinoma co-existing with gastric GIST in the absence of neurofibromatosis-1," *World Journal of Surgical Oncology*, vol. 7, no. 1, p. 18, 2009.

[16] A. Kanno, K. Ide, K. Kurita, T. Terano, and K. Yamamoto, "Octreotide LAR was useful for avoiding hypoglycemia in an elderly patient with insulinoma," *Nihon Ronen Igakkai Zasshi. Japanese Journal of Geriatrics*, vol. 54, no. 2, pp. 172–178, 2017.

[17] D. E. Jaroszewski, R. T. Schlinkert, G. B. Thompson, and D. K. Schlinkert, "Laparoscopic localization and resection of insulinomas," *Archives of Surgery*, vol. 139, no. 3, pp. 270–274, 2004.

34

Fast Clinical, but Long-Term, Biochemical Remission after Waterhouse–Friderichsen Syndrome

Igor Alexander Harsch

Department of Internal Medicine II, Division of Endocrinology and Metabolism, Rainweg 68, Saalfeld 07318, Germany

Correspondence should be addressed to Igor Alexander Harsch; iharsch@thueringen-kliniken.de

Academic Editor: Toshihiro Kita

Background. The Waterhouse–Friderichsen Syndrome (WFS) is a course of bacterial meningitis with a lethality rate that is still high today. One hallmark of the clinical course is intravascular coagulopathy. This causes hemorrhagic infarctions in the adrenal glands, rapidly causing a primary adrenal insufficiency. Only few reports highlight the course of the remaining adrenal insufficiency or adrenal restitution in survivors. *Case Presentation.* After 3 weeks in an intensive care unit, a 45-year-old male survived WFS with necroses on the legs and forefeet and with primary adrenal insufficiency confirmed by the ACTH stimulation test. The substitution therapy with hydrocortisone and fludrocortisone could be gradually discontinued after nine months due to a further positive clinical course. Although the patient reported good mental and physical performance further on, the cortisol response in ACTH testing showed tiny incremental rises of the stimulated serum cortisol, but to reach a formally normal level, it took about five years. *Discussion.* The report demonstrates a case with a relatively fast clinical remission. A remission of the corticotrophic response occurred in small increments during an observational period of five years. The data suggest that not only a clinical remission is possible but also a complete biochemical remission, although this process may take a much longer timespan.

1. Introduction

The Waterhouse–Friderichsen Syndrome (WFS) is a rare course of bacterial meningitis. The most common pathogen is the meningococcus *Neisseria meningitidis*. WFS occurs in about 15% of meningococcal septicemia. The clinical course is characterized not only by the neurological symptoms but also by septic shock with intravascular coagulopathy. Petechial and purpuric lesions of the skin are a classical sign of the disease. Furthermore, the coagulopathy typically causes hemorrhagic infarctions in the adrenal glands, rapidly causing a state of adrenal insufficiency [1]. The disorder typically affects young children [2] or people with functional or anatomical hyposplenia or asplenia [3]. With all options of contemporary intensive care medicine, the lethality is still reported at about 90% [4].

Survivors are often handicapped by the consequences of amputations of the extremities and the primary adrenal insufficiency. Adrenal crisis is reported to occur in about 8% of patients with primary adrenal failure, and such events are unpredictable [5]. We report our experience in a 45-year-old male. A Medline research showed no reports on course and expectable duration of adrenal replacement therapy or the chances for a biochemical remission after WFS.

2. Case Presentation

In October 2015, the patient was 45 years old and had been found unconscious but rousable by his colleagues at his workstation. In the emergency room of the nearest clinic, he showed fever, hypotension, and tachycardia, as well as petechiae at the extremities. His mental state soon changed from prostration to coma. He was transferred to the intensive care unit and developed septic shock and multiple organ failure. Vigorous therapy was instituted immediately. He required intubation and mechanical ventilation. Antibiotic therapy was begun with ampicillin/sulbactam; later on, he was treated with ceftriaxone and fosfomycin. High-dose hydrocortisone substitution was initiated, and an Adrenocorticotrophic Hormone (ACTH) test proved pathologic. For circulatory support, catecholamines were necessary for 8 days, and he was in dialysis care for 2 weeks. Meningococci serogroup B could be cultured from blood and cerebrospinal fluid. Necrosis due to the severe circulatory disorder was located at the lateral foot edge, the heels, the toes, and in the interdigital spaces. After one month, the patient could be transferred to a neurological rehabilitation clinic. At the time of transfer, he had a hydrocortisone substitution therapy (30-10-10 mg) and fludrocortisone at 0.1 mg once daily. The patient developed a progressive mummification of the toes. Unfortunately, forefoot amputations had to be performed on both sides.

In February 2016, he underwent plastic surgery of the forefeet with grafting with latissimus dorsi flaps to deal with the tissue necrosis. Apart from the functional limitations caused by the tissue necroses (see Figures 1 and 2; 7 months after the onset of the disease), the forefoot amputations, and consecutive reconstructive surgery, his mental and physical performance was good. Under endocrinological supervision, the cortisone replacement therapy was gradually reduced and halted in July 2016. In retrospect, the mode of infection in the patient remained unclear. There was also no evidence of an impairment of the immune system.

ACTH testing in our clinic was first performed in June 2016 with 250 μg corticotropin as recommended by the Endocrine Society [6]. The testing was always begun between 8.30 and 9.00 a.m. We always used 250 μg Tetracosactid (=25 I. E. ACTH) (Synacthen™, Alfasigma S. p. A., Bologna, Italy) for the testing and measured serum cortisol before, as well as 30 and 60 minutes after, ACTH stimulation. Serum cortisol is measured by an Electro-Chemiluminescence Immuno Assay (ECLIA) (Elecsys Cortisol II; COBAS®).

As established by our reference laboratory, a rise of serum cortisol >21 μg/dl is regarded significant. In June, the basal cortisol value was 9.43 μg/dl, 12.4 μg/dl after 30 minutes and 13.8 μg/dl after 60 minutes, respectively.

According to the recommendations of the Endocrine Society, peak cortisol levels below 500 nmol/l (~18 μg/dl) (assay and laboratory dependent) at 30 or 60 minutes indicate adrenal insufficiency. That being said, the patient was initially instructed to keep his emergency card and supply hydrocortisone in case of infection, trauma, and other situations prone to cause adrenal crisis. Such events did not occur in the further course. The patient reported a continuingly good mental and physical performance, and the ACTH test was repeated 4 months after cortisone withdrawal in October 2016 with a basal cortisol value of 10.7 μg/dl, of 16.5 μg/dl after 30 minutes and of 17.3 μg/dl after 60 minutes of ACTH stimulation. The overview of the further ACTH tests carried out shows that there were tiny incremental rises into the range of the normal stimulation values (>21 μg/dl) in a course of five years (Figure 3).

3. Discussion

Case reports about WFS focus more on the way the patient's life was saved than on the aftermath. Thus, there is only little published data about the chances of functional adrenocortical remission. The data from our repetitive ACTH-testing over 5 years suggest that a steady regeneration of the zona fasciculata (mainly responsible for cortisol production) after the adrenal trauma caused by WFS is possible.

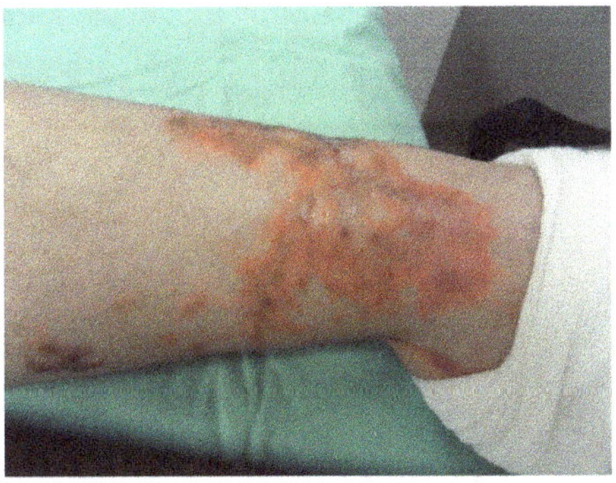

Figure 1: Residuum of tissue necrosis, anterior tibial margin, May 2016.

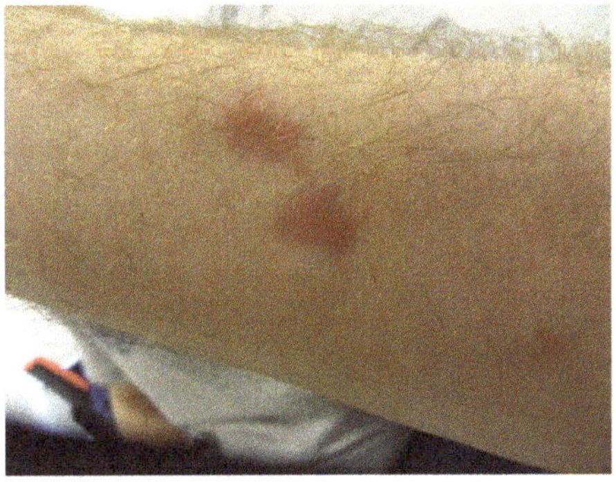

Figure 2: Residuum of skin necrosis, lower thigh, May 2016.

Slightly different normal ranges for cortisol increases 30 and/or 60 minutes after ACTH stimulation are established between different laboratories. Because of these discrepancies, we do not want to focus the discussion on when exactly a complete biochemical remission of the corticotrophic axis occurred again, but on the recognizable tendency towards an increasingly higher stimulability of the cortisol response, as can be seen in Figure 3. With consistent test conditions (i.e., ACTH from the same manufacturer and using the same measuring methods), a coincidence is largely eliminated. Rather, our observations suggest a very slow but steady reconstitution of the adrenal secretion capacity.

In agreement with this finding and according to the available literature, an "intrinsic plasticity" of adrenal tissue is regarded as established. This assumption is based on the presence of adrenal progenitor stem cells continuously repopulating in the adrenal cortex in a corticotropin-responsive pathway. The first studies on this issue stem from 1938 [7] and 1949 [8] with rat models. The experimental approach, also in more recent studies, is the study of rat adrenal secretion and growth during regeneration after adrenal enucleation [9]. However, this raises the issue of transferability of such results from animal to human.

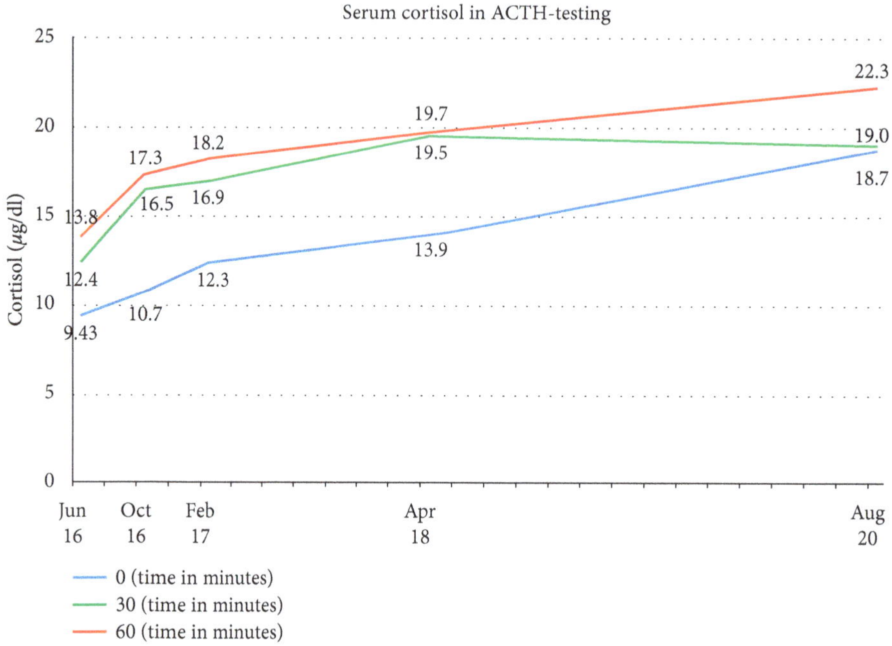

FIGURE 3: Course of serum cortisol in repetitive ACTH testing from June 2016 to August 2020 (x-axis). The blue lines stand for the basal serum cortisol level, the green line represents the serum levels 30 minutes after ACTH stimulation, and the red line represents the serum levels 60 minutes after ACTH stimulation.

In our attempt to gain recent data about humans, we found no publications on the issue of adrenal reconstitution after WFS in a Medline research. A largely comparable situation with no further pathogens influencing adrenal function is tuberculous Addison's disease. In a study of 4 cases, a lack of normalization of adrenocortical function after successful antituberculous chemotherapy has been described in a follow-up of 2–5 years [10]. Recently, patients with autoimmune Addison's disease were treated with Tetracosactide (ACTH 1–24) [11]. Only 2 of 11 patients achieved a clinical remission with peak serum concentrations greater than 400 nmol/l where cortisone replacement therapy could be stopped. One of the 2 patients achieved enduring remission; in the other, steroid replacement therapy had to be restarted after week 64. Two other case reports detail the remission of Addison's disease. In the first case of a 39-year-old male, clinical remission was achieved, but even years after withdrawal of hydrocortisone therapy, the rise of cortisol in an ACTH stimulation test was below the normal value [12].

In the second case, a 23-year-old female was on HC for 11 years, and about one year after withdrawal of HC, the stimulated cortisone was 580 nmol/l after 30 minutes [13].

Although the pathophysiology in autoimmune Addison's disease is different from the direct tissue destruction by hemorrhagic infarction or by tuberculosis, the sum of these data favors the hypothesis that the adrenals may be able to regenerate not only to a degree allowing normal mental and physical performance for the patients. This does not necessarily mean that the adrenal secretion is appropriate in situations of stress. However, our data suggest that not only a clinical remission is possible but also a complete biochemical remission, although this process may take a much longer timespan.

Consent

The patient gave informed consent to report his case.

Acknowledgments

The author is grateful to Andrea Ortloff for the help with the graphical presentation. The author is grateful to Roman Harsch (BA Translation) for language editing.

References

[1] J. Varon, K. Chen, and G. L. Sternbach, "Rupert waterhouse and carl friderichsen: adrenal apoplexy," *The Journal of Emergency Medicine*, vol. 16, no. 4, pp. 643–647, 1998.

[2] C. Friderichsen, "Nebennierenapoplexie bei kleinen Kindern," *Jb Kinderheilk*, vol. 87, pp. 109–125, 1918.

[3] Y. Hata, T. Chiba, M. Ohtani, S. Ishizawa, and N. Nishida, "An autopsy case of pneumococcal waterhouse-friderichsen syndrome with possible functional asplenia/hyposplenia," *International Journal of Clinical and Experimental Pathology*, vol. 8, no. 6, pp. 7518–7525, 2015.

[4] A. Skoczyńska, M. Kadłubowski, J. Knap, M. Szulc, M. Janusz-Jurczyk, and W. Hryniewicz, "Invasive meningococcal disease associated with a very high case fatality rate in the North-West of Poland," *FEMS Immunology and Medical Microbiology*, vol. 46, no. 2, pp. 230–235, 2006.

[5] S. Hahner, M. Loeffler, B. Bleicken et al., "Epidemiology of adrenal crisis in chronic adrenal insufficiency: the need for new prevention strategies," *European Journal of Endocrinology*, vol. 162, no. 3, pp. 597–602, 2010.

[6] S. R. Bornstein, B. Allolio, W. Arlt et al., "Diagnosis and treatment of primary adrenal insufficiency: an endocrine

society clinical practice guideline," *The Journal of Clinical Endocrinology & Metabolism*, vol. 101, no. 2, pp. 364–389, 2016.

[7] D. J. Ingle and G. M. Higgins, "Regeneration of the adrenal gland following enucleation," *The American Journal of the Medical Sciences*, vol. 196, no. 2, pp. 232–239, 1938.

[8] R. O. Greep and H. W. Deane, "Histological, cytochemical and physiological observations on the regeneration of the rat's adrenal gland following enucleation 1," *Endocrinology*, vol. 45, no. 1, pp. 42–56, 1949.

[9] A. Hochol, A. Markowska, V Meneghelli et al., "Effects of neurotensin and bombesin on the secretory and proliferative activity of regenerating rat adrenal cortex," *Histology and Histopathology*, vol. 14, no. 4, pp. 1073–1078, 1999.

[10] E. Bhatia, S. K. Jain, R. K. Gupta, and R. Pandey, "Tuberculous Addison's disease: lack of normalization of adrenocortical function after anti-tuberculous chemotherapy," *Clinical Endocrinology*, vol. 48, no. 3, pp. 355–359, 1998.

[11] E. H. Gan, K. MacArthur, A. L. Mitchell et al., "Residual adrenal function in autoimmune Addison's disease: improvement after Tetracosactide (ACTH1-24) treatment," *The Journal of Clinical Endocrinology & Metabolism*, vol. 99, no. 1, pp. 111–118, 2014.

[12] L. C. C. J. Smans and P. M. J. Zelissen, "Partial recovery of adrenal function in a patient with autoimmune Addison's disease," *Journal of Endocrinological Investigation*, vol. 31, no. 7, pp. 672–674, 2008.

[13] A. J. Chakera and B. Vaidya, "Spontaneously resolving Addison's disease," *QJM*, vol. 105, no. 11, pp. 1113–1115, 2012.

Rare Bilateral Adrenal Haemorrhage with Addisonian Crisis: When Risk Factors Come in Droves

Anders Boisen Jensen[1] **Elise Durand,**[2] **and Vojtech Pavlicek**[1]

[1]*Department of Endocrinology, Kantonsspital Münsterlingen, Spitalcampus 1, 8596 Münsterlingen, Switzerland*
[2]*Department of Radiology, Kantonsspital Münsterlingen, Spitalcampus 1, 8596 Münsterlingen, Switzerland*

Correspondence should be addressed to Anders Boisen Jensen; andersboisen.jensen@kssg.ch

Academic Editor: Carlo Capella

Addisonian crisis is the life-threatening acute manifestation of adrenal insufficiency due to absolute or relative glucocorticoid deficiency. Adrenal haemorrhage is a rare condition of unknown incidence with the risk of adrenal insufficiency and death, not uncommonly first being diagnosed on the pathologists table. We report the case of a 68-year-old female patient with respiratory tract infection suffering acute life-threatening adrenal insufficiency caused by bilateral adrenal haemorrhages following orthopedic surgery while taking anticoagulation therapy. The patient rapidly deteriorated with hypotension, showing how important it is to consider a possible Addisonian crisis when this scenario occurs, especially with precipitating factors such as anticoagulant therapy, sepsis, or surgery.

1. Introduction

Addisonian crisis is the life-threatening acute manifestation of adrenal insufficiency due to absolute or relative glucocorticoid deficiency. Adrenal insufficiency based on pathophysiology can be classified as primary, secondary, or tertiary, where the latter two, also called "central adrenal insufficiency," are caused by insufficient secretion of adrenocorticotropic hormone (ACTH) from the pituitary gland and corticotropin-releasing hormone (CRH) from the hypothalamus, respectively. Primary adrenal insufficiency (Addison's disease) results from destruction of the adrenal cortex and becomes manifest when at least 90% of the adrenal cortical tissue has been destroyed. In the developed countries, autoimmune disease accounts for approximately 80–90% of the cases, with metastatic disease, adrenal haemorrhage or infarction, drugs, and infections accounting for the rest. The yearly incidence in Europe is about 4.4–6.0 new cases per million with a prevalence of 93–144 cases per million [1].

Adrenal haemorrhage is rare with an unknown incidence but with the serious risk of adrenal insufficiency and death, not uncommonly first being diagnosed when an autopsy has taken place due to the nonspecific nature of the symptoms [2]. The diagnosis may be suspected or confirmed in a computed tomography (CT) or magnetic resonance imaging (MRI), demonstrating bilateral adrenal haemorrhage in about 20% of the total cases. The complete and potentially fatal loss of adrenal function after bilateral adrenal bleeding is practically given in every case. Risk factors for adrenal bleeding are advanced age, major surgery (especially cardiovascular and orthopedic surgery), infections (e.g., meningococcemia "Waterhouse-Friderichsen syndrome"), blunt abdominal trauma, significant hypotension, antiphospholipid syndrome, heparin-associated thrombocytopenia (HIT), anticoagulant use, and catecholamine excess (e.g., phaeochromocytoma) [3]. Kovacs et al. reported that, according to a case-control study with 23 patients with massive bilateral adrenal haemorrhage and 92 control patients, the variables with the strongest association with adrenal bleeding were hospital duration, thrombocytopenia, heparin use, sepsis, and hypotension [3]. The incidence of adrenal bleeding on anticoagulation therapy is rare and only a third of the patients with adrenal haemorrhage are anticoagulated [4].

We report the rare case of a patient with acute adrenal insufficiency caused by bilateral adrenal haemorrhage whilst on anticoagulation therapy following orthopedic surgery and a respiratory tract infection, demonstrating how the early diagnose and treatment of an Addisonian crisis can be lifesaving.

2. Case Presentation

A 68-year-old female was admitted to the emergency room from an orthopedic rehabilitation clinic with tiredness, vertigo, nausea, vomiting, and bilateral flank pain for the last three days. Eleven days earlier, she underwent a total knee prosthesis surgery on the left side. Before admission, her blood pressure values from the rehabilitation clinic showed no hypotensive episodes. Due to an atrial fibrillation, the patient was being anticoagulated with phenprocoumon. The phenprocoumon was stopped days prior to her surgery, during which she was anticoagulated with unfractioned heparin, and then restarted a few days postoperatively. There was no record of her suffering any blunt trauma or receiving corticosteroid therapy. Three days before admission, an abdominal ultrasound scan showed no abnormalities in the perirenal regions. Due to an aspiration pneumonia, piperacillin/tazobactam antibiotics had been started three days prior to admission. Clinically the patient was lethargic and apyrexial, her blood pressure hypotensive with 84/57 mm Hg, and her heart rate arrhythmic tachycardic with 138 BPM. No cutaneous or mucosal hyperpigmentation was evident. Her left knee was painless to palpation, slightly warm with swelling but no redness.

The key laboratory findings at admission were hypocortisolism with hypokalemia and hyponatraemia, further findings are listed in Table 1. Usually hypocortisolism causes hyperkaliemia, but our patient was at admission suffering from vomiting which speaks for the hypokaliemia being caused by gastrointestinal loss of potassium; the antibiotics of the patient piperacillin/tazobactam can however also cause this electrolyte disturbance. ACTH was unfortunately not measured until four days later at which time it was still elevated at 173 ng/l, consistent with a non-ACTH dependent adrenal aetiology of the hypocortisolism. Urine culture and serial blood cultures (all taken whilst on antibiotic therapy) were clear. Chest and left knee radiography were normal. A CT of her abdomen showed bilateral hyperdense oval enlargement of the adrenal glands (right 27 × 16 mm, left 32 × 21 mm) consistent with acute adrenal haemorrhages, no sign of malignant tumor was demonstrated (Figure 1).

Later the patient developed a severe anaemia (hemoglobin 70 g/l) without any clinical signs of blood loss, a gastroscopy revealed no signs of bleeding. The adrenal haemorrhages were, due to their moderate size on the CT, felt to not be the cause of her reduced hemoglobin why we interpreted the culprit to be a fluid shift in the context of the Addisonian crisis. The hemoglobin improved significantly to a value of 92 g/l at discharge without a blood transfusion. Before discharge, a HIT with positive platelet factor 4 antibodies was diagnosed due to falling thrombocyte count whilst on prophylactic unfractioned heparin, and heparin was replaced with fondaparinux and by discharge changed to rivaroxaban, when a therapeutic anticoagulation was deemed safe again after the adrenal haemorrhage. The 21-hydroxylase, antiadrenal antibody, and antiphospholipid syndrome antibody essays were negative, making an autoimmune cause of the primary adrenal insufficiency unlikely. An ACTH stimulation test was not performed given the clinical presentation, very low serum-cortisol, and CT-findings, leaving little doubt about the presence of an adrenal crisis and its aetiology.

With the clinical constellation at admission of acute flank pain, hypotension, hyponatremia, and radiological signs of an adrenal bleeding whilst on anticoagulation, an Addisonian crisis as the acute manifestation of primary adrenal insufficiency was strongly suspected. Intravenous hydrocortisone therapy and a saline infusion were immediately started, and phenprocoumon was stopped. The patient was referred to the intensive care unit (ICU) for circulatory support with norepinephrine and further intravenous fluids until her condition stabilised 4–6 hours later. The hydrocortisone was tapered down over the next 4-5 days until she was on a split dose of 30 mg/day per orally, and subsequently fludrocortisone 0.1 mg/day was initiated.

On review as an outpatient, the condition of the patient was back to baseline. A follow-up unenhanced CT (Figure 2) was performed 4 months later demonstrating no signs of malignant tumor and regression of the enlarged adrenal glands (right 22 × 12 mm, left 20 × 12 mm), a sign that the haematoma was slowly resolving [5]. It is important that patients should have follow-up scanning until resolution of the haematoma and that the possibility of underlying pathological processes such as malignancy is considered, especially in patients with unilateral adrenal haemorrhages.

After starting fludrocortisone 0.1 mg a day, the sodium level was 141 mmol/l, the potassium level 4.6 mmol/l (both in the normal range) and the renin level in the lower normal range with 4.8 m*U*/l, which could make one suspect that the patient may not have had aldosterone deficiency despite glucocorticoid deficiency or that the patient on her own had ingested more hydrocortisone than was prescribed, which through the mineralocorticoid effect of hydrocortisone would have lowered the renin level.

The continuous adjustment of the medication takes place in the outpatient setting. Five months after the first diagnosis of primary adrenal insufficiency, despite on several occasions being given verbal and written information about adrenal insufficiency and its medical management including an emergency card, the patient was again admitted to the intensive care unit with an Addisonian crisis due to an influenza-infection with fever up to 40°C having failed to increase her hydrocortisone dose. She survived after receiving high-dose intravenous hydrocortisone and fluid resuscitation in the ICU and was discharged after being

Table 1: Laboratory studies at admission.

Parameter	Result (CH units)	Normal range
Sodium	124 mmol/l	136–145 mmol/l
Potassium	2.6 mmol/l	3.4–5.0 mmol/l
Serum osmolality	258 mmol/kg	280–300 mmol/kg
Blood urea nitrogen	3.0 mmol/l	<11.9 mmol/l
Chloride	87 mmol/l	96–108 mmol/l
pH	7.40	7.37–7.45
Bicarbonate	27 mmol/l	21–26 mmol/l
Glucose	5.4 mmol/l	3.9–6.4 mmol/l
Creatinine	47 μmol/l	44–80 μmol/l
eGFR (CKD-EPI)	98 ml/min	>90 ml/min
Random serum-cortisol	39 nmol/l	80–690 nmol/l
ACTH (day 4)	173 ng/l	<61 ng/l
TSH	2.23 mU/l	0.27–4.2 mU/l
C-reactive protein	158 mg/l	<5 mg/l
Hemoglobin	118 g/l	120–160 g/l
Eosinophils	0.1 G/l (0.7%)	<0.7 G/l (2–4%)
Thrombocytes	135 G/l	150–375 G/l
INR (international normalized ratio)	2.8	2.0–3.0
Antiadrenal & 21-hydroxylase antibodies	Negative	
Antiphospholipid syndrome antibodies	Negative	
Platelet factor 4 IgG antibodies	24.6 U/ml	<1.0 U/ml
Urine culture	Negative	
Blood culture	Negative	

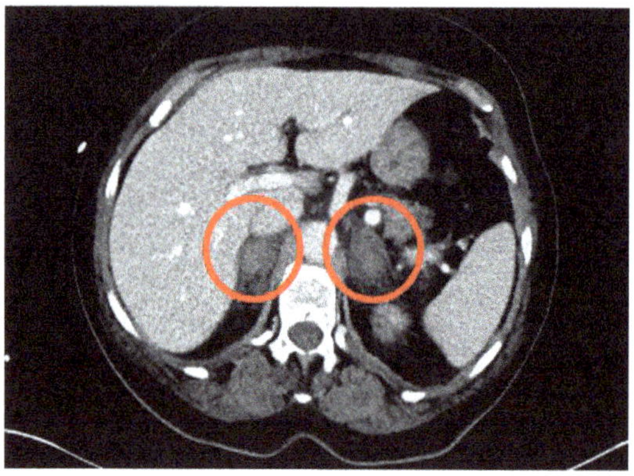

Figure 1: CT of the abdomen at admission (horizontal plane).

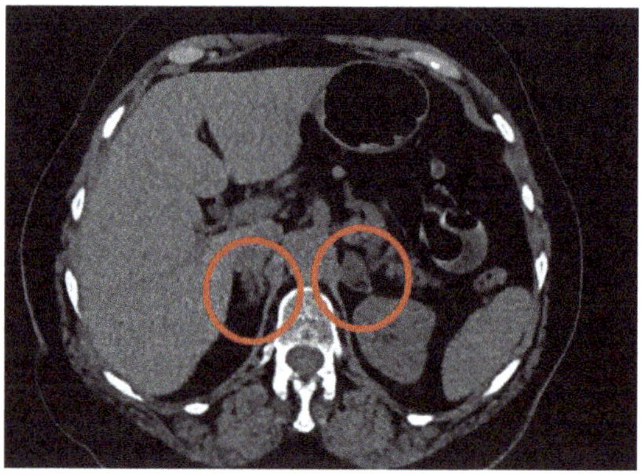

Figure 2: Follow up CT of the abdomen (horizontal plane).

given repeated information about sick day rules when experiencing stressful situations.

3. Discussion

The anatomy of the adrenal vasculature may play an important role in the development of adrenal haemorrhage. The adrenal glands are one of the best vascularised organs in the body; the adrenal vasculature is supplied through three arteries going into the adrenal tissues but at the same time having a limited venous drainage through only one adrenal vein. The arteries penetrate the surface of the adrenal gland; divide into 50–60 branches that form a vascular plexus around the zona reticularis. This rather abrupt arteriovenous transition zone constitutes a so called "vascular dam," with a propensity to cause congestion of the vasculature owing to the anatomical "bottleneck" when the blood is further drained into medullary sinusoids and ultimately into the single adrenal vein [3]. According to Fox, the eccentric longitudinal smooth muscle fibres of the adrenal vein could, in situation of vascular contraction, cause local stasis and pockets of turbulence, in which venous thrombosis would form, causing vascular wall necrosis leading to a secondary haemorrhagic event [6]. Dobbie and Symington suggested that this mechanism for build-up of venous stasis actually has a physiological role, allowing the adrenal cortex to become engorged with and, using the elastic fibres in the venous wall, subsequently explosively expel a large volume of blood containing adrenal cortical hormones out of the adrenal gland into the systemic circulation, allowing for an acute hormonal effect [7]. An additional thrombogenic factor in stressful situations is the ACTH and catecholamine secretion which increases the arterial blood flow to the adrenal glands, causing adrenal venous stasis and inducing platelet aggregation, both of which increase the risk of an infarction and secondary haemorrhage [2].

In our patient, several risk factors for an adrenal haemorrhage were identified: anticoagulation therapy, heparin induced thrombocytopenia, recent surgery, and infection. Most of the reported adrenal haemorrhage cases whilst on anticoagulant therapy occurred within the first 2–4 weeks after initiation [8, 9]. Our patient, however, had been using phenprocoumon for several years. In a review by Rao, after surgery, adrenal bleeding is most commonly seen in the first fifteen days postoperatively [10], which was also the case in our patient. She had no vasodilatory therapy, which could have had a protective effect against the development of adrenal haemorrhage by increasing the perfusion in ischemic vessels [3]. The administration of heparin before and after the knee surgery, in this patient with slightly decreased platelet count of 135 G/l on the day of admission, could have played a significant role in the development of the bilateral adrenal bleedings, since Kovacs defined heparin for a minimum of 4 days and thrombocytopaenia as high risk factors for adrenal haemorrhage [3]. Her platelet count on the day before admission was however normal at 173 G/l, which in our view excludes the weeks later established diagnosis of a HIT as precipitating factor of the adrenal bleeding.

In our opinion, the reason for the adrenal bleeding in this patient is most likely the stress induced by the surgery and the infection on top of the preexisting anticoagulation therapy. The anticoagulation therapy had been used for years and by admission, her INR-values were in the therapeutic range, which gives support to the notion of her infection and surgery as the main triggers for the adrenal bleeding.

Rapid clinical deterioration in hypotensive patient with hyponatremia should always lead to investigations for a possible Addisonian crisis, and the prompt intravenous administration of fluids and hydrocortisone can be lifesaving and should be given while awaiting diagnostic laboratory test results. An Addisonian crisis due to adrenal haemorrhage should be suspected in patients showing signs such as abdominal/flank/back pain, signs of occult haemorrhage, and adrenal insufficiency, especially in the presence of coinciding risk factors such as anticoagulation therapy, recent surgery, and infection. A CT of the adrenal glands can help to establish the diagnosis.

References

[1] E. Charmandari, N. C. Nicolaides, and G. P. Chrousos, "Adrenal insufficiency," *The Lancet*, vol. 383, no. 9935, pp. 2152–2167, 2014.

[2] R. H. Rao, "Bilateral massive adrenal hemorrhage," *Medical Clinics of North America*, vol. 79, no. 1, pp. 107–129, 1995.

[3] K. A. Kovacs, Y. M. Lam, and J. L. Pater, "Bilateral massive adrenal hemorrhage," *Medicine*, vol. 80, no. 1, pp. 45–53, 2001.

[4] V. P. Xarli, A. A. Steele, P. J. Davis, E. S. Buescher, C. N. Rios, and R. Garcia-Bunuel, "Adrenal hemorrhage in the adult," *Medicine*, vol. 57, no. 3, pp. 211–222, 1978.

[5] A. Kawashima, C. M. Sandler, R. D. Ernst et al., "Imaging of nontraumatic hemorrhage of the adrenal gland," *RadioGraphics*, vol. 19, no. 4, pp. 949–963, 1999.

[6] B. Fox, "Venous infarction of the adrenal glands," *The Journal of Pathology*, vol. 119, no. 2, pp. 65–89, 1976.

[7] J. W. Dobbie and T. Symington, "The human adrenal gland with special reference to the vasculature," *Journal of Endocrinology*, vol. 34, no. 4, p. 479, 1966.

[8] F. D. Mcdonald, A. R. Myers, and R. Pardo, "Adrenal hemorrhage during anticoagulant therapy," *JAMA: The Journal of the American Medical Association*, vol. 198, no. 10, pp. 1052–1056, 1966.

[9] A. Vella, T. B. Nippoldt, and J. C. Morris, "Adrenal hemorrhage: a 25-year experience at the Mayo clinic," *Mayo Clinic Proceedings*, vol. 76, no. 2, pp. 161–168, 2001.

[10] R. H. Rao, A. H. Vagnucci, and J. A. Amico, "Bilateral massive adrenal hemorrhage: early recognition and treatment," *Annals of Internal Medicine*, vol. 110, no. 3, pp. 227–235, 1989.

36

A Case of Successful Treatment with Unilateral Oophorectomy in a Patient with Resistant Polycystic Ovary Syndrome

S. Pathmanathan,[1] I. Ranathunga,[2] and N. P. Somasundaram[2]

[1]*Diabetes and Endocrinology Unit, District General Hospital-Kaluthara, Kaluthara, Sri Lanka*
[2]*Diabetes and Endocrinology Unit, National Hospital of Sri Lanka, Colombo, Sri Lanka0000*

Correspondence should be addressed to I. Ranathunga; ish_75@yahoo.com

Academic Editor: Wei Wu

Background. Polycystic ovary syndrome (PCOS) is a common endocrine disorder with heterogeneous etiology. Typical features consist of oligo/anovulation, polycystic ovaries, and features of hyperandrogenism. Pathogenesis is multifactorial, and positive family history may have a predisposition for disease development. The syndrome is associated with multiple metabolic and nonmetabolic entities. As the disease is involved with multiple adverse outcomes, the successful treatment is pivotal. Among the more advanced options, the unilateral oophorectomy is considered as a last resort to alleviate the symptoms. *Case Presentation.* A 29-year-old female presented to us with oligomenorrhea, severe hirsutism, androgenic pattern hair loss, acne, increased skin pigmentation, and secondary subfertility. On examination, she was obese with a body mass index (BMI) of 29.6 kg/m^2. She had evidence of acanthosis nigricans, androgenic pattern balding, acne, dorsal, supraclavicular fat deposition, and moderate-severe hirsutism. Investigations confirmed excess right ovarian testosterone secretion which led to the ultimate management with right oophorectomy with successful alleviation of clinical features. *Conclusions.* The multifaceted medical treatment comprises the first-line therapy in PCOS. Surgery is considered as a second-line option in resistant PCOS following failure of initial therapeutic options. We report a case of resistant polycystic ovary syndrome with secondary subfertility and moderate-to-severe hirsutism who was successfully treated with unilateral oophorectomy with favorable results.

1. Introduction

Polycystic ovary syndrome is a common endocrine disorder in premenopausal women. The prevalence of the disease varies depending on the population studied and ranges from 4–20% [1, 2]. The syndrome is characterized by the presence of oligo/anovulation, polycystic ovary appearance on imaging and clinical and biochemical features of hyperandrogenism. The diagnostic criteria had been evolved over past few decades, and many experts recommend the Rotterdam criteria in making the diagnosis at present [3]. The pathogenesis is thought to be multifactorial with possible involvement of genetic and environmental factors [4]. The disorder is associated with numerous other metabolic and nonmetabolic diseases which render to the increased morbidity and mortality linked to the disease [5–8]. Multiple treatment options are available for successful treatment of the disease which are mainly guided by the treatment goals [9]. Surgery has been used as a possible treatment option for infertility resistant to other treatment methods but is less popular as a method to treat hyperandrogenic symptoms resistant to other treatment [10].

2. Case Report

A 29-year-old previously healthy mother of one child presented with oligomenorrhea, severe hirsutism, androgenic pattern hair loss, acne, increased skin pigmentation, and secondary subfertility over five-year duration. Her cycles occurred once in every 3-4 months with bleeding lasting 5–7 days. She did not complain of associated dysmenorrhea. She has attained menarche at the age of 13 years and had regular menstrual cycles thereafter until five years back. A family history of a similar endocrinopathy was not evident.

On examination, she was obese with a body mass index (BMI) of 29.6 kg/m^2. She had evidence of acanthosis nigricans, androgenic pattern balding, acne, and dorsal and supraclavicular fat deposition without any other specific features of Cushing's syndrome (Figure 1). Skin had a generalized increased in pigmentation without any predisposition to specific areas. Ferriman–Gallwey score was sixteen out of thirty-three which was suggestive of moderate-severe disease. Her systemic examination was nonsignificant.

On laboratory evaluation, her total testosterone was 215 ng/dL, luteinizing hormone (LH) was 7.27 IU/L, and follicle-stimulating hormone (FSH) was 7.42 IU/L. The thyroid profile, serum prolactin, dehydroepiandrosterone sulfate (DHEAS), and stimulated 17-hydroxyprogesterone (OHP) were found to be normal. Imaging with transvaginal ultrasound scan and MRI-pelvis revealed enlarged ovaries with multiple peripheral cysts which was suggestive of bilateral polycystic ovary syndrome. CECT of adrenal glands was found to be normal. A summary of the investigations is depicted in Table 1.

3. Conclusion: Features Suggestive of Polycystic Ovaries

For further evaluation of markedly elevated serum total testosterone levels, she underwent bilateral adrenal and ovarian venous sampling which revealed a significant high testosterone levels being secreted from the right ovary (Figure 3, Table 2).

She was started on medical nutrition therapy, metformin, antiandrogen (spironolactone), local therapy, and later a trial of GnRH analogs which were all found to be ineffective. To improve fertility, she underwent bilateral ovarian drilling without any successful outcomes. Enlarged bilateral ovaries with typical polycystic appearance were evident on laparoscopy (Figure 4).

Failing all the above treatments, she underwent right-sided oophorectomy which was the culprit ovary for the highest testosterone production as the last resort. Histology was compatible with polycystic ovary disease with multiple ovarian follicles, some with luteinized cells and stromal hyperplasia (Figure 5). In contrast, the presence of steroidogenically active nests of luteinized theca cells scattered in the ovarian stroma is seen in ovarian hyperthecosis. These cell clusters arise from the differentiation of the ovarian interstitial cells into luteinized stromal cells [11]. The clinical presentation of the two conditions may be similar though PCOS is commonly seen in premenopausal females, while ovarian hyperthecosis is more prevalent in the postmenopausal age group.

Following surgery, she had improvement of her clinical symptoms including hirsutism, regularization of the menstrual cycles, and normalization of total serum testosterone levels (46 ng/dL) and is currently under our follow-up for more than one year without any clinical or biochemical deterioration.

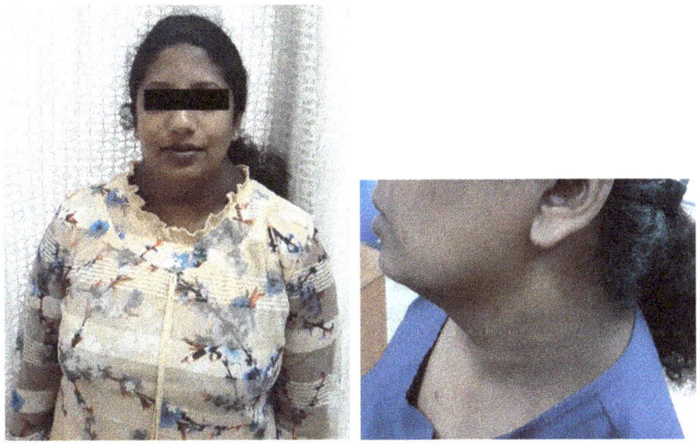

Figure 1: The index patient demonstrating central obesity and acanthosis nigricans.

4. Discussion

PCOS is mainly a clinical diagnosis made in conjunction with recommended diagnostic criteria. Though multiple diagnostic criteria are available at present, the commonly used is the criteria defined by the European Society for Human Reproduction and Embryology/American Society for Reproductive Medicine (ESHRE/ASRM), Rotterdam criteria [3]. Nevertheless, other supportive investigation including biochemistry, imaging, and histology contribute to the diagnostic accuracy. Selective venous catheterization, which is an invasive modality of investigation, has been successfully employed to aid in the localization and the diagnosis of the source of androgen secretion. Even though ovarian venous sampling is not used as a routine investigation, the utilization of the test can rule out possible malignant causes and plan more selective, third-line treatment options in the presence of significant hyperandrogenism as in the index patient [12]. Nonetheless, difficulty in catheterization and the invasiveness of the procedure may limit its successful use [13].

The treatment of the disease should be guided by the goals of therapy [9]. First-line treatment consists of lifestyle interventions including diet and exercise targeted in achieving significant weight loss [9]. Further treatment will depend on the fertility wishes which include hormonal contraceptives, metformin therapy, clomiphene citrate, letrozole, and gonadotrophin therapy [9]. Surgery has been rarely practiced as a possible treatment option for infertility resistant to other treatment methods [14]. Out of the available surgical options, laparoscopic ovarian drilling is an established treatment option for infertility for women resistant to medical therapy [15]. Though the exact mechanism is not clear, the destruction of ovarian follicles and stroma leading to a reduction in androgen and inhibin levels, which drives the pathogenesis and a subsequent rise in follicle-stimulating hormone (FSH) levels, is the most possible explanation [16]. Utilization of surgical options such as ovarian drilling, wedge resection, unilateral or bilateral oophorectomy is less considered for the management of resistant hyperandrogenism manifested by hirsutism, acne etc., though some studies have demonstrated improved clinical outcomes [10, 17, 18]. Literature suggests the

TABLE 1: Summary of investigations.

Investigation	Result	Reference range
Serum total testosterone	215 ng/dL	14–76 ng/dL
LH	7.27 IU/L	1.8–11.78 IU/L (follicular phase)
FSH	7.42 IU/L	3.03–8.08 IU/L (follicular phase)
17-Hydroxyprogesterone (17-OHP)	3.954 nmol/L	<2.1 nmol/L
Synacthen stimulated 17-OHP	4.915 nmol/L	<9.6 nmol/L
Dehydroepiandrosterone sulfate (DHEAS)	23.1 μg/dL	35–430 μg/dL
LDDST suppressed serum total testosterone	118.67 nmol/L	<50%
Low-dose dexamethasone suppression test (LDDST)	13.79 nmol/L	<50 nmol/L
Fasting blood glucose	86 mg/dL	<100 mg/dL
Oral glucose tolerance test (2 hour)	128 mg/dL	<140 mg/dL
Lipid profile	Cholesterol: 248 mg/dL HDL: 39 mg/dL LDL: 183 mg/dL TG: 132 mg/dL	<200 mg/dL >60 mg/dL < 130 mg/dL < 150 mg/dL
TSH/fT4	1.18 μIU/L/1.42 ng/dL	0.55–4.78 μIU/L/0.89–1.76 ng/dL
Postoperative serum total testosterone	46 ng/dL	14–76 ng/dL
Transvaginal scan	Both ovaries are enlarged, R/ovary: 14 ml, L/ovary: 17 ml, multiple small follicles are seen at the periphery of the ovary, prominent stroma is seen Features suggestive of polycystic ovaries (Figure 2)	
MRI-pelvis	Both ovaries are enlarged, R/ovary: 16 ml, L/ovary: 20 ml, multiple tiny follicles (>20) in both ovaries with a peripheral distribution. The size of the follicles is less than 10 mm. Prominent stroma is noted.	
CECT-adrenal glands	Normal	

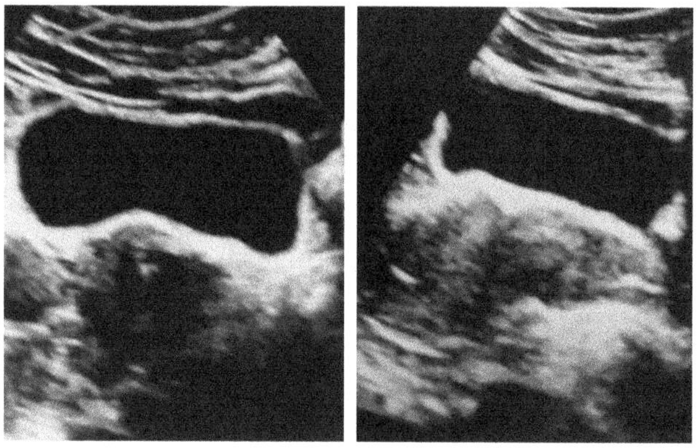

FIGURE 2: Both ovaries are enlarged; R/ovary: 14 ml; L/ovary: 17 ml; multiple small follicles are seen at the periphery of the ovary; prominent stroma seen.

possibility of decreased androgen and LH levels following surgery which may contribute the favorable clinical outcomes, though the results are inconsistent [10]. Unilateral oophorectomy remains an uncommon option that can be exerted in resistant patients who has undergone multiple medical and conservative surgical treatment. However, theoretically, removal of one ovary can lead to less production of androgens and can lead to improvement of clinical features and fertility [14]. Studies have demonstrated that unilateral oophorectomy can restore regular menstruation and fertility in majority [14]. Ovarian surgery has not generally been demonstrated to have an effect on the severity of hirsutism, but has been suggested to decrease hair growth rate in some women [19, 20]. There are insufficient and conflicting data to assess acne as an outcome [18, 21]. The possibility of the disease recurrence despite initial improvement at a later date remains a possibility, and active vigilance should be carried out indefinitely [14]. The index patient had a significant improvement in the androgenic features including hirsutism, acne, and androgenic pattern hair loss as well as regularization of menstrual cycles following surgery.

This case highlights the importance of further evaluation of resistant PCOS patients with more advanced investigations such as ovarian venous sampling and consideration of aggressive surgical interventions such as unilateral oophorectomy which can yield successful outcomes. Furthermore,

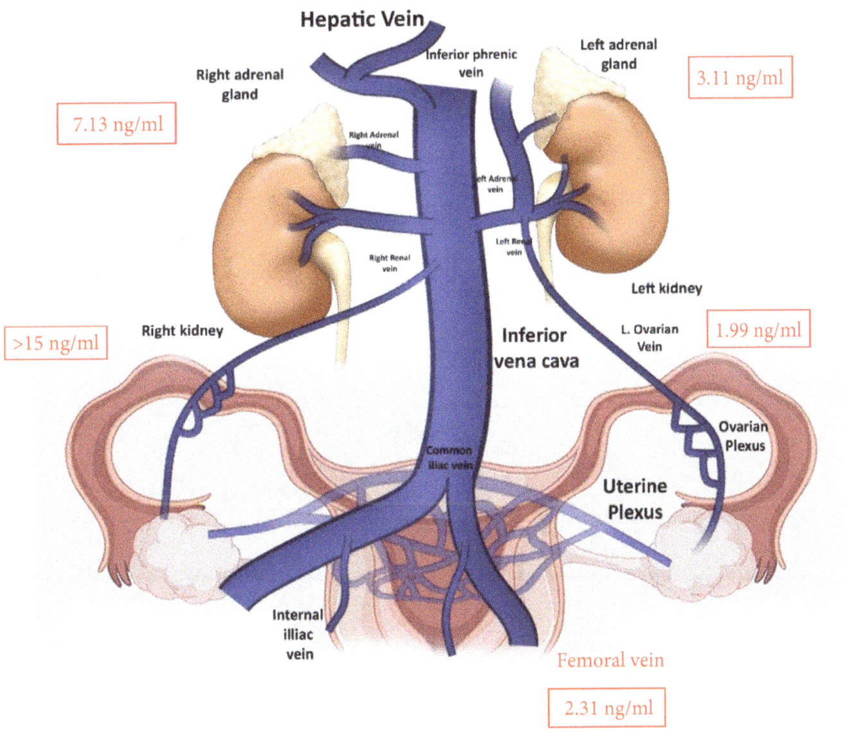

Figure 3: Bilateral ovarian/adrenal venous sampling: serum testosterone levels.

Table 2: Bilateral ovarian/adrenal venous sampling.

	Left ovary	Right ovary	Left adrenal	Right adrenal	Femoral vein
Serum total testosterone	1.99 ng/ml	>15 ng/ml	3.11 ng/ml	7.13 ng/ml	2.31 ng/ml
Serum cortisol			3820 nmol/L	303.5 nmol/L	348 nmol/L

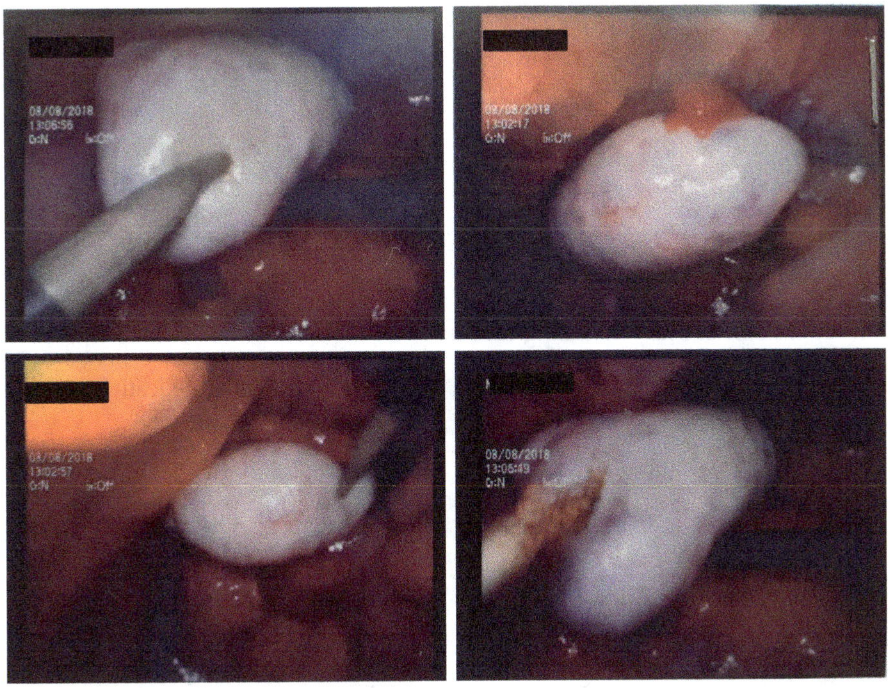

Figure 4: Enlarged bilateral ovaries with typical polycystic appearance.

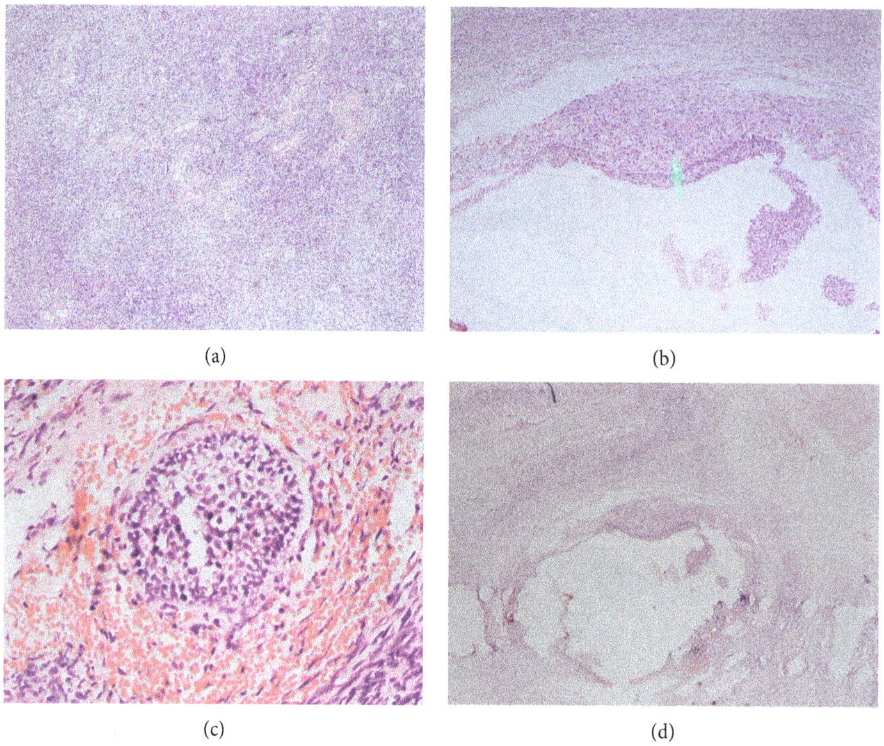

FIGURE 5: Right ovary histology: ovarian tissue comprises multiple ovarian follicles, some with luteinized cells. Areas of stromal hyperplasia are seen; however, luteinized cell collections are not seen. There is no evidence of hyperplasia or malignancy. Conclusion of histological features is consistent with polycystic ovary with stromal hyperplasia. (a) Stromal hyperplasia. (b) Ovarian follicle with luteinized cells. (c) Multiple follicles (400x). (d) Multiple follicles (40x).

consideration of unilateral oophorectomy in the event of unilateral testosterone hypersecretion can be limited in the reproductive age group due to concomitant fertility wishes. Nevertheless, further study of similar case reports and more detailed research will be beneficial in the future and will add up to the options available for treatment in the resistant patients for conventional treatment.

5. Conclusions

In conclusion, here, we have described a rare case of resistant polycystic ovary syndrome who presented to us with severe hirsutism and was found to have unilateral secretion of very high testosterone levels. She was successfully treated with unilateral oophorectomy of the culprit ovary indicating that surgery can be considered in resistant patients as a last resort.

Abbreviations

PCOS: Polycystic ovary syndrome
BMI: Body mass index
LH: Luteinizing hormone
FSH: Follicle-stimulating hormone
DHEAS: Dehydroepiandrosterone sulfate
17-OHP: 17-hydroxyprogesterone
MRI: Magnetic resonance imaging
CECT: Contrast-enhanced computed tomography
LDDST: Low-dose dexamethasone suppression test
THS: Thyroid stimulating hormone
ESHRE/ASRM: European Society for Human Reproduction and Embryology/American Society for Reproductive Medicine.

Consent

The authors have obtained informed written consent from the patient to report and publish about her illness anonymously.

Authors' Contributions

S. Pathmanathan, I. Ranathunga, and N. P. Somasundaram were involved in the history taking, examination, diagnosing, and management of patient's condition and prepared the manuscript for publication. All authors read and approved the final manuscript.

References

[1] R. Azziz, K. S. Woods, R. Reyna, T. J. Key, E. S. Knochenhauer, and B. O. Yildiz, "The prevalence and features of the polycystic ovary syndrome in an unselected population," *The Journal of Clinical Endocrinology & Metabolism*, vol. 89, no. 6, pp. 2745–2749, 2004.

[2] M. Asuncion, R. M. Calvo, J. L. San Millan, J. Sancho, S. Avila, and H. F. Escobar-Morreale, "A prospective study of the

prevalence of the polycystic ovary syndrome in unselected Caucasian women from Spain," *Journal of Clinical Endocrinology & Metabolism*, vol. 85, no. 7, pp. 2434–2438, 2000.

[3] H. J. Teede, M. L. Misso, M. F Costello et al., "Recommendations from the international evidence-based guideline for the assessment and management of polycystic ovary syndrome," *Fertility and Sterility*, vol. 110, no. 3, pp. 364–379, 2018.

[4] R. L. Rosenfield and D. A. Ehrmann, "The pathogenesis of polycystic ovary syndrome (PCOS): the hypothesis of PCOS as functional ovarian hyperandrogenism revisited," *Endocrine Reviews*, vol. 37, no. 5, pp. 467–520, 2016.

[5] A. Dunaif, K. R. Segal, W. Futterweit, and A. Dobrjansky, "Profound peripheral insulin resistance, independent of obesity, in polycystic ovary syndrome," *Diabetes*, vol. 38, no. 9, pp. 1165–1174, 1989.

[6] T. L. Setji, N. D. Holland, L. L. Sanders, K. C. Pereira, A. M. Diehl, and A. J. Brown, "Nonalcoholic steatohepatitis and nonalcoholic Fatty liver disease in young women with polycystic ovary syndrome," *The Journal of Clinical Endocrinology & Metabolism*, vol. 91, no. 5, pp. 1741–1747, 2006.

[7] E. S. Ford, W. H. Giles, and A. H. Mokdad, "Increasing prevalence of the metabolic syndrome among U.S. Adults," *Diabetes Care*, vol. 27, no. 10, pp. 2444–2449, 2004.

[8] A. A. Deeks, M. E. Gibson-Helm, and H. J. Teede, "Anxiety and depression in polycystic ovary syndrome: a comprehensive investigation," *Fertility and Sterility*, vol. 93, no. 7, pp. 2421–2423, 2010.

[9] R. S. Legro, S. A. Arslanian, D. A. Ehrmann et al., "Diagnosis and treatment of polycystic ovary syndrome: an Endocrine Society clinical practice guideline," *The Journal of Clinical Endocrinology & Metabolism*, vol. 98, no. 12, pp. 4565–4592, 2013.

[10] N. Johnson and K. Wang, "Is ovarian surgery effective for androgenic symptoms of polycystic ovarian syndrome?" *Journal of Obstetrics and Gynaecology*, vol. 23, no. 6, pp. 599–606, 2003.

[11] N. B. Judith, "Nonneoplastic disorders," *Pathology of the Ovary*, pp. 33–61, Springer, Berlin, Germany, 2004, https://www.springer.com/gp/book/9781475738896.

[12] G. A. Kaltsas, J. J. Mukherjee, B. Kola et al., "Is ovarian and adrenal venous catheterization and sampling helpful in the investigation of hyperandrogenic women?" *Clinical Endocrinology*, vol. 59, no. 1, pp. 34–43, 2003.

[13] A. C. Wentz, R. I. White, C. J. Migeon, T. H. Hsu, H. V. Barnes, and G. S. Jones, "Differential ovarian and adrenal vein catheterization," *American Journal of Obstetrics and Gynecology*, vol. 125, no. 7, pp. 1000–1007, 1976.

[14] E. M. Kaaijk, "Clinical outcome after unilateral oophorectomy in patients with polycystic ovary syndrome," *Human Reproduction*, vol. 14, no. 4, pp. 889–892, 1999.

[15] S. Mitra, P. K. Nayak, and S. Agrawal, "Laparoscopic ovarian drilling: an alternative but not the ultimate in the management of polycystic ovary syndrome," *Journal of Natural Science, Biology and Medicine*, vol. 6, no. 1, pp. 40–48, 2015.

[16] R. Flyckt and J. Goldberg, "Laparoscopic ovarian drilling for clomiphene-resistant polycystic ovary syndrome," *Seminars in Reproductive Medicine*, vol. 29, no. 2, pp. 138–146, 2011.

[17] O. G. J. Naether, V. Baukloh, R. Fischer, and T. Kowalczyk, "Surgery: long-term follow-up in 206 infertility patients with polycystic ovarian syndrome after laparoscopic electrocautery of the ovarian surface," *Human Reproduction*, vol. 9, no. 12, pp. 2342–2349, 1994.

[18] S. A. K. Amer, V. Gopalan, T. C. Li, W. L. Ledger, and I. D. Cooke, "Long term follow-up of patients with polycystic ovarian syndrome after laparoscopic ovarian drilling: clinical outcome," *Human Reproduction*, vol. 17, no. 8, pp. 2035–2042, 2002.

[19] H. Vejlsted and R. Albrechtsen, "Biochemical and clinical effect of ovarian wedge resection in the polycystic ovary syndrome," *Obstetrics and Gynecology*, vol. 47, no. 5, p. 575, 1976.

[20] J. Hamerlynck, "Polycystic ovaries disease: one ovary too many?" *Lancet (London, England)*, vol. 2, pp. 937-938, 1982.

[21] H. Gjönnaess, "Polycystic ovarian syndrome treated by ovarian electrocautery through the laparoscope," *Fertility and Sterility*, vol. 41, no. 1, pp. 20–25, 1984.

37

Type IV RTA in Chronic Adrenal Insufficiency and Concomitant Lisinopril Treatment

Francesca Galbiati

Department of Medicine, University of Pittsburgh Medical Center, 200 Lothrop Street, Suite N715, Pittsburgh, PA 15213, USA

Correspondence should be addressed to Francesca Galbiati; galbiatif@upmc.edu

Academic Editor: Osamu Isozaki

Type IV renal tubular acidosis (RTA) is the only RTA characterized by hyperkalemia, and it is caused by a true aldosterone deficiency or renal tubular aldosterone hyporesponsiveness. It is frequent among hospitalized patients as it is related to type 2 diabetes mellitus (T2DM) and common medications such as ACE-inhibitors (ACE-is) and trimethoprim-sulfamethoxazole (TMP-SMX). Drug-induced RTA commonly manifests in patients with predisposing conditions such as mild renal insufficiency and certain pharmacological therapies. ACE-i use and chronic adrenal insufficiency (cAI) are other significant risk factors. Chronic ACTH suppression is thought to induce global adrenal atrophy, including the zona glomerulosa, thus affecting aldosterone secretion as well. Furthermore, in the setting of cAI, treatment with ACE-is further suppresses aldosterone production. This case report describes a patient with cAI secondary to corticosteroid use for years who developed type IV RTA in the setting of lisinopril use. Potassium (K) elevation persisted despite removing underlying conditions and metabolic acidosis correction. The patient required long-term treatment with mineralocorticoids in addition to sodium bicarbonate to maintain normal K levels and acid-base status. Mineralocorticoid administration is a second-line treatment for type IV RTA, but it might be necessary for a subgroup of high-risk patients. In fact, it is important to consider patients with chronic adrenal insufficiency and on ACE-is treatment at increased risk for refractory hyperkalemia in the setting of type IV RTA. Indeed, this subgroup of patients can have severe hypoaldosteronism.

1. Introduction

Type IV renal tubular acidosis (RTA) is the only RTA characterized by hyperkalemia, and it is caused by a true aldosterone deficiency or renal tubular aldosterone hyporesponsiveness [1]. It is frequent among hospitalized patients as it is related to type 2 diabetes mellitus (T2DM) and common medications such as ACE-inhibitors (ACE-is) and trimethoprim-sulfamethoxazole (TMP-SMX), and it occurs more often in patients with chronic kidney disease (CKD) [2]. Drug-induced RTA commonly manifests in patients with predisposing conditions, for example, the use of diclofenac and mild renal insufficiency exacerbated the potassium-altering effect of trimethoprim [3]. ACE-i use °and chronic adrenal insufficiency (cAI) are other significant risk factors. It is well known that chronic steroid treatment is a major cause of ACTH suppression [4]. Chronic ACTH suppression is thought to induce global adrenal atrophy [4, 5], including the zona glomerulosa, thus affecting aldosterone secretion as well. In cAI, treatment with ACE-is further suppresses aldosterone production by inhibiting the angiotensin-converting enzyme (Figure 1). In the clinical setting of cAI and concomitant ACE-i treatment, type IV RTA can be refractory to first-line interventions with subsequent persistent hyperkalemia requiring treatment with mineralocorticoids in addition to sodium bicarbonate. The literature on type IV RTA in patients with secondary or iatrogenic causes of hypoaldosteronism is sparse and requires more data.

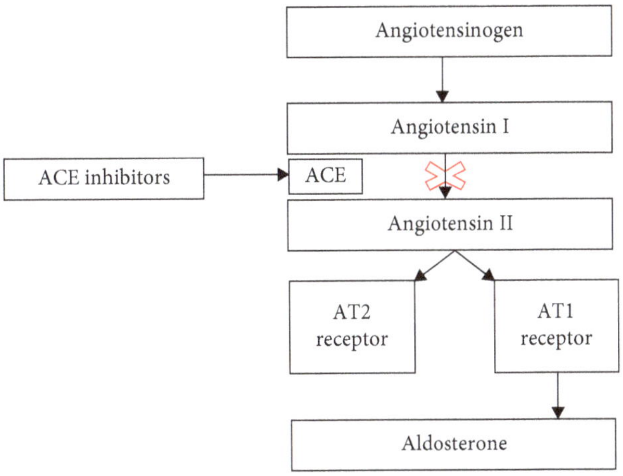

Figure 1: Effects of ACE-inhibitors on angiotensin conversion. ACE-inhibitors suppress the ACE enzyme action, thus blocking the conversion of angiotensin I to angiotensin II and its action on AT2 and AT1 receptors. The interaction between angiotensin II and AT1 receptors leads to aldosterone production.

2. Case Presentation

A 66-year-old female with a history of rheumatoid arthritis on prednisone 5 mg daily, T2DM, CKD, AI secondary to chronic steroid use, and recent hospitalization for methicillin-resistant *Staphylococcus aureus* (MRSA) osteomyelitis still on antibiotics, now admitted for cholangitis treatment, suddenly presents unexplained hyperkalemia. At the time of admission, the patient was started on piperacillin-tazobactam for cholangitis and on TMP-SFX for a history of MRSA osteomyelitis. She also received stress-dose steroids for 48 hours with immediate clinical improvement. The patient's hospitalization was prolonged (more than 30 days) and complicated by acute kidney injury, hyperkalemia, and nonanion gap metabolic acidosis (NAGMA) outlined as follows. The patient also had a history of hypertension treated with lisinopril 5 mg daily, which was initially discontinued and restarted during the hospitalization (day 30) at the increased dose of 10 mg daily given severe hypertension. On day 33, the patient's creatinine rose to 1.5 mg/dL from a baseline of 1.2 mg/dL, and her previously normal potassium (K) increased to 5.5 mmol/L (Table 1). This was thought to be related to lisinopril, which was discontinued. Off lisinopril, her kidney function recovered, but unexpectedly, hyperkalemia worsened to 6.3 mmol/L, and she presented a new-onset NAGMA with serum bicarbonate 17.5 mmol/L. The abnormally elevated K was then attributed to TMP-SMX-induced hyperkalemia, so TMP-SFX was switched to doxycycline, and the patient was given patiromer. Despite these interventions, both hyperkalemia and NAGMA persisted (K, 6.3 mmol/L and bicarbonate, 19.6 mmol/L on day 35). At that point, urine electrolytes and venous blood gas were obtained, demonstrating a positive urine anion gap and venous pH of 7.31. The urinalysis was normal with pH of 7, no evidence of infection, and absence of proteinuria, glycosuria, and microhematuria. Plasma renin activity was 0.95, and aldosterone levels were undetectable; however, the treatment with ACE-I could affect the interpretation of this test. The picture was now consistent with type IV RTA, so the patient was started on oral sodium bicarbonate 1300 mg three times a day with the resolution of NAGMA. Despite the discontinuation of possible culprit medications, the patient was still hyperkalemic. Finally, considering her cAI with a likely component of hypoaldosteronism worsened by lisinopril, fludrocortisone 0.1 mg was added daily with immediate normalization of K (from 5.2 mmol/L to 4.4 mmol/L). This happened the fourth day after stopping lisinopril (Table 1). The patient had to continue the daily therapy with both sodium bicarbonate and fludrocortisone to maintain normal K levels and acid-base status and did not experience any electrolyte imbalance or worsening hypertension, while on the mineralocorticoid replacement therapy, as a demonstration that, she was indeed aldosterone-deficient. Of note, cortisol and adrenocorticotropic hormone levels were not measured during this admission as the patient's diagnosis of adrenal insufficiency was well established, and she was on treatment.

3. Discussion

The classical manifestations of type IV RTA are hyperkalemia and NAGMA. In the inpatient setting, these are frequently primarily attributed to patients' comorbidities and polypharmacy, thus missing the correct diagnosis. The type IV RTA workup (serum K, urine electrolytes and anion gap, urine pH, and urine bicarbonate) is cost-effective and straightforward and should be included in first-line tests for hyperkalemia workup. It is, in fact, crucial to address diagnosis and treatment quickly, given the risk of hyperkalemia in hospitalized patients [6]. However, healthcare providers often prescribe expensive tests and medications (i.e., newer potassium binders) to address hyperkalemia with delays in the diagnosis and increase in healthcare expenses.

When approaching patients with cAI and on ACE-is presenting with hyperkalemia, it is important to consider a primary adrenal insufficiency-like picture. The chronic ACTH suppression by exogenous steroid medications can cause adrenal atrophy and subphysiological aldosterone

Table 1: Hospital course timeline starting from day 30; medication management; serum potassium, bicarbonate, and creatinine levels.

Day of admission	Potassium (mmol/L)	Bicarbonate (mmol/L)	Creatinine (mg/dL)
30	4.0	21.6	1.2
Lisinopril 10 mg daily was restarted on day 30			
31	3.6	21.9	1.3
32	3.9	21.3	**1.4**
33	**5.5**	**17.5**	**1.5**
Lisinopril discontinued due to acute kidney injury on day 33			
34	**5.9**	**19.1**	**1.7**
TMP-SMX was switched to doxycycline; the patient received patiromer on day 34			
35	**6**	**19.6**	**1.4**
35	**6.3**	**19.6**	**1.5**
Sodium bicarbonate 1300 mg three times a day was started on day 35			
36	**5.5**	20.5	1.2
Fludrocortisone 0.1 mg daily was started on day 36			
37	4.4	20.8	1.1
38	4.5	21.6	1.2
Discharge			

Values of serum potassium, serum bicarbonate, and serum creatinine levels over the course of admission and treatment modifications secondary to acute kidney injury, hyperkalemia, and NAGMA. Based on our laboratory normal range, abnormal values are highlighted in bold.

levels in addition to hypocortisolemia. The additive inhibition of the angiotensin-converting enzyme by ACE-is further affects aldosterone production, thus inducing significant hypoaldosteronism.

The limitations of this case report are that, with only one patient, we cannot formulate robust evidence-based guidance on the treatment of type IV RTA in the particular condition of concomitant cAI and ACE-is use. Also, we do not have a documented measure of cortisol and ACTH in our patient at the time of presentation. Last, a combination of medications, such as bactrim and lisinopril, and cAI can explain type IV RTA in this patient; however, the prompt response to fludrocortisone and the absence of side effects on a long-term mineralocorticoid replacement therapy is indicative of a true aldosteronism deficiency.

4. Conclusion

In patients with unexplained hyperkalemia and underlying predisposing conditions, type IV RTA must always be considered. In particular, the index of suspicion must be high in patients with cAI and on concomitant ACE-I treatment leading to further suppression of aldosterone activity. Occasionally, in secondary or iatrogenic hypoaldosteronism, refractory hyperkalemia responds only to sodium bicarbonate and fludrocortisone given in combination.

Abbreviations

RTA: Renal tubular acidosis
T2DM: Type 2 diabetes mellitus
ACE-is: Angiotensin-converting enzyme inhibitors
TMP-SMX: Trimethoprim sulfamethoxazole
CKD: Chronic kidney disease
cAI: Chronic adrenal insufficiency
MRSA: Methicillin-resistant *Staphylococcus aureus*
NAGMA: Nonanion gap metabolic acidosis
K: Potassium.

References

[1] F. E. Karet, "Mechanisms in hyperkalemic renal tubular acidosis: figure 1," *Journal of the American Society of Nephrology*, vol. 20, no. 2, pp. 251–254, 2009.
[2] D. Batlle and J. Arruda, "Hyperkalemic forms of renal tubular acidosis: clinical and pathophysiological aspects," *Advances in Chronic Kidney Disease*, vol. 25, no. 4, pp. 321–333, 2018.
[3] M. A. Perazella, "Trimethoprim-induced hyperkalaemia," *Drug Safety*, vol. 22, no. 3, pp. 227–236, 2000.
[4] A. K. Younes and N. K. Younes, "Recovery of steroid induced adrenal insufficiency," *Translational Pediatrics*, vol. 6, no. 4, pp. 269–273, 2017.
[5] N. El Ghorayeb, I. Bourdeau, and A. Lacroix, "Role of ACTH and other hormones in the regulation of aldosterone production in primary aldosteronism," *Frontiers in Endocrinology*, vol. 7, no. 72, 2016.
[6] M. S. Stevens and R. W. Dunlay, "Hyperkalemia in hospitalized patients," *International Urology and Nephrology*, vol. 32, no. 2, pp. 177–180, 2000.

38

Acute Sheehan's Syndrome Presenting with Hyponatremia Followed by a Spontaneous Pregnancy

Maria M. Pineyro, Leonardo Diaz, Macarena Guzzetti, Mariana Risso, and Jimena Pereda

Clinica de Endocrinología y Metabolismo, Hospital de Clínicas, Facultad de Medicina, Universidad de la República, Montevideo, Uruguay

Correspondence should be addressed to Maria M. Pineyro; mercepin@gmail.com

Academic Editor: Toshihiro Kita

Background. Acute Sheehan's syndrome is rare, as well as hyponatremia as its initial manifestation. In addition, spontaneous pregnancy in patients after Sheehan's syndrome is unusual. To our knowledge, no cases of spontaneous pregnancy after acute Sheehan's syndrome have been reported. We describe a case of Sheehan's syndrome that presented with acute hyponatremia and a spontaneous pregnancy. *Case.* A 34-year-old female developed blood loss during delivery, which required a blood transfusion. On day seven postpartum, she presented with headaches, lethargy, and difficulty in breastfeeding. The workup showed hyponatremia (118 mEq/l), secondary hypothyroidism, and low prolactin levels. Magnetic resonance imaging showed pituitary necrosis. She was treated with NaCl, hydrocortisone (cortisol results were not available), and levothyroxine. Laboratory tests six weeks after discharge showed low IGF-1 and 8 AM cortisol and normal FT4, LH, FSH, and PRL levels. She was able to partially breastfeed until 4 months postpartum. Regular menstrual cycles started three months later. She became spontaneously pregnant one year later. *Conclusion.* Acute Sheehan's syndrome should be considered in the evaluation of postpartum patients with suggestive symptoms. Physicians should be aware that hyponatremia could be an initial manifestation of Sheehan's syndrome, which requires a high index of suspicion for diagnosis. Spontaneous pregnancy can occur after acute Sheehan's syndrome.

1. Introduction

Sheehan's syndrome is a well-known cause of hypopituitarism resulting from postpartum pituitary ischemic necrosis after massive blood loss during delivery [1, 2]. Its frequency has recently declined due to modern obstetric care, more so in developed countries. It is usually diagnosed several years postpartum. Acute presentation is extremely rare and can be life-threatening. Moreover, hyponatremia in the acute form of Sheehan's syndrome is also exceptional. In addition, spontaneous pregnancy in patients with Sheehan's syndrome is very rare [3]. To our knowledge, there are only two reported cases of acute Sheehan's syndrome with a successful pregnancy, one after ovulation induction and the other after in vitro fertilization [1, 4].

We described an extremely rare case of Sheehan's syndrome that presented postpartum with acute severe hyponatremia and a spontaneous pregnancy one year after diagnosis.

2. Case Presentation

A 34-year-old female (with 2 previous pregnancies and 1 delivery) with no significant past medical history delivered a healthy, normal-weight male infant at 40 weeks of gestation. At delivery (via the vaginal route), she developed significant blood loss, which required a transfusion of two units of blood. She was discharged 72 hours postpartum. On day seven postpartum, she presented to the emergency department because of headaches, blurred vision, paresthesias, lethargy, and difficulty breastfeeding. On physical

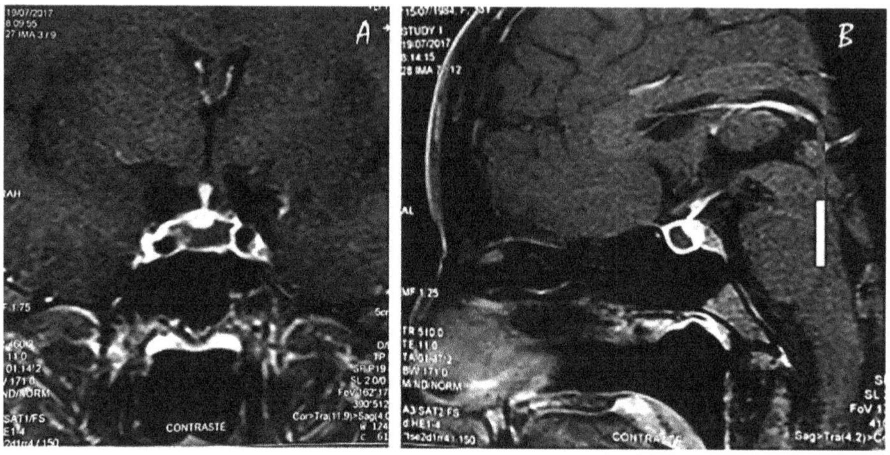

FIGURE 1: Coronal (a) and sagittal (b) postcontrast MRI at diagnosis. It shows an enlarged pituitary gland with suprasellar extension, peripheral enhancement of the pituitary gland, and irregular and poorly enhanced central portion after gadolinium injection.

examination, she appeared confused, was hypotensive (80/60 mmHg), and was tachycardic.

Laboratory tests showed hyponatremia of 118 mEq/l (normal range (NR): 138–145) and normocytic normochromic anemia with hemoglobin of 9.7 g/dl (NR: 11.3–14.7). Sheehan's syndrome was suspected based on her clinical presentation with a significant postpartum hemorrhage. Hormone workup revealed secondary hypothyroidism with low free T4 (0.58 ng/dl, NR 0.89–1.76) and normal TSH (0.35 μIU/ml, NR 0.35–5.5) and relatively low prolactin levels (PRL) of 7.12 ng/ml for the early postpartum period (NR for adult women 1.9–25; for women in the third trimester of pregnancy, NR is 84–232). Pituitary MRI showed an enlarged pituitary gland with suprasellar extension, with peripheral enhancement of the pituitary gland, and an irregular and poorly enhanced central portion after gadolinium injection (Figure 1).

She was treated with NaCl replacement to increase her Na levels by 8 mEq/day. Serum 8 AM cortisol was drawn, and as the results were not readily available, treatment with hydrocortisone was initiated with the suspicion of secondary adrenal insufficiency. In addition, levothyroxine treatment was started. Her sodium levels returned to normal, and she was discharged on hormonal replacement therapy (levothyroxine 100 mcg/day, hydrocortisone 15 mg in two divided doses: 10 mg at 8 a.m. and 5 mg at 16:00 pm).

Laboratory tests six weeks after discharge of the diagnosis of Sheehan's syndrome showed low IGF-1, normal free T4 and LH and FSH levels, PRL levels of 10.2 ng/ml, and serum 8 AM cortisol 24 hours after the last dose of hydrocortisone of 1.72 μg/dl (she did not take the evening dose and took the morning dose after blood was drawn). Cortisol levels at the time of hospitalization before hydrocortisone treatment were 36.2 μg/dl. Table 1 shows a summary of her hormonal workup. She was able to breastfeed partially until 4 months.

Regular menstrual cycles started three months after delivery. A repeat MRI performed seven months later showed a smaller pituitary gland with peripheral enhancement after gadolinium injection (Figure 2).

Doses of levothyroxine were gradually decreased with normal FT4 levels when she became spontaneously pregnant one year after the previous delivery. The lowest dose of L-thyroxin on which she became pregnant was 50 mcg 2 days a week and 75 mcg 5 days a week. The dose was increased during pregnancy to 75 mcg per day. The cortisol level was rechecked before pregnancy 24 hours after the last dose of hydrocortisone and was still low (2.54 μg/dl).

She had an uneventful pregnancy on levothyroxine 75 mcg/day and hydrocortisone 15 mg/day in two divided doses. She delivered a healthy, normal-weight female at 39 weeks of gestation.

3. Discussion

A diagnosis of Sheehan's syndrome is rarely made in the acute postpartum state. Sheehan's syndrome's true incidence is unknown, and it has been reported to occur in 1%–3.1% of women who lose 1–2 liters of blood associated with hypotension in developed countries [1, 2, 5]. However, prevalence has been reported to be higher in undeveloped countries (3.1%–27.6%) [6–8].

Sheehan's syndrome is generally diagnosed several years postpartum with chronic manifestations such as failure to lactate, amenorrhea, symptoms of hypothyroidism, and adrenal insufficiency. The time between postpartum hemorrhage and symptom onset can be several years. The diagnostic delay is variable. An average delay of 20 ± 8.3 years with a range of 2–36 years was reported in 124 patients with Sheehan's [9]. Ramiandrasoa et al. reported a mean diagnostic delay of 9 ± 9.7 years in 39 women diagnosed with Sheehan's syndrome [10]. Also, Kristjansdottir et al. reported a diagnostic delay from 1 month to 20 years in 8 patients [11].

Acute Sheehan's syndrome is rare, with only 27 cases reported in the literature [1, 3, 12–35] (Table 2).

The first symptoms were reported between 6 hours and 20 days postpartum. Most occur after a massive postpartum hemorrhage and moderate to severe anemia. In one case, severe hypotension was reported at the beginning of the

Table 1: Hormonal workup.

Date	FT4 (0.89–1.76 mU/ml)	Cortisol (5–25 μg/dl)	LH (2.4–12.6 IU/L)	FSH (2.11–11.3 IU/L)	Prolactin (0.15–25 ng/ml)	Na (135–145 mEq/l)	K (3.5–5.5 mEq/l))
07/18/17	0.58	36.2			7.12	118	4.0
07/28/17						138	4.1
08/05/17						137	
09/02/17		1.72	4.11	7.65	10	143	4.0
05/08/18							
07/04/18	1.05						

Delivery date: 07/11/2017.

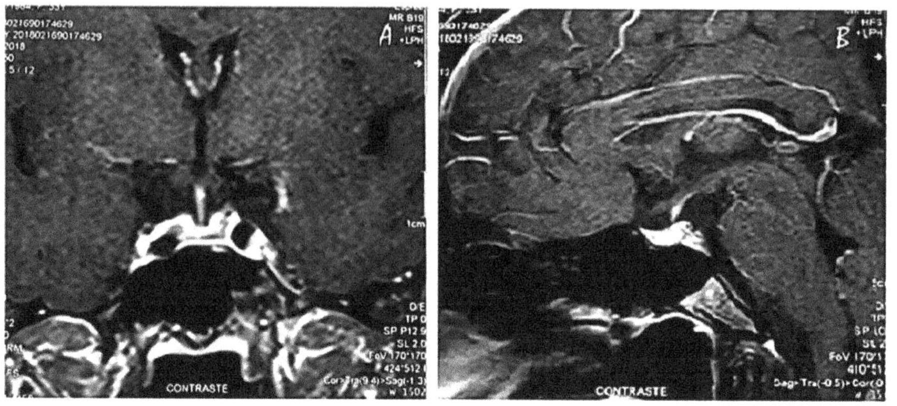

Figure 2: Coronal (a) and sagittal (b) postcontrast MRI 7 months after diagnosis showed a smaller pituitary gland with peripheral enhancement after gadolinium injection.

epidural anesthesia without postpartum hemorrhage, followed by panhypopituitarism and diabetes insipidus [15]. In 16 cases, the main presentation was hyponatremia, with a few also presenting with diabetes insipidus, hypothyroidism, panhypopituitarism, and headache. Acute Sheehan's syndrome usually presents with hypotension, tachycardia, failure to lactate, hypoglycemia, fatigue, lethargy, nausea, and vomiting. In the acute phase, hypopituitarism can include ACTH deficiency, which can be fatal if not treated [7].

Hyponatremia is an initial symptom of acute Sheehan's syndrome in approximately 60% of the reported cases. In addition, it is a common electrolyte disturbance in the chronic presentation (33% to 69%) [36–38]. Acute hyponatremia can be life-threatening because it can cause cerebral edema. There are several proposed pathophysiological mechanisms for the development of hyponatremia in this syndrome. It may be due to diminished free water clearance caused by hypothyroidism and adrenal insufficiency [2, 39]. Moreover, a glucocorticoid deficit may enhance the inappropriate secretion of vasopressin. The hypersecretion of vasopressin could be due to the reduction in cardiac output and systemic blood pressure induced by the absence of cortisol. In addition, cortisol deficiency results in increased hypothalamic secretion of corticotropin-releasing hormone (CRH), a vasopressin secretagogue [39, 40]. Furthermore, the negative feedback of cortisol on CRH and ACTH is removed with adrenal insufficiency [41]. Our case presented with secondary hypothyroidism, which may also produce hyponatremia due to reduced free-water clearance.

Cortisol levels were initially normal, but she was pregnant, a condition known to increase CBG levels due to high estrogen levels. In the third trimester of pregnancy, total cortisol levels are increased 2 to 3-fold compared to those of nonpregnant women, which is equivalent to the CBG increase during pregnancy [42]. Cortisol-binding globulin has been reported to normalize between 3 and 6 weeks postpartum [43]. However, others have reported that it remains elevated for 3–6 months [44]. This may be due to its increased half-life. Cortisol levels were low when retested on several occasions. Gonadotropin function was not affected or restored.

Recovery of hormonal function has been reported in the first postpartum year in 2 cases of acute Sheehan's syndrome [13, 22]. In one case, although panhypopituitarism persisted, diabetes insipidus resolved within two years of diagnosis [14]. In our case, while prolactin levels were initially relatively low for the early postpartum period, she was able to partially breastfeed. The latter may be due to a partial lactotroph deficiency or recovered function. This patient had partial hypopituitarism because the gonadotrophic axis was not affected or restored.

The preservation of some hormonal axes could be explained because pituitary necrosis is frequently incomplete, with selective loss of hormone secretion [25]. There can be remnant intact pituitary tissue that continues to receive blood supply from alternative arteries of the neurohypophysis if there is a stop in flow in the superior artery and continues to produce hormones, leading to a selective loss of hormone secretion.

Sheehan's syndrome early MRI findings include a nonhemorrhagic enlargement of the pituitary gland with a thin rim of peripheral enhancement after gadolinium, an intrasellar mass with suprasellar extension, and a lack of enhancement of the pituitary gland [13, 15, 19, 21, 24, 25, 29, 30]. However, in some cases, normal scans were reported in the acute period [1, 22, 23, 26, 27, 33, 34]. After subsequent involution with pituitary shrinkage, atrophic glands and an empty sella are reported in late scans [1, 7, 13, 19, 23–25, 29]. The pituitary gland during pregnancy increases in size and can reach a maximum size of 10 mm during the last trimester and 12 mm in the immediate postpartum period, with an upward symmetric convexity. There is an increase in the T1 signal intensity of the pituitary gland, more so during the third trimester. After the first week postpartum, the pituitary gland returns to its normal size [45].

Sheehan's syndrome pathogenesis is not yet fully understood, with the principal proposed factor being an ischemia of the enlarged anterior pituitary gland during severe peripartum hemorrhage. Due to lactotroph hyperplasia, there is a physiological enlargement of the pituitary gland during pregnancy, reaching 120–136% of its original size [46]. This pituitary hyperplasia is not accompanied by an

Table 2: Reported cases of acute Sheehan's syndrome.

Authors	Age (y)	Time of diagnosis related to delivery	Symptoms at presentation	Hypo natremia	Hormone deficit at diagnosis	Hormone recovery	CT scan at diagnosis	CT scan at F/U	Pituitary MRI at diagnosis	Pituitary MRI at follow-up
Putterman et al. [3]	27	7 days	Paresthesia, headache, weakness, somnolence	Yes	LH/FSH, TSH, ACTH	No	Pituitary infarction, increased CSF surrounding gland	Empty sella (6 months postpartum)		
Zuker [12]	20	14 hours	Hypoglycemia	No	ACTH	No	No enhancing pituitary (ischemia)	Small, well enhancing pituitary (3 months after postpartum)		
Lavalle et al. [13]	30	6 hours	Seizures	Yes	TSH, ACTH	TSH, ACTH	Normal	Peripherally enhancing sellar mass with suprasellar extension (5 days after delivery)	Intrasellar mass with suprasellar extension with peripheral enhancement	Atrophic gland (48 days after delivery)
Kan and Calligerous [14]	32	24 hours	Polydipsia and polyuria	No	FSH/LH, TSH, ACTH, ADH	ADH	Normal pituitary gland			
Dejager et al. [15]	32	3 days	Headache, polydipsia, and polyuria	No	GH, LH/FSH, PRL, ADH	No			Holosellar 11-mm mass, pituitary gland did not enhance with contrast, peripheral rim	Shrinkage of pituitary mass of 4 mm, and dissappearance of bright neurophypophysis spot (30 days after delivery
Boulanger et al [16]	30	10 days	Asthenia, failure to lactate	Yes	LH/FSH, TSH, ACTH, PRL	Not reported				
Kale et al. [17]	23	20 days	Psychosis	No	FSH/LH, TSH, ACTH	Not reported		Empty sella		
Schrager et al. [18]	39	12 days	Nausea, vomiting, fatigue, dizziness, diarrhea	Yes	TSH, ACTH	Not reported				

Table 2: Continued.

Authors	Age (y)	Time of diagnosis related to delivery	Symptoms at presentation	Hypo natremia	Hormone deficit at diagnosis	Hormone recovery	CT scan at diagnosis	CT scan at F/U	Pituitary MRI at diagnosis	Pituitary MRI at follow-up
Lust et al. [19]	32	3 days	Headache, failure to lactate	Yes	TSH, ACTH	No			Enlarged pituitary isointense T1 abutting optic chiasm with peripheral gland enhancement	Empty sella (4 months after delivery)
Wang et al. [20]	32	7 days	Polyuria, renal insufficiency	Yes	LH/FSH, TSH, ACTH	Not reported				
Bunch et al. [21]	23	6 days	Fatigue, diffuse abdominal pain, weakness, hypoglycemia	Yes	TSH, ACTH	Not reported			Enlarged pituitary gland, peripheral enhancement	Normal-sized pituitary gland with heterogen-eous uptake of contrast (1 month after delivery)
Munz et al. [22]	33	6 days	Stupor, headache, nausea, vomiting	Yes	TSH, ACTH, PRL	Yes	Normal		Normal	
Wang et al. [23]	33	19 days	Respiratory distress	No	LH/FSH, TSH, ACTH, PRL	Not reported			Normal	Empty sella (day 32 after delivery)
Kaplun et al. [24]	29	17 days	Fatigue, failure to lactate, fever, postural syncope	Yes	GH, LH/ FSH, TSH, ACTH, PRL	No			Nonenhancing minimally hypointense lesion in pituitary gland	Empty sella (6 months after delivery)
Kaplun et al. [24]	21	3 days	Headache, fever	Yes	GH, LH/ FSH, TSH, ACTH, PRL	No			Enlarged pituitary gland with suprasellar extension, peripheral enhancement with an irregular and poorly enhanced central portion	Empty sella (11 months after delivery)
Anfuso et al. [25]	35	8 days	Asthenia, headache, abdominal pain	Yes	GH, LH/ FSH, TSH, ACTH, PRL	No			Lack of enhancement of pituitary gland	Atrophy of adenohypophysis
Kumar et al. [26]	36	4 days	Polyuria	No	TSH, ACTH, PRL, ADH	No			Normal	Normal

Table 2: Continued.

Authors	Age (y)	Time of diagnosis related to delivery	Symptoms at presentation	Hypo natremia	Hormone deficit at diagnosis	Hormone recovery	CT scan at diagnosis	CT scan at F/U	Pituitary MRI at diagnosis	Pituitary MRI at follow-up
Robalo et al. [27]	45	15 days	Headache, fatigue, polydipsia olyuria	No	GH, LH/ FSH, TSH, ACTH, PRL, ADH	No	Discrete enlargement of anterior pituitary lobe, hypointense after contrast		Normal pituitary Ectopic posterior pituitary	
Shoib et al. [28]	31	16–18 days	Psychosis, failure to lactate	No	LH/FSH, TSH, ACTH	Not reported		Empty sella		
Sasaki et al. [29]	37	4–6 days	Failure to lactate	Yes	GH, LH/ FSH, TSH, ACTH, PRL	No			Slight swelling of anterior lobe and pituitary stalk. There was no enhancement of central portion but a peripheral rim of enhancement	Empty sella
Hale et al. [30]	31	6 days	Severe headaches, failure to lactate, orthostatic hypotension, nausea and vomiting	Yes	TSH, ACTH, PRL, ADH	No			Infarcted enlarged pituitary with an expanded sella, with peripheral rim enhancement after contrast	NA
Matsuzaki et al. [1]	27	8 days	Seizure	Yes	GH, FSH/ LH, TSH, ACTH, PRL	No			No abnormalities	Atrophic pituitary gland
Windpessl et al. [31]	31	8 days	Headache, lethargy, postural light-headedness, failure to lactate	Yes	TSH, ACTH	No			Pituitary hyperintense	Pituitary infarction
Rahim et al. [32]	27	2 days	Severe bifrontal headache and photophobia, failure to lactate	No	No	No	Subtly enlarged pituitary gland with an area of focal hypodensity		Acute pituitary infarction	
Meregildo-Rodriguez [33]	24	4 days	Hypoglycemia, seizures	No	GH, FSH/ LH, ACTH, TSH, PRL	No	Normal		Normal	

Table 2: Continued.

Authors	Age (y)	Time of diagnosis related to delivery	Symptoms at presentation	Hypo natremia	Hormone deficit at diagnosis	Hormone recovery	CT scan at diagnosis	CT scan at F/U	Pituitary MRI at diagnosis	Pituitary MRI at follow-up
Rahmani Tzvi-Ran et al. [34]	24	1 day	Headache, fatigue, and failure to lactate	Yes	GH, FSH/LH, TSH, ACTH, PRL, ADH	No			Normal pituitary with circumferential enhancement	
Olmes et al. [35]	28	2 days	Failure to lactate, polyuria.	No	FSH/LH, TSH, ACTH, ADH	No				

increase in vascular supply. There is an interruption of arterial blood flow to the gland that may result from arterial spasm due to hypotension resulting from postpartum hemorrhage. In addition, there may be compression of the superior hypophyseal artery because of pituitary enlargement. Moreover, due to hypercoagulation, thrombosis in the pituitary arteries might contribute [7].

Spontaneous pregnancy rarely occurs in patients with Sheehan's syndrome because most patients have hypogonadotropic hypogonadism [47]. Hypogonadotropic hypogonadism has been reported in 67%–100% of patients with Sheehan's syndrome [48, 49]. To our knowledge, no cases of spontaneous pregnancy after acute Sheehan's syndrome have been reported. There are only two reported cases of acute Sheehan's syndrome with a successful pregnancy. One case had ovulation induction, the other in vitro fertilization [1, 4]. In our case, the gonadotropin axis was functional, so pregnancy was a possibility. In a recent review by Zhan et al., 27 patients with Sheehan's syndrome and 32 pregnancies were reported in the literature [4]. Of these pregnancies, 19 (59.4%) were conceived spontaneously, whereas 11 (34.4%) were induced by ovulation. One reported case was due to egg donation [50]. The case reported by Zhan et al. achieved a successful pregnancy by in vitro fertilization and embryo transfer [4].

In this case, we do not believe a lymphocytic hypophysitis complicated with postpartum hemorrhage can be a differential diagnosis, as she did not have symptoms of hypopituitarism and/or of mass lesions prior to the obstetric hemorrhage [51]. In addition, pituitary MRI did not show an enlarged triangular- or dumbbell-shaped gland with a thickened stalk, nor did it enhance homogenously after contrast [52].

In addition, we believe the pituitary apoplexy of an asymptomatic, nonfunctioning pituitary adenoma is not a differential diagnosis either. It presents as sudden and severe headache in more than 80% of cases, with variable degrees of visual-field impairment and ocular palsy in more than 50% of cases (III cranial nerve, most often). Moreover, there were no predisposing risk factors for pituitary apoplexy such as hypertension, coagulopathy, surgery, dynamic testing, or use of dopamine agonists. In addition, an MRI, 7 months later, did not show a residual pituitary adenoma [53]. Furthermore, we do not believe that Rathke's cleft cyst can be a diagnosis either. They are cystic remnants of the craniopharyngeal duct, usually asymptomatic, but they can present with headache, endocrine dysfunction, diabetes insipidus, and visual impairment. In addition, MRI shows a midline cyst usually with T1-hyperintense signal due to proteinaceous mucinous cyst contents [54].

During pregnancy, appropriate hormonal replacement in patients with hypopituitarism is required. Hydrocortisone is the preferred glucocorticoid replacement during pregnancy, as it does not cross the placenta due to its degradation by the 11β-hydroxysteroid dehydrogenase 2 enzyme [55]. Higher doses of hydrocortisone may be required during the third trimester.

4. Conclusion

Acute presentation of Sheehan's syndrome should be considered in the evaluation of postpartum patients with suggestive symptoms such as hypotension, tachycardia, failure to lactate, hypoglycemia, fatigue, lethargy, nausea, and vomiting. Physicians should be aware that hyponatremia might be an initial manifestation of this entity, which requires a high index of suspicion for diagnosis. Spontaneous pregnancy after acute Sheehan's syndrome is exceedingly rare but can happen in women with preserved gonadal function.

References

[1] S. Matsuzaki, M. Endo, Y. Ueda et al., "A case of acute Sheehan's syndrome and literature review: a rare but life-threatening complication of postpartum hemorrhage," *BMC Pregnancy and Childbirth*, vol. 17, p. 188, 2017.

[2] F. Kelestimur, "Sheehan's syndrome," *Pituitary*, vol. 6, pp. 181–188, 2003.

[3] C. Putterman, Y. Almog, Y. Caraco, D. J. Gross, and E. Ben-Chetrit, "Inappropriate secretion of antidiuretic hormone in Sheehan's syndrome: a rare cause of postpartum hyponatremia," *American Journal of Obstetrics and Gynecology*, vol. 165, pp. 1330–1333, 1991.

[4] Y. Zhan, T. Xu, X. Wang, and D. Shi, "Perinatal management and outcomes of pregnancy following sheehan syndrome: a case report and literature review," *Maternal-Fetal Medicine*, vol. 03, pp. 213–220, 2021.

[5] R. Abs, B. A. Bengtsson, E. Hernberg-Stahl et al., "GH replacement in 1034 growth hormone deficient hypopituitary adults: demographic and clinical characteristics, dosing and safety," *Clinical Endocrinology*, vol. 50, pp. 703–713, 1999.

[6] F. Tanriverdi, H. S. Dokmetas, N. Kebapci et al., "Etiology of hypopituitarism in tertiary care institutions in Turkish population: analysis of 773 patients from Pituitary Study Group database," *Endocrine*, vol. 47, pp. 198–205, 2014.

[7] H. Diri, Z. Karaca, F. Tanriverdi, K. Unluhizarci, and F. Kelestimur, "Sheehan's syndrome: new insights into an old disease," *Endocrine*, vol. 51, pp. 22–31, 2016.

[8] A. H. Zargar, B. Singh, B. A. Laway, S. R. Masoodi, A. I. Wani, and M. I. Bashir, "Epidemiologic aspects of postpartum pituitary hypofunction (Sheehan's syndrome)," *Fertility and Sterility*, vol. 84, pp. 523–528, 2005.

[9] D. Gokalp, G. Alpagat, A. Tuzcu et al., "Four decades without diagnosis: Sheehan's syndrome, a retrospective analysis," *Gynecological Endocrinology*, vol. 32, pp. 904–907, 2016.

[10] C. Ramiandrasoa, F. Castinetti, I. Raingeard et al., "Delayed diagnosis of Sheehan's syndrome in a developed country: a retrospective cohort study," *European Journal of Endocrinology*, vol. 169, pp. 431–438, 2013.

[11] H. L. Kristjansdottir, S. P. Bodvarsdottir, and H. A. Sigurjonsdottir, "Sheehan's syndrome in modern times: a nationwide retrospective study in Iceland," *European Journal of Endocrinology*, vol. 164, pp. 349–354, 2011.

[12] N. Zuker, M. Bissessor, M. Korber et al., "Acute hypoglycaemic coma--a rare, potentially lethal form of early onset Sheehan syndrome," *The Australian and New Zealand Journal of Obstetrics and Gynaecology*, vol. 35, pp. 318–320, 1995.

[13] G. Lavallee, R. Morcos, J. Palardy, M. Aube, and D. Gilbert, "MR of nonhemorrhagic postpartum pituitary apoplexy," *AJNR. American journal of neuroradiology*, vol. 16, pp. 1939–1941, 1995.

[14] A. K. Kan and D. Calligerous, "A case report of Sheehan syndrome presenting with diabetes insipidus," *The Australian and New Zealand Journal of Obstetrics and Gynaecology*, vol. 38, pp. 224–226, 1998.

[15] S. Dejager, S. Gerber, L. Foubert, and G. Turpin, "Sheehan's syndrome: differential diagnosis in the acute phase," *Journal of Internal Medicine*, vol. 244, pp. 261–266, 1998.

[16] E. Boulanger, D. Pagniez, S. Roueff et al., "Sheehan syndrome presenting as early post-partum hyponatraemia," *Nephrology Dialysis Transplantation*, vol. 14, pp. 2714-2715, 1999.

[17] K. Kale, N. Nihalani, N. Karnik, and N. Shah, "Postpartum psychosis in a case of sheehan's syndrome," *Indian Journal of Psychiatry*, vol. 41, pp. 70–72, 1999.

[18] S. Schrager and L. Sabo, "Sheehan syndrome: a rare complication of postpartum hemorrhage," *Journal of the American Board of Family Practice*, vol. 14, pp. 389–391, 2001.

[19] K. Lust, H. D. McIntyre, and A. Morton, "Sheehan's syndrome--acute presentation with hyponatraemia and headache," *The Australian and New Zealand Journal of Obstetrics and Gynaecology*, vol. 41, pp. 348–351, 2001.

[20] H. Y. Wang, C. T. Chang, and M. S. Wu, "Postpartum hemorrhage complicated with irreversible renal failure and central diabetes insipidus," *Renal Failure*, vol. 24, pp. 849–852, 2002.

[21] T. J. Bunch, W. F. Dunn, A. Basu, and R. I. Gosman, "Hyponatremia and hypoglycemia in acute Sheehan's syndrome," *Gynecological Endocrinology*, vol. 16, pp. 419–423, 2002.

[22] W. Munz, R. Seufert, P. G. Knapstein, and K. Pollow, "Early postpartum hyponatremia in a patient with transient Sheehan's syndrome," *Experimental and Clinical Endocrinology and Diabetes Official Journal German Society of Endocrinology and German Diabetes Association*, vol. 112, pp. 278–280, 2004.

[23] S. Y. Wang, S. R. Hsu, S. L. Su, and S. T. Tu, "Sheehan's syndrome presenting with early postpartum congestive heart failure," *Journal of the Chinese Medical Association Journal of the Chinese Medical Association*, vol. 68, pp. 386–391, 2005.

[24] J. Kaplun, C. Fratila, A. Ferenczi et al., "Sequential pituitary MR imaging in Sheehan syndrome: report of 2 cases," *AJNR. American journal of neuroradiology*, vol. 29, pp. 941–943, 2008.

[25] S. Anfuso, T. S. Patrelli, E. Soncini, P. Chiodera, G. M. Fadda, and G. B. Nardelli, "A case report of Sheehan's syndrome with acute onset, hyponatremia and severe anemia," *Acta Bio-Medica Atenei Parmensis*, vol. 80, pp. 73–76, 2009.

[26] S. Kumar, D. Burrows, S. Dang, and D. Simmons, "Sheehan syndrome presenting as central diabetes insipidus: a rare presentation of an uncommon disorder," *Endocrine Practice*, vol. 17, pp. 108–114, 2011.

[27] R. Robalo, C. Pedroso, A. Agapito, and A. Borges, "Acute Sheehan's syndrome presenting as central diabetes insipidus," *BMJ Case Reports*, vol. 17, no. 1, pp. 1-4, 2012.

[28] S. Shoib, M. M. Dar, T. Arif, H. Bashir, M. H. Bhat, and J. Ahmed, "Sheehan's syndrome presenting as psychosis: a rare clinical presentation," *Medical Journal of the Islamic Republic of Iran*, vol. 27, pp. 35–37, 2013.

[29] S. Sasaki, I. Fujisawa, T. Ishihara et al., "A novel hook-shaped enhancement on contrast-enhanced sagittal magnetic resonance image in acute Sheehan's syndrome: a case report," *Endocrine Journal*, vol. 61, pp. 71–76, 2014.

[30] B. Hale and A. S. Habib, "Sheehan syndrome: acute presentation with severe headache," *International Journal of Obstetric Anesthesia*, vol. 23, pp. 383–386, 2014.

[31] M. Windpessl, A. Karrer, and C. Schwarz, "Acute hyponatremia in puerperium: Sheehan's syndrome," *The American Journal of Medicine*, vol. 131, pp. e147–e148, 2018.

[32] A. Rahim, J. Baird-Gunning, D. E. Ashton, T. Angstmann, and R. Lahoria, "Acute Sheehan syndrome manifesting as unremitting headache," *Neurohospitalist*, vol. 8, pp. NP1–NP2, 2018.

[33] E. M. Rodriguez, "Acute sheehan's syndrome: a case and an updated literature review," *Revista Mexicana de Endocrinologia, Metabolismo y Nutricion*, vol. 5, pp. 72–74, 2018.

[34] I. Rahmani Tzvi-Ran, J. Olchowski, M. Fraenkel, A. Bashiri, and L. Barski, "A rare cause of postpartum acute hyponatremia," *Endocrinol Diabetes Metabolism Case Reports*, vol. 2019, pp. 18–0124, 2019.

[35] G. L. Olmes, E. F. Solomayer, J. C. Radosa et al., "Acute sheehan's syndrome manifesting initially with diabetes insipidus postpartum: a case report and systematic literature review," *Archives of Gynecology and Obstetrics*, vol. 306, no. 3, pp. 699–706, 2021.

[36] Y. Y. Huang, M. K. Ting, B. R. Hsu, and J. S. Tsai, "Demonstration of reserved anterior pituitary function among patients with amenorrhea after postpartum hemorrhage," *Gynecological Endocrinology*, vol. 14, pp. 99–104, 2000.

[37] C. Ratarasarn, R. Rajatanavin, and T. Himathongkam, "Salient clinical features of Sheehan's syndrome," *Journal of the Medical Association of Thailand = Chotmaihet thangphaet*, vol. 72, pp. 41–47, 1989.

[38] P. C. Pham, P. A. Pham, and P. T. Pham, "Sodium and water disturbances in patients with Sheehan's syndrome," *American Journal of Kidney Diseases The Official Journal of the National Kidney Foundation*, vol. 38, p. E14, 2001.

[39] R. W. Schrier, "Body water homeostasis: clinical disorders of urinary dilution and concentration," *Journal of the American Society of Nephrology Journal of the American Society of Nephrology*, vol. 17, pp. 1820–1832, 2006.

[40] B. Wolfson, R. W. Manning, L. G. Davis, R. Arentzen, and F. Baldino Jr., "Co-localization of corticotropin releasing factor and vasopressin mRNA in neurones after adrenalectomy," *Nature*, vol. 315, pp. 59–61, 1985.

[41] H. Raff, "Glucocorticoid inhibition of neurohypophysial vasopressin secretion," *American Journal of Physiology*, vol. 252, pp. R635–R644, 1987.

[42] B. I. St-Jean and A. Lacroix, "Adrenal cortex and medulla physiology during pregnancy, labor, and puerperium," in *Maternal-Fetal and Neonatal Endocrinology*, E. C. S. Kovacs and C. L. Deal, Eds., Academic Press, Cambridge, Massachusetts, 2020.

[43] E. Demey-Ponsart, J. M. Foidart, J. Sulon, and J. C. Sodoyez, "Serum CBG, free and total cortisol and circadian patterns of adrenal function in normal pregnancy," *Journal of Steroid Biochemistry*, vol. 16, pp. 165–169, 1982.

[44] C. Jung, J. T. Ho, D. J. Torpy et al., "A longitudinal study of plasma and urinary cortisol in pregnancy and postpartum," *Journal of Clinical Endocrinology & Metabolism*, vol. 96, pp. 1533–1540, 2011.

[45] J. F. Bonneville, "Normal pituitary gland and pregnancy," in *MRI of the Pituitary Gland*, B. F. Bonneville JF, F. Cattin, and S. Naggi, Eds., Springer, Heidelberg, Germany, 2016.

[46] J. G. Gonzalez, G. Elizondo, D. Saldivar, H. Nanez, L. E. Todd,

and J. Z. Villarreal, "Pituitary gland growth during normal pregnancy: an in vivo study using magnetic resonance imaging," *The American Journal of Medicine*, vol. 85, pp. 217–220, 1988.

[47] H. G. Grimes and M. H. Brooks, "Pregnancy in Sheehan's syndrome. Report of a case and review," *Obstetrical and Gynecological Survey*, vol. 35, pp. 481–488, 1980.

[48] O. Gei-Guardia, E. Soto-Herrera, A. Gei-Brealey, and C. H. Chen-Ku, "Sheehan syndrome in Costa Rica: clinical experience with 60 cases," *Endocrine Practice*, vol. 17, pp. 337–344, 2011.

[49] H. Diri, F. Tanriverdi, Z. Karaca et al., "Extensive investigation of 114 patients with Sheehan's syndrome: a continuing disorder," *European Journal of Endocrinology*, vol. 171, pp. 311–318, 2014.

[50] T. A. O. Adedugbe, S. O. Iwuala, O. A. Fasanmade, A. Ajayi, and A. E. Ohwovoriole, "Successful pregnancy using ovum donation in sheehan's syndrome: a case report," in *Proceedings of the 96th Annual Meeting and Expo of the Endocrine Society Chicago, EUU*, Chicago, IL, USA, June 2014.

[51] Z. Karaca, F. Tanriverdi, K. Unluhizarci, and F. Kelestimur, "Pregnancy and pituitary disorders," *European Journal of Endocrinology*, vol. 162, pp. 453–475, 2010.

[52] F. Caranci, G. Leone, A. Ponsiglione et al., "Imaging findings in hypophysitis: a review," *La Radiologia medica*, vol. 125, pp. 319–328, 2020.

[53] G. Barkhoudarian and D. F. Kelly, "Pituitary apoplexy," *Neurosurgery Clinics of North America*, vol. 30, pp. 457–463, 2019.

[54] R. Trifanescu, O. Ansorge, J. A. Wass, A. B. Grossman, and N. Karavitaki, "Rathke's cleft cysts," *Clinical Endocrinology*, vol. 76, pp. 151–160, 2012.

[55] M. Fleseriu, I. A. Hashim, N. Karavitaki et al., "Hormonal replacement in hypopituitarism in adults: an endocrine society clinical practice guideline," *Journal of Clinical Endocrinology & Metabolism*, vol. 101, pp. 3888–3921, 2016.

A Novel Mutation of the Calcium-Sensing Receptor Gene Causing Familial Hypocalciuric Hypercalcemia Complicates Medical Followup after Roux-en-Y Gastric Bypass: A Case Report and a Summary of Mutations Found in the Same Hospital Laboratory

Elin Rebecka Carlsson[1] **Mai-Britt Toft Nielsen,**[2] **Anne Mette Høgh,**[1] **Rikke Veggerby Grønlund,**[3] **Mogens Fenger,**[1] **and Louise Ambye**[1]

[1]*Department of Clinical Biochemistry, Copenhagen University Hospital Hvidovre, Denmark*
[2]*Department of Endocrinology, Copenhagen University Hospital Hvidovre, Denmark*
[3]*Gubra, Hørsholm, Denmark*

Correspondence should be addressed to Elin Rebecka Carlsson; elin.rebecka.carlsson@regionh.dk

Academic Editor: Eli Hershkovitz

Heterozygous inactivating mutations in the calcium-sensing receptor (CaSR) gene are known to cause familial hypocalciuric hypercalcemia (FHH), usually a benign form of hypercalcemia without symptoms of a disrupted calcium homeostasis. FHH can be mistaken for the more common primary hyperparathyroidism (PHPT), for which surgical treatment may be needed. We describe a case of a 36-year-old woman with hypercalcemia and elevated PTH, initially suspected of having PHPT. Sequencing of the CaSR-gene revealed a mutation in nucleotide 437, changing the amino acid in position 146 from Glycine to Aspartate. The mutation was previously undescribed in the literature, but a very low calcium:creatinine clearance ratio supported the diagnosis FHH. A few years later, the patient's two daughters were tested and the association between mutation and hypercalcemia could be confirmed. The patient was gastric bypass-operated and therefore, due to malabsorption and increased risk of fracture, was in need of adequate calcium supplementation. The chronically elevated calcium levels challenged medical followup, as calcium sufficiency could not be monitored in a traditional manner. Eventually the patient developed elevated alkaline phosphatase, a further increased PTH and a decreased DXA T-score indicating calcium deficiency and bone resorption. As a supplement, all CaSR-mutations found at our hospital, 2005-2018.

1. Introduction

Calcium homeostasis is crucial for many biological functions and is regulated by direct and indirect effects of parathyrine (PTH) on kidney, bone, and intestine, released as a reaction to sensing of hypocalcemia in the parathyroid gland, mediated through the calcium-sensing receptor (CaSR) [1]. Calcium is usually absorbed throughout the whole intestine, where an adequate vitamin D-level is required for optimal uptake [2]. If the supply is insufficient, increased PTH stimulates urinary calcium reabsorption and resorption of calcium from the skeleton. In addition, through their own calcium-sensing receptors, the kidneys promote urinary calcium reabsorption independently of PTH [1].

Heterozygous inactivating mutations in the CaSR-gene are known to cause familial hypocalciuric hypercalcemia (FHH), also called benign hypercalcemia due to its mild, often asymptomatic phenotype [3, 4]. Neonatal severe hyperparathyroidism and autosomal dominant hypocalcemia (ADH) are other more severe clinical manifestations of mutations in the same gene. So far, more than 130 FHH-causing mutations of the CaSR-gene have been described and novel mutations keep being reported [1].

In patients with hypercalcemia, the main reason for sequencing the CaSR-gene in search for mutations is to distinguish patients with FHH from patients with primary hyperparathyroidism (PHPT), who otherwise have a similar presentation biochemically [4, 5]. Parathyroidectomy, a removal of one or several of the parathyroid glands is needed to treat symptomatic PHPT that typically arises as a sporadic mutation in an adenoma [6], while FHH rarely requires treatment and cannot be cured surgically, unless a total parathyroidectomy is performed [7]. Most patients with FHH have a mutation in the CaSR-gene (FHH 1) but occasionally the cause is a mutation in two other genes, GNA11 (FHH2) or AP2S1 (FHH3), the latter associated with a more severe phenotype [1, 5, 8, 9]. A similar clinical presentation in patients without mutations related to the CaSR-gene may also be caused by CaSR-blocking autoantibodies, as seen in autoimmune hypocalciuric hypercalcemia (AHH) [3]. Apart from genetic sequencing, the calcium:creatinine clearance ratio is important in distinguishing between PHPT and FHH [10].

Calcium deficiency and secondary hyperparathyroidism are also problematic and commonly seen in patients treated for obesity with Roux-en-Y gastric bypass, where a part of the stomach and proximal intestine is excluded from food passage [11]. These patients are at increased risk of getting a fracture compared to the general population [12] and an adequate supplementation of calcium and vitamin D, monitored by measurements of calcium-ion, 25-hydroxy-vitamin D, and PTH, is important to reduce this risk [13].

We describe a case of a 36-year-old gastric bypass-operated woman with hypercalcemia and elevated PTH. Sequencing of the CaSR-gene revealed a previously undescribed mutation in nucleotide 437, changing the amino acid in position 146 from Glycine to Aspartate. Six years later, her two daughters were tested. One of the daughters was found to carry the same mutation.

2. Case Presentation

A 36-year-old woman was referred to the department of endocrinology for further examination of hypercalcemia, which was discovered during routine blood tests after gastric bypass operation 1 year earlier. There was no history of kidney stones, fractures, or osteoporosis that may be a result of hypercalcemia, and she had no known hyperthyroidism, Addison's disease, malignancy, sarcoidosis, or any other granulomatous disease that could explain the hypercalcemia. She had lost contact with her mother and sister, her only living relatives. Thus, a family history of hypercalcemia could not be investigated.

The patient inconsistently took calcium and vitamin D3 supplements in addition to iron, cobalamine, and multivitamins after the gastric bypass operation. She did not take thiazide diuretic or any other medications. She had symptoms of depression, anxiety, and tiredness and was later prescribed antidepressant medication. She also had recurrent episodes of dizziness, tremor, sweating, and fatigue, which resolved with the ingestion of carbohydrate and was related to hypoglycemia. Reactive hypoglycemia is a known late complication of gastric bypass operation induced by inappropriate hyperinsulinemia after the intake of rapidly absorbed carbohydrates [13]. The reactive hypoglycemia responded to dietitian instructions.

Repeated blood tests showed Ca-ion between 1.42 and 1.47 mmol/l (ref: 1.18 – 1.32 mmol/l), PTH between 6.3 and 8.9 pmol/l (ref: 1.7 – 7.1 pmol/l), and 25-hydroxy vitamin D between 43 and 58 nmol/l (ref: > 50 pmol/l). Alkaline phosphatase and thyroid function were normal. Dual-energy X-ray absorptiometry (DXA) showed T= -0.6 and T= -0.2 at the lumbar spine and total hip, respectively (Table 1).

Based on the mild hypercalcemia and the high normal to slightly elevated PTH, the patient was suspected of having primary PHPT. Before referral to a surgeon, FHH, the rare differential diagnosis to PHPT, had to be excluded. Genetic testing for mutations in the CaSR-gene showed a heterozygous mutation in nucleotide 437, changing the amino acid in position 146 from Glycine (G) to Aspartate (D) (c.[437G>A];[=], p.[(G146D)];[=]), reference sequence NM_000388.3 OMIM 601199), here called G146D. The found mutation was not formerly associated with FHH. However, urine calcium:creatinine clearance ratio was very low, 0.0029 and 0.0017 on two occasions, which verified the diagnosis of FHH, at the same time excluding the more common PHPT.

The CaSR is a member of the subfamily C of G-protein-coupled receptors which have seven transmembrane domains and function as disulfide-linked homodimers [14]. Its gene is located on chromosome 3q13.3-21.1 [15] and includes seven exons where exon 2-7 are protein coding [1]. The mutation G146D is located in exon three, in the coding region of the receptor's extracellular Venus flytrap domain, more specifically as a part of LB1, a domain important for the ligand binding of calcium ions (Ca^{2+}) and the amino acid L-tryptophan (L-Trp) that functions as an allosteric activator, enhancing the sensitivity of the receptor towards Ca^{2+} [14]. The binding of Ca^{2+} at this position seems to be important for maintaining the structural integrity of the receptor whereas other binding positions for Ca^{2+} are of more importance for receptor activity. Mutations in amino acids positioned as number 145 and 147, flanking number 146 on each side, have both been shown to eliminate the Ca^{2+} induced receptor activity. Based on this and the fact that the amino acid in position 146 is a part of the L-Trp binding cleft, it is likely that a mutation in position 146 reduces the receptor activity. Indeed, predictions from public *in silico* evaluation tools (Mutation Taster, PolyPhen, Provean) that were used to assist in the interpretation of the DNA-variant G146D all predicted a homozygous mutation G146D to be disease causing when factors like the location of the mutation regarding change of splice site, active site, or amino acid, as well as the nucleotide conservation between species, were taken into consideration. This knowledge about the CaSR-structure and consequence of mutations in neighboring amino acid positions was however not available at the time the patient was diagnosed.

Table 1: Results from biochemical analysis and measures of bone mineral density.

		I		II_1	II_2
CaSR mutation		+/-		+/-	-/-
		at presentation	at time for II_1's and II_2's testing	at diagnosis	at testing
Age		36	42	17	12
Biochemical analyses:	Reference:				
25-hydroxy vitamin D (nmol/L)	> 50	53	40 ↓	25 ↓	24 ↓
Calcium ion, ionized (mmol/L)	1.18 – 1.32	1.47 ↑	1.46 ↑	1.45 ↑	1.15
Parathyrine (pmol/L)	1.1 – 7.1	8.9 ↑	10.9 ↑	4.2	14.1 ↑
Alkaline Phosphatase (U/L)	35 - 105[a]	89	118 ↑	91	213
Calcium:Creatinine clearance ratio	> 0.010	< 0.003 ↓	not measured		
Measure of bone mineral density:		Result	Result		
DXA Lumbar spine (T-score)	> - 1.0	-0.6	-1.2 ↓		
DXA Total hip (T-score)	> - 1.0	-0.2	0.1		

For the patient (I), results are shown at presentation, as well as at the time for testing of her two daughters (II_1 and II_2) whose results at testing are shown. Apart from CaSR-gene sequencing and results from I's presentation, all blood samples from all three patients are drawn and analyzed at the same day.
[a]Reference range for Alkaline Phosphatase differs with age; the one for adults is shown in the table, for the girl aged 17 years reference range is 42-102, and for the girl aged 12 it is 143-396. ↑ indicates that the result is above upper reference limit. ↓ indicates that the result is below lower reference limit. +/-, heterozygous mutation in the CaSR-gene; -/-, no mutation in the CaSR-gene.

Six years later, the patient's two daughters, 12 and 17 years old, were tested for the mutation. The youngest daughter did not have any mutation in the CaSR-gene, but she had a low level of D-vitamin associated with secondary hyperparathyroidism, low Ca-ion and elevated alkaline phosphatase. The eldest daughter was found to be carrying the same mutation in the CaSR-gene as her mother, associated with hypercalcemia and inappropriately high PTH. She, too, had a low level of D-vitamin. Both daughters had normal thyroid and liver function tests. The patient at this point had an unchanged mild hypercalcemia, but additionally she had developed elevated alkaline phosphatase, a further increased PTH-level and a decreased DXA T-score (lumbar spine) indicating FHH accompanied by calcium deficiency and bone resorption (Table 1).

3. Discussion

We have described a case story of a woman with hypercalcemia and permanently elevated PTH, where sequencing of the CaSR-gene revealed a probable disease-causing mutation in nucleotide 437, changing the amino acid in position 146 from Glycine to Aspartate. Mutations in the same locus had not been previously described, but the clinical presentation with a low calcium:creatinine clearance strongly supported the diagnosis FHH. Six years later, following CaSR-gene sequencing in two daughters, we were finally able to confirm that the novel mutation found most likely is the cause of the hypocalciuric hypercalcemic phenotype in this family. At this time, updated mutation databases and a better understanding of CaSR-structure and function were helpful in predicting the mutation to be disease causing, inactivating the CaSR.

In hyperparathyroidism, a correct diagnosis is important for several reasons. For our patient, the diagnosis of FHH1 ensured that she avoided unnecessary parathyroidectomy and finally enabled prescription of the proper vitamin and mineral supplementations. For the eldest daughter, who is a carrier of the same mutation, the diagnosis meant that she, like her mother, was not considered for surgery. In general, it is important to test females of FHH families, because calcium gets across the placenta and, in FHH mothers, leads to fetal hypercalcemia with a subsequent suppression of fetal parathyroid function resulting in the risk of transient, neonatal, hypocalcemic tetanus [16]. Apart from this, FHH is usually asymptomatic with rarely seen complications such as pancreatitis, gallstones, or chondrocalcinosis [3, 4, 10]. As complications are correlated to the degree of hypercalcemia, most distinctly in patients with FHH3 [1], simply monitoring the calcium level without treatment often suffice. Extreme values or symptoms of hypercalcemia might be treated with calcimimetics [17].

Chronic hypercalcemia is associated with kidney stones and osteoporosis (the latter not in FHH), but also neuromuscular and psychiatric symptoms [6]. The patient in the case vignette reported fatigue and depression, which could be caused by hypercalcemia. To our knowledge, this is the first case report of a patient with FHH treated for obesity with gastric bypass surgery, a combination that challenges medical investigation and followup. Especially, monitoring of calcium homeostasis needs a broader approach, as plasma levels of calcium and PTH are chronically elevated. In this case, malabsorption after gastric bypass surgery resulting in calcium deficiency could be identified by an increased level of PTH, compared to the habitual level of PTH, eventually combined with an increased level of alkaline phosphatase and a reduced bone mineral density (BMD). This complexity emphasizes the importance of qualified medical followup after gastric bypass surgery.

Interestingly, this case report also illustrates another complexity, namely, the large variation within the spectrum of hyperparathyroidism, here with several variants seen in the same family. First, we have our patient with FHH and calcium deficiency, second the eldest daughter with FHH and normal level of PTH, and last the youngest daughter with secondary hyperparathyroidism due to deficiency of vitamin D and calcium. In common, all family members have low levels of D-vitamin.

Compared to the relatively high prevalence of PHPT, FHH is rare [4]. At our hospital, we started in 2005 to perform genetic testing by polymerase chain reaction (PCR) and Sanger sequencing of the six protein coding exons (exon 2-7) and intron boundaries of the CaSR-gene. Since the beginning, we have sequenced DNA from 822 patients suspected of having a parathyroid adenoma. Altogether, we have found 56 different mutations in heterozygous form (Supplementary Table S1), a majority of which as of September 2018 had been described in the medical literature [5, 18–26] and/or reported in mutation databases like ClinVar [27]. Most of the mutations found were inactivating mutations. In total, a mutation was found in 91 (11%) of the patients tested. The real mutation prevalence in this population is, although, most certainly higher. This is due to the limitations of the method that only sequence the coding exons and the intron boundaries of the CaSR-gene but not the promoter region, the deep intron regions, and the 3′untranslated region. Moreover, large genomic deletions and sequence variants in primer binding sites can be missed, resulting in false-negative test results. Mutations in other genes, for example, GNA11 or AP2S1 where mutations can result in FHH2 and FHH3, are not examined.

Important to note and as illustrated in this case report is that the interpretation of the clinical consequence of the mutation can change depending on the data available for a found mutation at the given time. The clinical picture, supported by results from routine biochemical analyses and diagnostic imaging, will always be of great value in diagnosis.

Consent

Informed consent for publication was obtained from the patient involved.

Authors' Contributions

Elin Rebecka Carlsson collected and interpreted the biochemical data and wrote the article. Mai-Britt Toft Nielsen collected the clinical data, wrote parts of the case report section, and contributed to discussion. Anne Mette Høgh and Rikke Veggerby Grønlund interpreted mutation analysis results. Mogens Fenger was medically responsible for the analysis and contributed to discussion. Louise Ambye was responsible for the analytical method and quality of the analysis, contributed with information about the CaSR-receptor and mutation data and contributed also to discussion. All authors read and approved the final manuscript.

Acknowledgments

We would like to thank Bente Elmfeldt Madsen, for performing the PCR and sequencing analysis.

References

[1] F. M. Hannan, V. N. Babinsky, and R. V. Thakker, "Disorders of the calcium-sensing receptor and partner proteins: Insights into the molecular basis of calcium homeostasis," *Molecular Endocrinology*, vol. 57, no. 3, pp. R127–R142, 2016.

[2] R. H. Wasserman, "Vitamin D and the intestinal absorption of calcium: a view and overview," in *Vitamin D*, pp. 411–428, Elsevier Inc., 2nd edition, 2005.

[3] F. M. Hannan and R. V. Thakker, "Calcium-sensing receptor (CaSR) mutations and disorders of calcium, electrolyte and water metabolism," *Best Practice & Research Clinical Endocrinology & Metabolism*, vol. 27, no. 3, pp. 359–371, 2013.

[4] S. E. Christensen, P. H. Nissen, P. Vestergaard, and L. Mosekilde, "Familial hypocalciuric hypercalcaemia: a review," *Current Opinion in Endocrinology & Diabetes and Obesity*, vol. 18, no. 6, pp. 359–370, 2011.

[5] R. Vargas-Poussou, L. Mansour-Hendili, S. Baron et al., "Familial hypocalciuric hypercalcemia types 1 and 3 and primary hyperparathyroidism: similarities and differences," *The Journal of Clinical Endocrinology & Metabolism*, vol. 101, no. 5, pp. 2185–2195, 2016.

[6] W. D. Fraser, "Hyperparathyroidism," *The Lancet*, vol. 374, no. 9684, pp. 145–158, 2009.

[7] M. Shinall, K. Dahir, and J. Broome, "Differentiating familial hypocalciuric hypercalcemia from primary hyperparathyroidism," *Endocrine Practice*, vol. 19, no. 4, pp. 697–702, 2013.

[8] S. J. Marx, "Familial hypocalciuric hypercalcemia as an atypical form of primary hyperparathyroidism," *Journal of Bone and Mineral Research*, vol. 33, no. 1, pp. 27–31, 2018.

[9] S. Hovden, L. Rejnmark, S. A. Ladefoged, and P. H. Nissen, "AP2S1 and GNA11 mutations - not a common cause of familial hypocalciuric hypercalcemia," *European Journal of Endocrinology*, vol. 176, no. 2, pp. 177–185, 2017.

[10] D. A. Heath, "Familial hypocalciuric hypercalcemia," *Reviews in Endocrine and Metabolic Disorders*, vol. 1, no. 4, pp. 291–296, 2000.

[11] S. Hewitt, T. T. Søvik, E. T. Aasheim et al., "Secondary hyperparathyroidism, vitamin D sufficiency, and serum calcium 5 years after gastric bypass and duodenal switch," *Obesity Surgery*, vol. 23, no. 3, pp. 384–390, 2013.

[12] K. M. Nakamura, E. G. C. Haglind, J. A. Clowes et al., "Fracture risk following bariatric surgery: a population-based study," *Osteoporosis International*, vol. 25, no. 1, pp. 151–158, 2014.

[13] G. Mingrone, S. Bornstein, and C. W. Le Roux, "Optimisation of follow-up after metabolic surgery," *The Lancet Diabetes & Endocrinology*, vol. 8587, no. 17, pp. 1–13, 2018.

[14] Y. Geng, L. Mosyak, I. Kurinov et al., "Structural mechanism of ligand activation in human calcium-sensing receptor," *ELife*, vol. 5, Article ID e13662, pp. 1–25, 2016.

[15] N. Janicic, E. Soliman, Z. Pausova et al., "Mapping of the calcium-sensing receptor gene (CASR) to human chromosome 3q13.3-21 by fluorescence in situ hybridization, and localization to rat chromosome 11 and mouse chromosome 16," *Mammalian Genome*, vol. 6, no. 11, pp. 798–801, 1995.

[16] A. K. Thomas, R. McVie, and S. N. Levine, "Disorders of maternal calcium metabolism implicated by abnormal calcium metabolism in the neonate," *American Journal of Perinatology*, vol. 16, no. 10, pp. 515–520, 1999.

[17] S. J. Marx, "Calcimimetic use in familial hypocalciuric hypercalcemia—a perspective in endocrinology," *The Journal of Clinical Endocrinology & Metabolism*, vol. 102, no. 11, pp. 3933–3936, 2017.

[18] S. Pidasheva, L. Canaff, W. F. Simonds, S. J. Marx, and G. N. Hendy, "Impaired cotranslational processing of the calcium-sensing receptor due to signal peptide missense mutations in familial hypocalciuric hypercalcemia," *Human Molecular Genetics*, vol. 14, no. 12, pp. 1679–1690, 2005.

[19] P. H. Nissen, S. E. Christensen, S. A. Ladefoged, K. Brixen, L. Heickendorff, and L. Mosekilde, "Identification of rare and frequent variants of the CASR gene by high-resolution melting," *Clinica Chimica Acta*, vol. 413, no. 5-6, pp. 605–611, 2012.

[20] P. H. Nissen, S. E. Christensen, L. Heickendorff, K. Brixen, and L. Mosekilde, "Molecular genetic analysis of the calcium sensing receptor gene in patients clinically suspected to have familial hypocalciuric hypercalcemia: phenotypic variation and mutation spectrum in a danish population," *The Journal of Clinical Endocrinology & Metabolism*, vol. 92, no. 11, pp. 4373–4379, 2007.

[21] A. Q. Rasmussen, N. R. Jørgensen, and P. Schwarz, "Identification and functional characterization of a novel mutation in the human calcium-sensing receptor that co-segregates with autosomal-dominant hypocalcemia," *Front Endocrinol (Lausanne)*, vol. 9, pp. 1–10, 2018.

[22] V. Guarnieri, L. Canaff, F. H. J. Yun et al., "Calcium-sensing receptor (CASR) mutations in hypercalcemic states: studies from a single endocrine clinic over three years," *The Journal of Clinical Endocrinology & Metabolism*, vol. 95, no. 4, pp. 1819–1829, 2010.

[23] S. Fukumoto, N. Chikatsu, R. Okazaki et al., "Inactivating mutations of calcium-sensing receptor results in parathyroid lipohyperplasia," *Diagnostic Molecular Pathology*, vol. 10, no. 4, pp. 242–247, 2001.

[24] K. Frank-Raue, G. Leidig-Bruckner, C. Haag et al., "Inactivating calcium-sensing receptor mutations in patients with primary hyperparathyroidism," *Clinical Endocrinology*, vol. 75, no. 1, pp. 50–55, 2011.

[25] C. Leech, P. Lohse, V. Stanojevic, A. Lechner, B. Göke, and C. Spitzweg, "Identification of a novel inactivating R465Q mutation of the calcium-sensing receptor," *Biochemical and Biophysical Research Communications*, vol. 342, no. 3, pp. 996–1002, 2006.

[26] F. M. Hannan, M. A. Nesbit, C. Zhang et al., "Identification of 70 calcium-sensing receptor mutations in hyper- and hypocalcaemic patients: evidence for clustering of extracellular domain mutations at calcium-binding sites," *Human Molecular Genetics*, vol. 21, no. 12, pp. 2768–2778, 2012.

[27] M. J. Landrum, J. M. Lee, M. Benson et al., "ClinVar: public archive of interpretations of clinically relevant variants," *Nucleic Acids Research*, vol. 44, no. D1, pp. D862–D868, 2016.

40

A Case Report of Mixed Osteomalacia and Low Bone Density from Vitamin D Deficiency as a Cause of Bilateral Tibial Stress Fractures in a Young Male Military Recruit from Singapore

Wann Jia Loh,[1] **Louise Hughes**,[2] **David Thai Chong Chua**,[3] **and Linsey Gani**[1]

[1]*Department of Endocrinology, Changi General Hospital, 2 Simei Street, Singapore 529889*
[2]*Department of Anatomical Pathology, Concord Hospital, Hospital Road, Concord West, New South Wales 2139, Australia*
[3]*Department of Orthopaedics, Changi General Hospital, 2 Simei Street, Singapore 529889*

Correspondence should be addressed to Wann Jia Loh; loh.wann.jia@singhealth.com.sg

Academic Editor: Michael P. Kane

Despite being a tropical country, vitamin D deficiency is common in Singapore. All young Singaporean males between the age of 18 and 21 years have to undergo mandatory military service. Stress fractures occur in military recruits, and risk factors include a sudden increase in physical activity and vitamin D deficiency. We report the bone histomorphometry findings from a case of bilateral tibial stress fractures in an 18-year-old military recruit who had vitamin D deficiency. The histomorphometry showed a mixed osteomalacia and osteoporosis pattern. This case is unique as it shows that stress fractures from a marching exercise can occur in apparently healthy well young man with vitamin D deficiency despite living in a tropical country.

1. Introduction

Stress fractures in military recruits are not uncommon with rapid increase in physical activity and low vitamin D level being major risk factors [1–3]. Despite a tropical country, vitamin D deficiency is common in Singapore [4, 5]. All young Singaporean males between the age of 18–21 years have to undergo 2 years of mandatory military service. We describe the bone histomorphometry finding of an 18-year--old military recruit who sustained bilateral tibial fractures in his initial basic military training course and findings of a mixed osteomalacia and low bone density with improvement in his bone density after 2 years of adequate vitamin D replacement.

2. Case Presentation

Our patient is an 18-year-old man of Chinese ethnicity who presented with bilateral leg pain after a short march of 200 meters during his first marching session. He has no other significant past medical history, in particular he had completed his puberty normally, and there was no previous history of GI malabsorption. There was no history of any long-term medication administration. There was no family history of osteoporosis or fractures. He did not smoke or drink alcohol. His body mass index (BMI) was 24.6 kg/m^2 (weight 73.5 kg, height 1.73 m). Further history revealed that the acute severe bilateral leg pain started after taking part in a marching session of 200 meters during his 1st week of basic military training. Initially, he had pain in his left shin after the march, and this was followed by pain in his right shin a day later. Because of the pain, he was unable to walk. The march was not a particularly stressful exercise, and he was not carrying any weights. However, this was his first marching session, and he has always been very physically inactive throughout his childhood and does not exercise regularly.

On examination, there was tenderness on palpation of the both proximal tibias. There were no blue sclerae or hypermobile joints. He was at Tanner stage 5 for puberty. An X- ray of his legs showed cortical irregularity and lucency with sclerotic margins in the proximal shaft of the tibia, confirming stress fractures (Figure 1(a)). The radiograph did not show features of bowing. Magnetic resonance imaging (MRI) of both calves confirmed transverse fractures of the bilateral proximal tibial metaphysis associated with bone marrow oedema and periosteal reaction (Figure 1(b)). His bone mineral density (BMD) using dual energy X-ray absorptiometry (DEXA) showed that he had lower bone mass and density expected for his age; his BMD of the lumbar spine measured 0.751 g/cm^2, with a corresponding Z score of −2.4. The BMD of the left hip measured 0.847 g/cm^2, corresponding to a Z score of −1.8; whereas, the BMD of the left femoral neck was 0.789 g/cm^2, corresponding to a Z score of −1.5. Secondary causes of osteoporosis were investigated for and were negative apart from a low vitamin D level of 10.7 μg/L (Table 1). Although coeliac screening is part of young osteoporosis workup, coeliac screening was not performed because he did not have predilection for autoimmune disease and the rarity of this disease in a person of Chinese ethnicity. The chest radiograph was normal. The X-ray of the pelvis did not show any features of hip deformity seen in osteomalacia such as coxa profunda or coxa vara.

Double tetracycline labelled qualitative bone histomorphometry was performed from the iliac crest with administration of tetracyline at day 1, 2, 15, and 16 followed by a bone biopsy at day 22. The results showed delay in mineralization, with increase in osteoid and blurred tetracycline labelling, as seen in osteomalacia (Figure 2). However, unlike osteomalacia, there was not a significant increase in the number of osteoblasts. There was also some degree of variability, thinning, and loss of connectivity of trabeculae (Figure 2), which are seen in osteoporosis. This was significant for his age. Therefore, the bone biopsy suggested a mixed picture of osteomalacia and osteoporosis. He was treated conservatively, given vitamin D supplementation, and advised adequate calcium intake.

2.1. Outcome and Follow-Up. With vitamin D replacement, the vitamin D level of the patient improved from 10.7 to 41.4 μg/L after 3 months. He was continued on maintenance vitamin D3 cholecalciferol 1000 international units per day to maintain a vitamin D level of >30 μg/L. Two years later, a repeat BMD performed using the DEXA scan showed significant improvement of BMD; 5.4% increase in the lumbar spine which represents a significant change (least significant change (LSC) = 0.22 g/cm^2) and 3.2% increase in BMD of the hip, which does not represent a significant change (LSC = 0.034 g/cm^2). He has not sustained any further fractures for the last 3 years since then.

3. Discussion

Despite being a tropical country (1°18′N 103°51É with mean sunshine 2022.4 h/y), vitamin D deficiency is prevalent. A previous study found 42.1% of young healthy adults in Singapore were found to have vitamin D levels of less than 20 ng/ml, although its prevalence in females was higher [1]. This in combination with increasing lack of physical activity in the young may herald an increase in the prevalence of poor bone health in the population [2]. Our case report demonstrates histology-proven osteomalacia due to vitamin D deficiency in an otherwise healthy young man. Of note, he has had no previous fractures, and his investigations did not reveal typical radiological abnormalities of osteomalacia. This emphasizes the importance of vitamin D in the maintenance of bone health especially in the young.

Osteomalacia is a disorder of bone characterized by delayed mineralization of newly formed osteoid at sites of bone turnover. Several different disorders may cause vitamin D deficiency leading to osteomalacia such as gastrointestinal malabsorption, liver disease, and renal disease [3]. Osteomalacia may be asymptomatic and present radiologically as osteopenia and Looser zones. Symptoms include bone pain, muscle weakness, fracture, and muscle cramps [3]. Osteomalacia is believed to be rare in developed nations due to the adequate nutrition, and previous cases of osteomalacia reported in the literature are mostly in the elderly or those with gastrointestinal malabsorption [3]. In this case, the bone histomorphometry showed that although there was delay in mineralization, unlike in osteomalacia, there was not a significant increase in the number of osteoblasts. We hypothesized that this may be due to the delay in bone biopsy which was performed about 6 weeks after the fracture, and the patient was already commenced on vitamin D replacement. Hence, the appearance of osteomalacia on bone histomorphometry may be attenuated.

The incidence of stress fractures has been reported to be as high as 20% in runners and accounts for 10–20% of consultations in a sports medicine clinic [4]. While the true incidence of stress fractures of the military recruits in our country is unknown, it is worthwhile to note that the incidence of stress fractures in U.S. military recruits was estimated to be 38 to 77 per 1000 person-years in 2009 [4] and reported to occur in 7.2% of UK Royal Marine military recruits [5]. The most common site of stress fractures is the tibia, followed by tarsals and metatarsals [6]. Bilateral femoral fractures have also been reported in young military recruits [4, 7]. While most stress fractures are uncomplicated and can be managed conservatively, there are some with high-risk stress fractures that have delayed recovery, chronic pain, and increased risk of progression to complete fracture. This usually affects specific sites which have a maximal tensile load in regions of hypovascularity and hence potentially reduces healing such as femoral neck, patella, anterior tibia, and medial malleolus [6]. Stress fractures occur more commonly at cortical bone instead of cancellous bone likely because of the slower remodeling rate of cortical bone [6].

The pathogenesis of stress fractures is suspected to be due to the imbalance between bone resorption and bone formation, in the setting of repeated mechanical loading without adequate rest. This leads to microfractures, bone oedema, and subsequently stress fractures [6].

The known risk factors predisposing to stress fractures include female gender, vitamin D deficiency, secondary causes of osteoporosis (e.g., malabsorption and hyperthyroidism), previous stress fracture, and excessive training

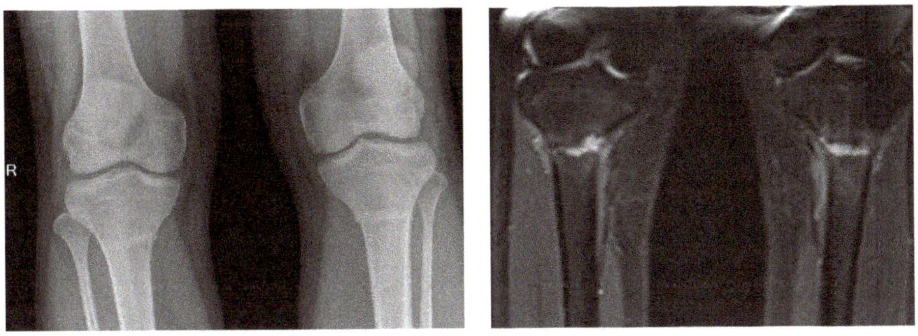

(a) (b)

FIGURE 1: X-ray and MRI. (a) X-ray of the patient's legs showed cortical irregularity and lucency with sclerotic margins in the proximal shaft of the tibia, confirming stress fractures. (b) MRI of the calves of the patient showed increased signal at linear T1RM sequence which suggests fluid clefs at both fracture sites.

TABLE 1: The summary of investigations performed to evaluate secondary causes of osteoporosis.

Blood tests	Patient	Reference range
Free thyroxine (pmol/L)	12.16	10–20
Thyroid stimulating hormone (mIU/L)	0.733	0.4–4
Albumin (g/L)	39	37–51
Haemoglobin (g/dL)	12.8	13–17
Creatinine (μmol/L)	59	65–125
25-Hydroxy vitamin D (μg/L)	10.7	
Calcium (mmol/L)	2.23	2.1–2.6
Phosphate (mmol/L)	1.3	0.65–1.65
Parathyroid hormone (pmol/L)	6.55	1.3–7.6
Alkaline phosphatase (U/L)	94	32–103
Total testosterone (nmol/L)	11.65	9.9–27.8
24-Hour urine free cortisol (nmol/day)	245	59–413
Urine calcium (mmol/L)	0.3	<0.6

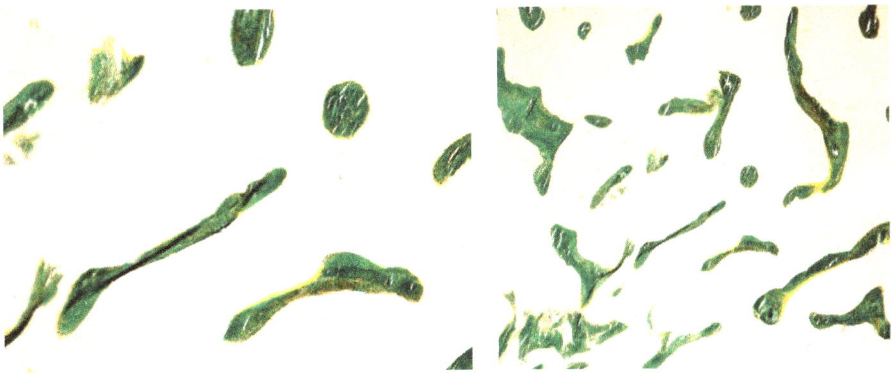

(a) (b)

FIGURE 2: Continued.

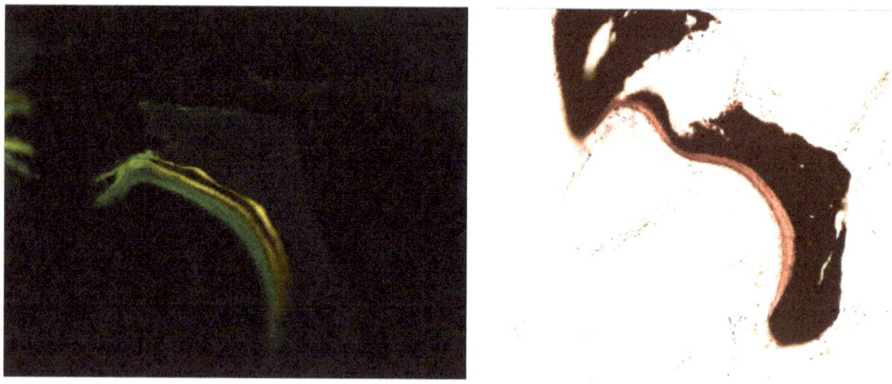

(c) (d)

Figure 2: Bone biopsy. (a) High resolution (alkaline phosphatase staining). (b) Low resolution (alkaline phosphatase staining). Both low and high power showed irregularity, variability, and loss of connectivity of bone trabeculae, with some thinning and scattered bone nubbins. (c) Unstained bone biopsy. (d) The Von Kossa (calcium) stain showed the thickened osteoid seam (red) with the calcified bone (black).

intensity, frequency, or duration [5, 6]. Females are at higher risk than men to suffer from stress fractures among both runners (9.2% in females and 3% in males) and military recruits (9.7% vs 6.5%, respectively) [8]. This may be explained by their smaller muscle size, dietary difference, and bone anatomy [8]. Vitamin D deficiency also increases the risk of stress fractures [9]. In a study of 1082 Royal Marine military recruits, vitamin D deficiency below 20 μg/L has been associated with increased risk of stress fractures in military recruits [5]. It is often misconceived that a tropical country has low rates of vitamin D deficiency. Recent studies reported that vitamin D deficiency (<20 μg/dL) was present in 13.4% of pregnant women [9] and 42% of healthy individuals [1]. In Singapore, the enrollment for compulsory national service is 18 years old which is a critical time of accruing bone mass, as peak bone mass range from early to late 20s [10].

Interventions to identify high-risk individuals and prevent fractures can be successful. For example, the U.S. Armed Forces successfully reduced the stress fracture rate by almost 60% by identifying individuals with slower run times, reducing frequency of running in less-fit individuals, and ensuring that every trainee receives adequate nutrition including vitamin D and calcium [4]. Individuals with vitamin D deficiency should be replaced with adequate vitamin D to ensure peak bone mass and may benefit from higher vitamin D load (e.g., 2000IU) [11] although clinical evidence for this is lacking. Our patient showed improvement of his bone mineral density with vitamin D repletion. Further studies are required to show if vitamin D supplementation at a younger age may help to ensure adequate peak bone mass, prior to the enlistment for national service.

4. Conclusion

This case demonstrates the importance of vitamin D repletion and possibility of osteomalacia presenting in an otherwise healthy young patient without typical symptoms, biochemical, and radiology findings due to inadequate vitamin D. Further studies should look into regular vitamin D supplementation especially in young patients with previous minimal sunlight exposure and regular physical activity who are entering into military service.

Disclosure

This case report was presented as a poster abstract in "World Congress on Osteoporosis, Osteoarthritis and Musculoskeletal Diseases (WCO-ICF-ESCEO 2019)."

References

[1] X. Bi, S. L. Tey, C. Leong, R. Quek, and C. J. Henry, "Prevalence of vitamin D deficiency in Singapore: its implications to cardiovascular risk factors," *PloS One*, vol. 11, no. 1, 2016.

[2] J. B. Koedijk, J. van Rijswijk, W. A. Oranje et al., "Sedentary behaviour and bone health in children, adolescents and young adults: a systematic review," *Osteoporosis International*, vol. 28, no. 9, pp. 2507–2519, 2017.

[3] B. Basha, D. S. Rao, Z.-H. Han, and A. M. Parfitt, "Osteomalacia due to vitamin D depletion: a neglected consequence of intestinal malabsorption," *The American Journal of Medicine*, vol. 108, no. 4, pp. 296–300, 2000.

[4] B. J. Webber, W. E. Trueblood, J. N. Tchandja, S. P. Federinko, and T. L. Cropper, "Concurrent bilateral femoral neck stress fractures in a military recruit: a case report," *Military Medicine*, vol. 180, no. 1, pp. e134–e137, 2015.

[5] T. Davey, S. A. Lanham-New, A. M. Shaw et al., "Low serum 25-hydroxyvitamin D is associated with increased risk of stress fracture during Royal Marine recruit training," *Osteoporosis International*, vol. 27, no. 1, pp. 171–179, 2016.

[6] K. C. McInnis and L. N. Ramey, "High-risk stress fractures: diagnosis and management," *PM&R*, vol. 8, no. 3S, pp. S113–S124, 2016.

[7] H. Fonte and R. Rodrigues-Pinto, "Femoral neck stress fracture in a young female recruit: case report," *SICOT-J*, vol. 4, p. 16, 2018.

[8] L. Wentz, P.-Y. Liu, E. Haymes, and J. Z. Ilich, "Females have a greater incidence of stress fractures than males in both military and athletic populations: a systemic review," *Military Medicine*, vol. 176, no. 4, pp. 420–430, 2011.

[9] T. Cheng, S. Loy, Y. Cheung et al., "Plasma vitamin D deficiency is associated with poor sleep quality and night-time eating at mid-pregnancy in Singapore," *Nutrients*, vol. 9, no. 4, p. 340, 2017.

[10] J. Lu, Y. Shin, M.-S. Yen, and S. S. Sun, "Peak bone mass and patterns of change in total bone mineral density and bone mineral contents from childhood into young adulthood," *Journal of Clinical Densitometry*, vol. 19, no. 2, pp. 180–191, 2016.

[11] M. P. McCabe, M. P. Smyth, and D. R. Richardson, "Current concept review: vitamin D and stress fractures," *Foot & Ankle International*, vol. 33, no. 6, pp. 526–533, 2012.

41

Testosterone Replacement Therapy and the Risk of Hypoglycemia

Analía Verónica Yamaguchi,[1] Pablo René Costanzo,[2] Verónica Andrea Peuchot,[1] and Pablo Knoblovits[2]

[1]*Clinical Medicine Department, Metabolism and Nuclear Medicine, Hospital Italiano de Buenos Aires, Buenos Aires, Argentina*
[2]*Department of Endocrinology, Metabolism and Nuclear Medicine, Hospital Italiano de Buenos Aires, Buenos Aires, Argentina*

Correspondence should be addressed to Pablo René Costanzo; tenetir@yahoo.com.ar

Academic Editor: Eli Hershkovitz

We report the case of a 45-year-old man with a history of Klinefelter syndrome undergoing testosterone replacement therapy, and with type 2 diabetes treated with metformin with poor metabolic control. When vildagliptin was added to his treatment, he presented hypoglycemia after the testosterone injection. We highlight this not widely reported drug interaction between hypoglycemic agents and testosterone.

1. Introduction

The use of testosterone as replacement therapy in patients with hypogonadism induces metabolic changes that lead to higher insulin sensitivity (decreased fat mass and increased lean mass, less insulin resistance and higher insulin secretion) [1, 2]. In addition, there is an increased glucose uptake by muscle cells [3]. This effect of testosterone therapy may be associated with a higher risk of hypoglycemia in patients with type 2 diabetes (DM2) under treatment. The interaction of testosterone with insulin has been frequently reported, while little is known about the interaction between testosterone and oral hypoglycemic agents when these drugs are concomitantly administered in hypogonadal men with DM2 [4].

A drug–drug interaction is defined as a change in the effect of a drug by the action of another drug when both are administered together. This action may be synergistic (when the effect is enhanced) or antagonistic (when the effect is decreased). An interaction is considered clinically relevant when the therapeutic activity and/or toxicity of a drug is changed to such an extent that a dosage adjustment of the drug or any other medical intervention is required because of the adverse reactions or significant lack of efficacy caused by such interaction [5, 6]. It should be noted that drug–drug interactions account for 2-3% of hospital admissions in patients older than 50 years of age who are taking medication [7, 8]. The likelihood of a relevant interaction is 50% in patients receiving 5 medications, increasing to 100% in patients receiving 7 drugs simultaneously [9]. In addition, it is important to highlight that oral hypoglycemic agents are a group of drugs with high potential for drug–drug interaction, since they have a narrow therapeutic window; i.e., the therapeutic dose is close to the toxic dose; these drug–drug interactions account for 3.3% of hospitalizations for hypoglycemia [10].

The aim of the publication of this case is to report the risk of hypoglycemia in hypogonadal diabetic patients treated with oral hypoglycemic agents and testosterone.

2. Case Report

A forty-five-year-old male patient presented to the clinical medicine department at Hospital Italiano with a 1-year history of DM2 with no medical controls since diagnosis. Personal history: Klinefelter syndrome (KS) diagnosed 4 years ago when the patient consulted for infertility (karyotype 47XXY), with no hormonal replacement, DM2, hypertension (HTN), dyslipidemia (DLD), obesity, sleep apnea treated with continuous positive airway pressure (CPAP). Usual medication: Metformin 1000 mg/day, enalapril 10 mg/day. Physical examination: weight: 110 kg, height: 1.70 m, body mass index (BMI): 38.1 kg/m^2, sagittal index: 27 cm. Ancillary tests: Labs: blood

TABLE 1: Results of prolonged 75-g OGTT with measurements at timepoints before and after TU administration.

Timepoints	Blood glucose before TU (mg/dL)	Insulin before TU (μIU/mL)	Blood glucose 48 hours after TU (mg/dL)	Insulin after TU (μIU/mL)
Baseline	106	25.6	91	13.8
30 min	190	63.3	180	80.8
60 min	226	88.7	167	71.4
90 min	181	125.6	142	68.5
120 min	120	74.9	113	38.6
180 min	104	31.9	80	16.1
240 min	77	15.7	74	14.3

TU: Testosterone Undecanoate.

glucose 89 mg/dL, glycosylated hemoglobin A1c (HbA1c) 8.5%, urea 30 mg/dL, creatinine 0.7 mg/dL, GGT 60 IU/L, total cholesterol 210 mg/dL, triglycerides 173 mg/dL, no-HDL-C 172 mg/dl, LDL-C 137 mg/dL, HDL-C 38 mg/dL, TSH 1.85 μIU/mL (normal: 0.40–4.94 μIU/mL), LH 31.7 mIU/mL (normal: 1.5–9.2 mIU/mL), FSH 26.5 mIU/mL (normal: 1.0–14.0 mIU/mL), prolactin 9.78 ng/mL (normal: 3.0–17.0 ng/mL), estradiol 31.3 pg/mL (normal: 30.0–90.0 pg/mL), total testosterone (TT) 0.79 ng/mL (normal: 3.0–8.8 ng/mL), bioavailable testosterone (BT) 0.21 ng/mL (normal: 1.20–4.80 ng/mL). Testicular ultrasound: both testes of normal shape, with diffuse hypoechogenicity and markedly reduced volume. Ambulatory blood pressure monitoring (ABPM): adequately controlled HTN. Diagnoses: DM2 with poor metabolic control, grade 2 obesity, hypergonadotropic hypogonadism, HTN, DLD, sleep apnea–hypopnea. During the medical interview, the patient reported decreased libido and erectile dysfunction. He was prescribed replacement therapy with testosterone undecanoate (TU) 1000 mg every 12 weeks (the patient was no longer seeking fertility), metformin 1500 mg/day, vildagliptin 100 mg/day and rosuvastatin 10 mg/day.

Forty-eight hours after the administration of the first intramuscular dose of TU 1000 mg, the patient reported symptoms of hypoglycemia (HG) (obnubilation, dizziness, chills), which was not objectively confirmed. At 3 months, the patient complained of the same symptoms 48 hours after the second injection of TU 1000 mg; on this occasion, HG was confirmed by capillary blood glucose levels of 50 mg/dL measured with the Accu-chek Performa® blood glucose meter. Given the low frequency of hypoglycemic events reported with the use of metformin and vildagliptin and the close time relation between the occurrence of clinical symptoms and the intramuscular administration of testosterone, such symptoms were interpreted as a potential drug–drug interaction between testosterone and vildagliptin, since metformin, unlike other oral hypoglycemic agents, does not stimulate insulin secretion, and metformin overdose does not cause hypoglycemia [11]. The patient had no other HG record of capillary blood glucose measurements or laboratory tests.

At nine months of clinical follow-up (before the third dose of TU) the patient had good adherence to treatment. Physical examination: weight 95.5 kg (13% loss from baseline weight), BMI: 33.0 kg/m^2 and good metabolic control: total cholesterol 121 mg/dL, HDL-C 34 mg/dL, triglycerides 104 mg/dL, LDL-C 66 mg/dL, blood glucose 98 mg/dL, GGT 36 IU/L, HbA1c 5.6%, TT 2.15 ng/mL, BT 0.7 ng/mL (15 weeks after the last injection of TU), PSA 0.54 ng/mL, 24-h microalbuminuria: 248.8 mg/24 h (normal: 0–30.0 mg/24 h). Vildagliptin was discontinued and the patient was asked to undergo a prolonged oral glucose tolerance test (OGTT) with blood glucose measurements at various timepoints, prior to and 48 hours after the next administration of testosterone. (Table 1, Figure 1).

The patient made good progress; 3 months after discontinuation of vildagliptin, a new dose of testosterone undecanoate was administered and the patient had no symptoms of HG. Follow-up labs were: blood glucose 88 mg/dL, HbA1c 5.5%, TT 2.5 ng/mL, BT 1.2 ng/mL, SHBG 27 mMol/L.

3. Methods

Blood samples were taken at 8:00 AM after 12-hour nocturnal fasting.

Insulin: Chemiluminescence (Architect I2000-Abbott). Reference range: 2.7–10.4 μIU/mL. Analytical sensitivity: <1.0 μIU/mL, with intra-assay and inter-assay coefficient of variation (CV) below 7.0%.

Total Testosterone: Chemiluminescence on the Immulite 2000 (Siemens) analyzer, laboratory reference ranges: 1.3–8.5 ng/mL for adult males; the intra-assay CV was 9.8% and the inter-assay CV was 14.4%.

Bioavailable Testosterone: Vermeulen calculation.

Glucose: UV enzymatic hexokinase method (AU5800 Beckman coulter).

OGTT: The patient arrived at the laboratory between 7 AM and 8.30 AM in an 8-hour fasting state. A baseline sample was collected after the 8-hour fast for blood glucose and insulin measurement, and the patient was asked to drink 75 g of glucose in 375 ml of water independent of his baseline fasting glucose levels. Samples were collected for blood glucose and insulin measurements at 30, 60, 90, 120, 180 and 240 min after intake, according to the World Health Organization criteria [12].

Pharmacokinetics and pharmacodynamics of the drugs used by this patient.

Testosterone Undecanoate: Pharmacodynamic properties: TU is an ester of the naturally occurring androgen, testosterone. The active form is formed by cleavage of the side chain. Pharmacokinetic properties: *Absorption:* TU is administered

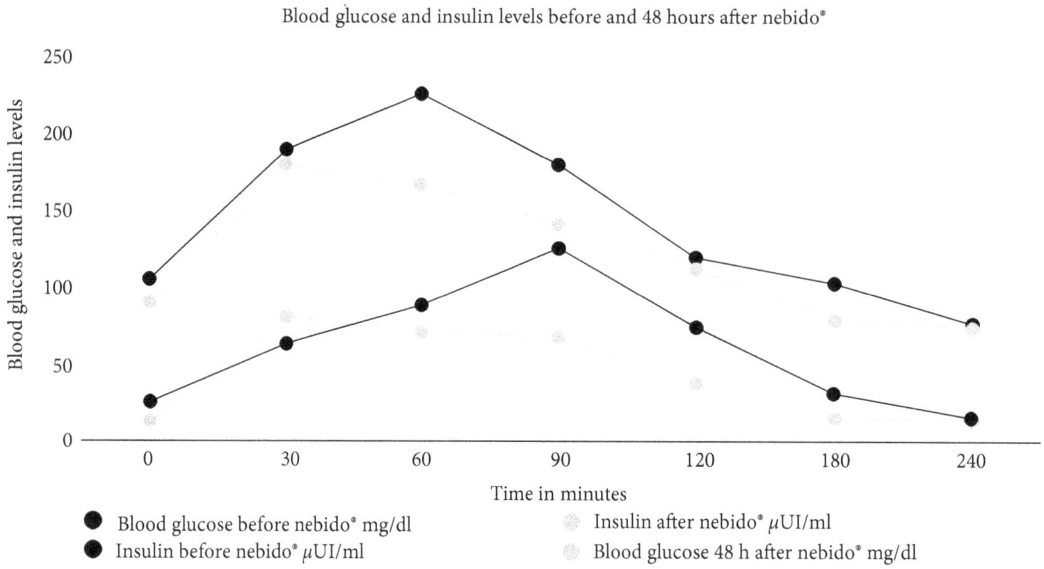

FIGURE 1: Results of prolonged 75-g OGTT with measurements at timepoints before and after TU administration.

intramuscularly, thus avoiding the first-pass effect of the liver. Following intramuscular injection, it is gradually released from the depot and almost completely cleaved by serum esterases into testosterone and undecanoic acid. An increase in serum testosterone concentrations above basal values may be measured one day after administration. *Distribution:* In two separate studies, mean maximum concentrations of testosterone of 6.92 and 12.97 ng/mL were measured about 7 and 14 days, respectively, after single IM administration of 1000 mg of testosterone undecanoate to hypogonadal men. Post-maximum testosterone concentrations decreased with an estimated half-life of approximately 53 days. *Metabolism:* Testosterone generated by ester cleavage from testosterone undecanoate is metabolized and excreted in the same way as endogenous testosterone (extensive hepatic and extrahepatic metabolism). The undecanoic acid is metabolized by β-oxidation in the same way as other aliphatic carboxylic acids.

Vildagliptin is a dipeptidyl-peptidase-4 (DPP-4) inhibitor. This inhibitory activity results in an increase in the levels of incretin hormones, among them GLP-1 (glucagon-like peptide 1) and GIP (glucose-dependent insulinotropic peptide), which stimulates insulin secretion and reduces glucagon secretion in a glucose-dependent manner [13]. Hypoglycemia does not appear to be a serious problem when vildagliptin is used as monotherapy (0.4% of patients treated with 100 mg/day of vildagliptin compared to 0.2% of patients treated with an active comparator or placebo) or as dual therapy in combination with metformin versus placebo (0.55% vs. 0.54%, respectively) or with pioglitazone versus placebo (0.3% vs. 1.9%, respectively). No serious hypoglycemic events were reported with vildagliptin therapy [14]. Interactions: Vildagliptin has a low potential for interactions with other drugs. Since vildagliptin is not a cytochrome P (CYP) 450 enzyme substrate, does not inhibit or induce CYP 450 enzymes, and is a weak substrate of *P*-glycoprotein, no relevant pharmacokinetic interactions have been observed after the concomitant administration of vildagliptin with pioglitazone, metformin, glyburide, amlodipine, ramipril, valsartan and simvastatin in healthy subjects.

Metformin: Unlike sulfonylureas, metformin does not stimulate insulin secretion; therefore it is more appropriate to refer to it as an insulin-sensitizing agent or antidiabetic drug. In overdose, metformin does not cause hypoglycemia.

4. Discussion

Men with KS have an increased mortality risk, probably due to their higher predisposition to develop congenital malformations, cardiovascular disease and endocrine-metabolic disorders, compared to age-matched controls [15].

Our patient had several cardiovascular risk factors, including HTN, DM2, DLD and obesity, the most commonly reported comorbidities in patients with this type of karyotypic abnormality. The prevalence of metabolic disorders in men with KS is associated with insulin resistance and DM2, and with an increased mortality from these causes [16]. Furthermore, hypogonadism per se is a risk factor for metabolic disorders and cardiovascular disease.

Patients with KS have a high prevalence of hypogonadism due to Leydig cell dysfunction, but in addition, metabolic abnormalities in this patient may contribute to a decline in testosterone levels. Insulin resistance-associated hyperglycemia (or hyperinsulinemia) contributes to a lower hypothalamic activity with a decrease in the number of gonadotropin-releasing factor pulses [17, 18]. However, other studies have shown a decreased testicular response to chorionic gonadotropin stimulation in patients with insulin resistance (IR), evidencing testicular function impairment in metabolic disorders [19]. In support of these findings, it has been demonstrated that in the presence of obesity and IR, Leydig cell steroidogenesis may be impaired due to IR at this level or to the action of hormones or cytokines from visceral fat [20–22].

Since hypogonadism in KS is a hormone deficiency of primary (testicular) origin, it could be stated that this condition might have been in our patient the initial manifestation in the development of metabolic disorder, and the development of metabolic disease might have subsequently further impaired testosterone production by mechanisms directly affecting the testicles. However, as patients with KS are, per se, more prone to the development of metabolic syndrome independently of their testosterone levels, it is highly likely that in our patient both syndromes might have influenced each other in a positive feedback manner, leading to the current medical condition.

Testosterone replacement therapy in hypogonadal patients leads to changes in body composition with a decrease in fat mass and an increase in lean mass, and it induces changes in insulin sensitivity [1]. After replacement therapy, there is a decline in insulin secretion and less IR, and an increase in the expression of the glucose transporter Glut4 and enhancement of its translocation, resulting in increased glucose uptake by muscle cells [2, 3]. These changes determine that long-term treatment with testosterone is associated with weight loss, improves glycemia, lipids and prevents the evolution of prediabetes to DM2 [23, 24]. In addition, complete remission of DM2, risk reduction of cardiovascular disease and mortality was reported with TU treatment [25–28].

Thus, in this case, in order to evaluate the insulin-sensitizing response of testosterone, a prolonged OGTT was performed with glucose and insulin measurements at 0, 30, 60, 120, 180 and 240 minutes before and after the administration of TU. The curve shows an insulin-sensitizing effect after TU administration, with a decrease in blood glucose and insulin levels.

We think that in this case there was no effect of one drug on the other drug's metabolism (vildagliptin and testosterone), but a synergistic action of both in the decrease of blood glucose levels. This explanation is reinforced by the fact that there is not demonstration that testosterone alone is capable of producing HG.

Metabolic disorders, especially DM2 and IR are really frequent in patients with KS [16]. Testosterone replacement or treatment with hypoglycemic agents or insulin is unavoidable, but before the initiation of therapy, it is important to be aware of the fact that androgens may enhance the hypoglycemic effect of blood glucose-lowering agents. Patients should be monitored for hypoglycemia so that, if needed, changes may be made in prescription or doses of hypoglycemic agents when administered in combination with androgens.

Even if for testosterone interactions with insulin have been most frequently reported [4] and little evidence is available on interactions between testosterone and oral hypoglycemic drugs, particularly DPP4 inhibitors, such interactions, especially hypoglycemic events as the case reported in this paper, should not be ruled out. This synergism resulting in hypoglycemia occurred in an acute manner 48 hours after the administration of testosterone and it did not recur when vildagliptin was discontinued. However, after testosterone administration, there was an improvement in basal and post-load levels of insulin and blood glucose. It is important that treating physicians be aware of this potential interaction so that they may adjust the doses of oral hypoglycemic agents, if needed.

References

[1] A. M. Isidori, E. Giannetta, E. A. Greco et al., "Effects of testosterone on body composition, bone metabolism and serum lipid profile in middle-aged men: a meta-analysis," *Clinical Endocrinology*, vol. 63, no. 3, pp. 280–293, 2005.

[2] X. Y. Wu, J. F. Mao, S. Y. Lu, Q. Zhang, and Y. F. Shi, "Testosterone replacement therapy improves insulin sensitivity and decreases high sensitivity C-reactive protein levels in hypogonadotropic hypogonadal young male patients," *Chinese Medical Journal*, vol. 122, no. 23, pp. 2846–2850, 2009.

[3] K. Sato, M. Iemitsu, K. Aizawa, and R. Ajisaka, "Testosterone and DHEA activate the glucose metabolism-related signaling pathway in skeletal muscle," *American Journal of Physiology-Endocrinology Metabolism*, vol. 294, no. 5, pp. E961–E968, 2008.

[4] D. Kapoor, E. Goodwin, K. S. Channer, and T. H. Jones, "Testosterone replacement therapy improves insulin resistance, glycaemic control, visceral adiposity and hypercholesterolaemia in hypogonadal men with type 2 diabetes," *European Journal of Endocrinology*, vol. 154, no. 6, pp. 899–906, 2006.

[5] M. S. F. Alfonso and M. R. Gayo, *Fundamentals of basic and clinical pharmacology*, Panamericana Editorial, Buenos Aires, 2nd edition, 2013.

[6] G. R. Wilkinson, "Drug metabolism and variability among patients in drug response," *New England Journal of Medicine*, vol. 352, no. 21, pp. 2211–2221, 2005.

[7] J. Talbot and P. Waller, *Stephens' Detection of New Adverse Drug Reactions*, John Wiley & Sons, Hoboken, NJ, USA, 5th edition, 2004.

[8] R. E. Grymonpre, P. A. Mitenko, D. S. Sitar, F. Y. Aoki, and P. R. Montgomery, "Drug-associated hospital admissions in older medical patients," *Journal of American Geriatrics Society*, vol. 36, no. 12, pp. 1092–1098, 1988.

[9] J. C. Delafuente, "Understanding and preventing drug interactions in elderly patients," *Critical Review in Oncology/Hematology*, vol. 48, pp. 133–143, 2003.

[10] L. Mallet, A. Spinewine, and A. Huang, "The challenge of managing drug interactions in elderly people," *The Lancet*, vol. 370, no. 9582, pp. 185–191, 2007.

[11] C. J. Bailey and R. C. Turner, "Metformin," *New England Journal of Medicine*, vol. 334, no. 9, pp. 574–579, 1996.

[12] World Health Organization, "Diabetes Mellitus. Report of a WHO study group," *World Health Organization Technical Report Series*, vol. 727, pp. 1–113, 1985.

[13] T. D. Filippatos, V. G. Athyros, and M. S. Elisaf, "The pharmacokinetic considerations and adverse effects of DDP-4 inhibitors," *Expert Opinion Drug Metabolism & Toxicology*, vol. 10, no. 6, pp. 787–812, 2014.

[14] E. Bosi, R. Camisasca, P. Collober, C. E. Rochotte, and A. J. Garber, "Effects of vildagliptin on glucose control over 24 weeks in patients with type 2 diabetes inadequately controlled with metformin," *Diabetes Care*, vol. 30, no. 4, pp. 890–895, 2007.

[15] A. Bojesen, S. Juul, N. Birkebæk, and C. H. Gravholt, "Increased mortality in Klinefelter syndrome," *The Journal of Clinical Endocrinology Metabolism*, vol. 89, no. 8, pp. 3830–3834, 2004.

[16] M. J. O'Connor, E. A. Snyder, and F. J. Hayes, "Klinefelter syndrome and diabetes," *Current Diabetes Reports*, vol. 19, no. 9, p. 71, 2019.

[17] P. Knoblovits, P. R. Costanzo, G. J. Valzacchi et al., "Erectile dysfunction, obesity, insulin resistance, and their relationship with testosterone levels in eugonadal patients in an andrology

clinic setting," *Journal of Andrology*, vol. 31, no. 3, pp. 263–270, 2009.

[18] P. R. Costanzo, S. M. Suárez, H. E. Scaglia, C. Zylbersztein, L. E. Litwak, and P. Knoblovits, "Evaluation of the hypothalamic-pituitary-gonadal axis in eugonadal men with type 2 diabetes mellitus," *Andrology*, vol. 2, no. 1, pp. 117–124, 2014.

[19] A. Iranmanesh, D. Lawson, and J. D. Veldhuis, "Glucose ingestion acutely lowers pulsatile LH and basal testosterone secretion in men," *American Journal of Physiology-Endocrinology and Metabolism*, vol. 302, no. 6, pp. E724–E730, 2012.

[20] N. Pitteloud, M. Hardin, A. Dwyer et al., "Increasing insulin resistance is associated with a decrease in Leydig cell testosterone secretion in men," *The Journal of Clinical Endocrinology & Metabolism*, vol. 90, no. 5, pp. 2636–2641, 2005.

[21] P. R. Costanzo and P. Knoblovits, "Male gonadal axis function in patients with type 2 diabetes," *Hormone Molecular Biology and Clinical Investigation*, vol. 26, no. 2, pp. 129–134, 2016.

[22] G. Dimopoulou, D. Goulis, G. G. Corona, and M. Maggi, "The complex association between metabolic syndrome and male hypogonadism," *Metabolism*, vol. 86, pp. 61–68, 2018.

[23] A. Yassin, A. Haider, K. Haider et al., "Testosterone therapy in men with hypogonadism prevents progression from prediabetes to type 2 diabetes: eight-year data from a registry study," *Diabetes Care*, vol. 42, no. 6, pp. 1104–1111, 2019.

[24] G. Hackett, "Metabolic effects of testosterone therapy in men with type 2 diabetes and metabolic syndrome," *Sexual Medicine Review*, vol. 7, no. 3, pp. 476–490, 2019.

[25] A. Haider, K. Haider, F. Saad, and M. Hanefeld, "Remission of type 2 diabetes and pleiotropic effects of long-term testosterone treatment for "late-onset" hypogonadism: a case report," *SAGE Open Medical Case Reports*, vol. 7, p. 2050313X18823454, 2019.

[26] A. Haider, K. S. Haider, and F. Saad, "Remission of type 2 diabetes in a hypogonadal man under long-term testosterone therapy," *Endocrinology Diabetes & Metabolism Case Reports*, vol. 2017, no. 1, pp. 17–0084, 2017.

[27] A. M. Traish, A. Haider, K. S. Haider, G. Doros, and F. Saad, "Long-term testosterone therapy improves cardiometabolic function and reduces risk of cardiovascular disease in men with hypogonadism: a real-life observational registry study setting comparing treated and untreated (control) groups," *Journal of Cardiovascular Pharmacology and Therapeutics*, vol. 22, no. 5, pp. 414–433, 2017.

[28] F. Saad, M. Caliber, G. Doros, K. S. Haider, and A. Haider, "Long-term treatment with testosterone undecanoate injections in men with hypogonadism alleviates erectile dysfunction and reduces risk of major adverse cardiovascular events, prostate cancer, and mortality," *The Aging Male*, vol. 20, pp. 1–12, 2019.

42

Vitamin D Toxicity Managed with Peritoneal Dialysis

Krystel Feghali ,[1] Kostas Papamarkakis,[2] Jackson Clark,[3] Neha Malhotra,[1] Lanu Stoddart,[4] and Ibitoro Osakwe[1]

[1]*Department of Endocrinology, Diabetes and Metabolism, University of Massachusetts Medical School, Baystate Medical Center, Springfield, MA, USA*
[2]*Division of Nephrology, University of Massachusetts Medical School, Baystate Medical Center, Springfield, MA, USA*
[3]*Division of Internal Medicine, University of Massachusetts Medical School, Baystate Medical Center, Springfield, MA, USA*
[4]*Division of Pathology, University of Massachusetts Medical School, Baystate Medical Center, Springfield, MA, USA*

Correspondence should be addressed to Krystel Feghali; krystel.feghalimd@baystatehealth.org

Academic Editor: Suat Simsek

Vitamin D deficiency is a global health issue that afflicts more than one billion children and adults worldwide. Vitamin D supplementation has increased over the years, whether through medical prescriptions, over-the-counter, or online purchasing. This is driven by a more recognized association between vitamin D sufficiency status and lower risk of cancer. In addition, more recently, it is used as a potential prophylactic and treatment for COVID-19 infection. This can lead to toxicity from over-ingestion. While rare, it has been reported in the literature. In this case report, we present a 75-year-old man with severe hypercalcemia secondary to vitamin D toxicity managed with peritoneal dialysis. He presented with biochemical evidence of hypercalcemia, acute kidney injury, and pancreatitis. Workup for his hypercalcemia led to the diagnosis of vitamin D toxicity as shown by a level greater than 200 ng/dL (Ref: 20–50 ng/mL) was confirmed by liquid chromatography-mass spectroscopy. Cornerstone medical management of hypercalcemia was provided which included aggressive intravenous fluid hydration, intravenous diuretics, calcitonin, bisphosphonate, and corticosteroid therapy. At every interruption of therapy, calcium levels trended upward. A thorough literature review yielded the finding of a sole case report from 1966 presented at the Third International Congress of Nephrology, in which peritoneal dialysis was used in the management of vitamin D toxicity and hypercalcemia. This modality is established to cause vitamin D deficiency. In collaboration with the nephrology team, 10 sessions of peritoneal dialysis were undertaken with resolution of hypercalcemia and downtrend in 25-hydroxyvitamin D levels as measured by dilution.

1. Introduction

Vitamin D deficiency and insufficiency are a global health issue that afflicts children and adults worldwide [1]. About 1 billion people have vitamin D deficiency, while 50% of the world's population has vitamin D insufficiency [2]. In the United States (US), the overall prevalence of vitamin D deficiency is estimated at 41.6% [3]. This global health issue has garnered medical attention for years, resulting in increased use of vitamin D supplementation. In 2013-2014, around 3.2% of the US adult population reported taking 4000 IU or more of vitamin D [4]. This may be due partly to the fact that vitamin D supplementation is readily available over-the-counter and through online purchasing. This upward trend in supplementation is also likely driven by a number of reasons, including the recognized association between vitamin D sufficiency status and lower risk of cancer [5–7]. More recently, vitamin D supplementation is used as potential prophylaxis and treatment for COVID-19 [8–10]. This raises the risk of complications including toxicity from overingestion. While rare, vitamin D toxicity has been reported in the literature. Herein, we present the case of a 75-year-old man with severe hypercalcemia secondary to vitamin D toxicity managed with peritoneal dialysis.

2. Case

A 75 year-old male with a medical history significant for coronary artery disease, chronic kidney disease, hypertension, hyperlipidemia, heart failure with preserved ejection fraction, and a history of stroke presented to the emergency room with a two-week history of progressive altered mental status, generalized weakness, and confusion. On arrival, he was found to be profoundly hypertensive, with laboratory data showing an acute kidney injury, an elevated lipase above 2000, and a serum calcium of 15.0 (Ref: 8.6–10.5 mg/dL). Workup for his hypercalcemia revealed a normal intact parathyroid hormone (PTH) level of 20 pg/mL (Ref: 15–65 pg/mL), though repeat PTH following zoledronic acid infusion was low at 10 pg/mL (Ref: 15–65 pg/mL). While PTH-mediated hypercalcemia was initially entertained given the first nonsuppressed PTH, a sestamibi scan showed no evidence of parathyroid adenoma. The 25-hydroxyvitamin D level was elevated >200 ng/mL (Ref: 20–50 ng/mL), confirmed by liquid chromatography-mass spectroscopy, and the 1, 25-hydroxyvitamin D level obtained by immunochemiluminometric assay was elevated at 345 pg/mL (Ref: 19.9–79.3). 24-hour urine calcium was elevated at 0.34 gm/24 hours (Ref: 0.05–0.30 gm/24 hours). Other workup including an angiotensin-converting enzyme level, serum immunofixation, and parathyroid hormone related peptide levels were all within normal limits. A CT scan revealed no obvious evidence of sarcoidosis or lymphadenopathy. He was initially treated with intravenous fluids and diuretics, with initial transient improvement in his serum calcium levels. By hospital day 4, there was worsening of his hypercalcemia, and the endocrine service was consulted. More careful history revealed that the patient had bottles for both 5,000 IU and 50,000 IU of vitamin D at his home that were purchased over-the-counter, which he had been consuming daily for the past two years, consistent with the diagnosis of hypercalcemia secondary to vitamin D toxicity. He was given a dose of zoledronic acid 4 mg on hospital day 8 as well as a total of 7 doses of calcitonin, while maintaining normal saline infusions and furosemide, again with modest improvement in his serum calcium levels. Despite an initial response, the patient's calcium started to uptrend, and he was started on high-dose prednisone 60 mg daily and placed on a calcium restricted diet on hospital day 11. He received a total of around 63 liters of intravenous fluids throughout his 42 days hospitalization. Despite these measures, when trialed off fluids and diuretics, his calcium would uptrend. After a thorough review of the literature and an interdisciplinary consensus with the nephrology and transfusion medicine teams and discussion of the risk and benefits with the patient and his family, decision was made to start the patient on continuous cycling peritoneal dialysis (CCPD) to treat his vitamin D toxicity. After the patient provided informed consent, a peritoneal dialysis catheter was placed on hospital day 27, and he was started on peritoneal dialysis. He completed 10 sessions of CCPD. His progress was monitored with total serum calcium, ionized calcium, and both 25-hydroxyvitamin D by dilution and 1, 25-hydroxyvitamin D levels after each dialysis session (Figures 1 and 2). The nephrology team measured 25-hydroxyvitamin D and 1, 25-hydroxyvitamin D levels in the peritoneal dialysis effluent fluid.

We used 24 hours CCPD with 1.5% dextrose solutions with 1.25 liters dwells cycling every 4 hours for a total of 10 sessions over 10 days. Our patient had a serum 25-hydroxyvitamin D level of about 400 ng/mL. Considering that an estimated 30% of total body vitamin D is circulating in the serum (with the rest distributed in adipose tissue, muscles, and other tissues) [11] and assuming a total blood volume of 4.0 liters, the patient at any one time had about 1,600,000 ng of circulating 25-hydroxyvitamin D.

His peritoneal dialysis effluent 25-hydroxyvitamin D ranged 60–77.8 ng/mL of effluent. With a fixed effluent of 1.25 liters, we effectively cleared about 75,000–97,000 ng of 25-hydroxyvitamin D with each exchange, corresponding to about 3,000–3,880 IU.

Eight days following discharge, blood work revealed a calcium level maintained in the normal range at 9.4 mg/dL and a 25-hydroxyvitamin D level of 461 ng/mL. His kidney function had also returned to baseline.

3. Discussion

Vitamin D was first described as a vitamin in the 20th century and is now recognized as a prohormone. A unique feature of vitamin D is that it is synthesized by the human body through direct sunlight exposure. Interestingly, prolonged exposure to UV light does not lead to toxic amounts of vitamin D3 because previtamin D3 and vitamin D3 are photoconverted to inactive metabolites [12, 13]. As shown in Figure 3, 7-dehydrocholesterol is converted to previtamin D3 through UVB in the skin. Previtamin D3 is then converted to vitamin D3 (cholecalciferol) through the effects of heat. Vitamin D3 is converted by 25-hydroxylase (CYP2R1) in the liver to 25-hydroxyvitamin D, the major circulating form of vitamin D. It circulates and binds to the vitamin D binding protein (DBP). In the kidney, 1α-hydroxylase converts 25-hydroxyvitamin D to 1,25-dihydroxyvitamin D (calcitriol), the active form. The renal synthesis of 1, 25-dihydroxyvitamin D is counter regulated by 24-hydroxylase that converts 25-hydroxyvitamin D into inactive 24, 25-dihydroxyvitamin D. Vitamin D is a fat-soluble vitamin and stored in adipose tissue. Reuptake of vitamin D in the kidneys occurs through binding to vitamin D binding protein. Thus, the excretion of vitamin D metabolites is primarily through the bile into the feces [14].

Vitamin D excess is described with certain inactivating mutations of CYP24A1 encoding vitamin D-24-hydroxylase [15], and more commonly, although infrequently, in situations of exogenous supplementation.

The daily upper limits for vitamin D supplementation are outlined in Table 1 [14]. From the year 2000 through June 30th, 2014, the National Poison Data System received reports of 25,397 human exposures to vitamin D. Between the years

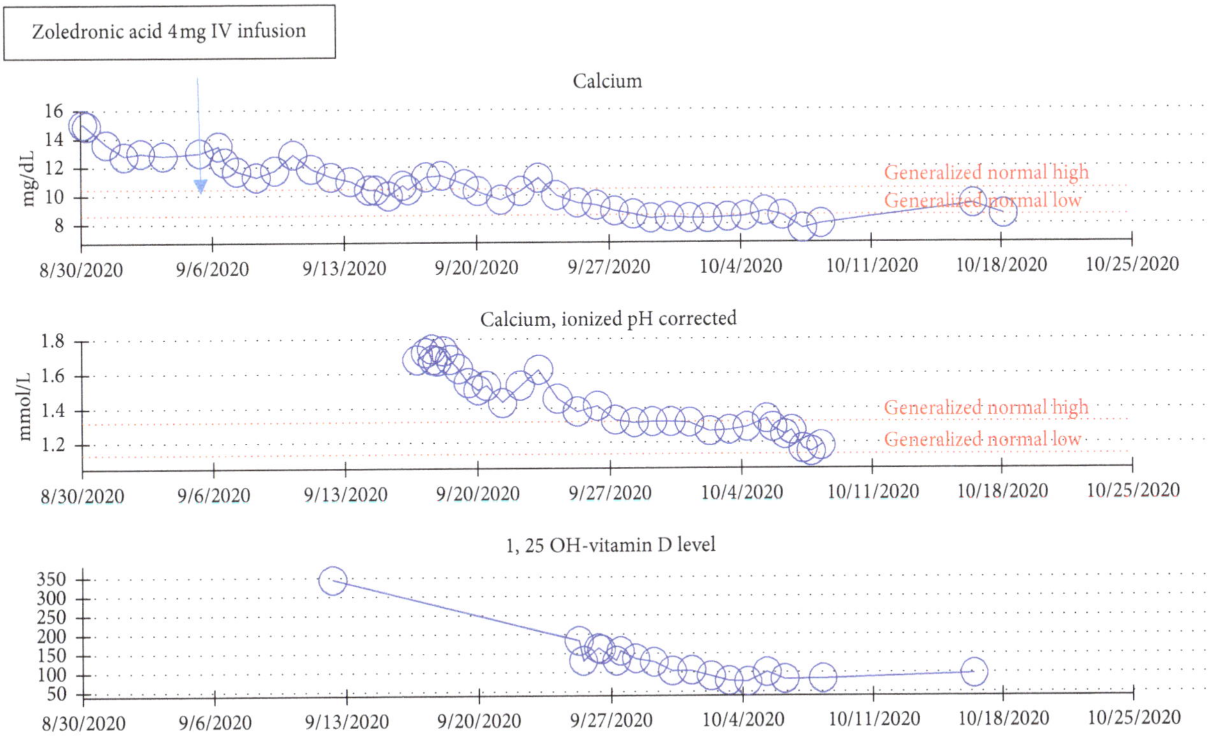

FIGURE 1: Trends of total serum calcium, ionized calcium, and 1,25-dihydroxyvitamin D levels during hospitalization.

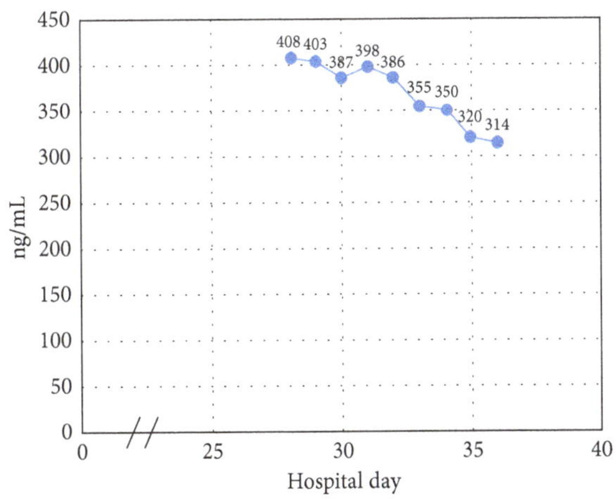

FIGURE 2: Serum 25-hydroxyvitamin D levels by dilution during hospitalization.

2000 and 2005, there was an average of 196 reported cases per year. By the end of 2014, there was a 1600% increase in exposure, with 4535 cases recorded [16].

Hypercalcemia is a biochemical manifestation of vitamin D toxicity (VDT). Signs and symptoms of VDT are due to the underlying hypercalcemia and include confusion, polyuria, polydipsia, anorexia, vomiting, and muscle weakness. Chronic intoxication may cause nephrocalcinosis, bone demineralization, and pain. The therapeutic approach to this non-PTH dependent hypercalcemia is universal. Consistently seen across several case reports and case series over the past 5 years [17–23], management of hypercalcemia secondary to hypervitaminosis D consisted of aggressive intravenous fluid resuscitation, diuretic therapy, calcitonin, and bisphosphonate therapy (alendronate, pamidronate, or zoledronic acid). Corticosteroid therapy (prednisone or prednisolone) has also been the cornerstone of management of 1,25-dihydroxyvitamin mediated hypercalcemia. It lowers the calcium level by reducing intestinal calcium absorption by decreasing transcellular active transport processes, increasing urinary excretion of calcium and altering the hepatic vitamin D metabolism to favor synthesis of inactive metabolites [24]. Second line therapy of VDT includes phenobarbital, ketoconazole, or aminoquinolones [24]. In

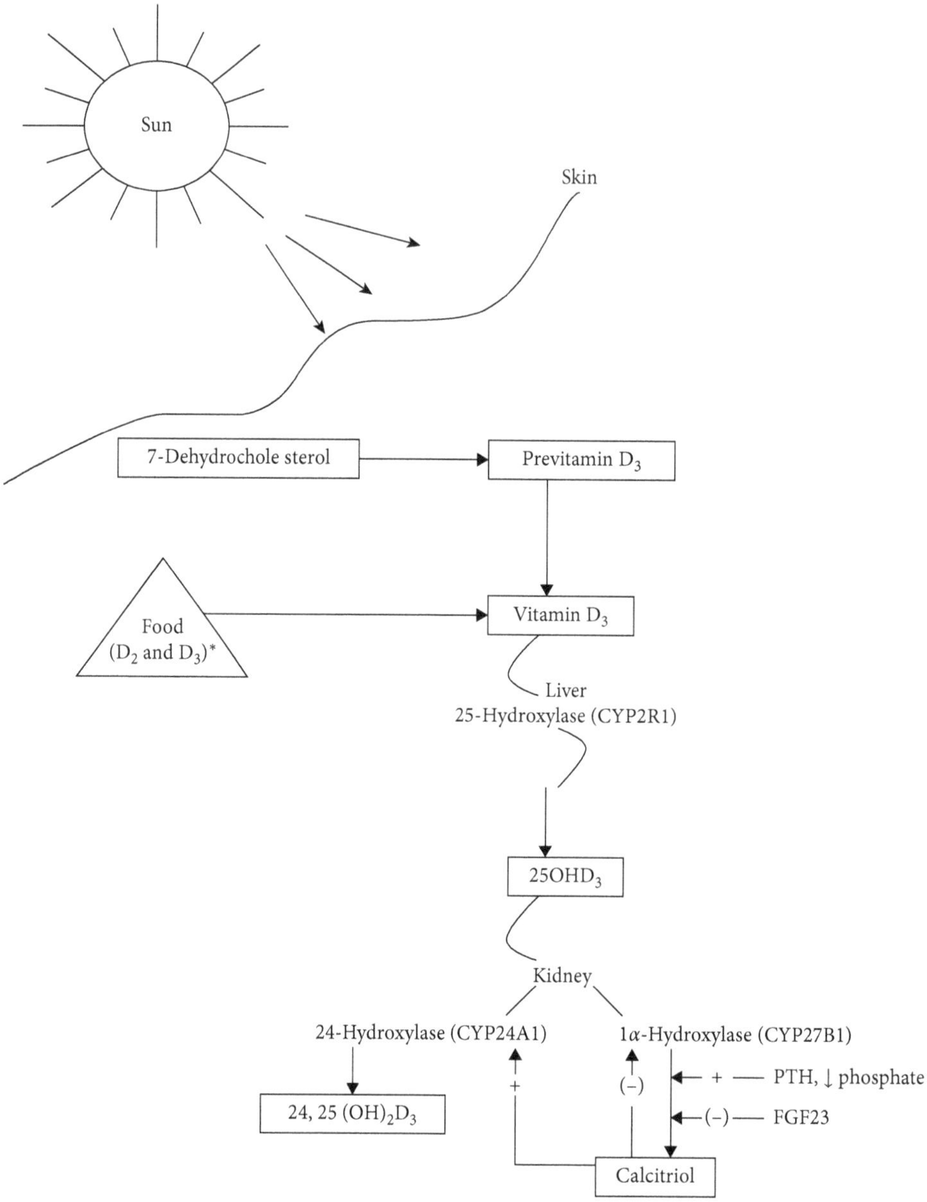

Figure 3: Pathway of vitamin D synthesis and metabolism (adapted from dietary reference intakes for calcium and vitamin D [14]).

addition, August et. al described the use of hydroxychloroquine 400 mg daily for hypercalcemia secondary to VDT in a 54-year-old man with kidney failure [25]. Rifampin and phenytoin have also been used in the management of VDT as they both induce CYP3A4 which metabolizes 25-hydroxyvitamin D into inactive 4β,25-dihydroxyvitamin D. This is the alternative pathway for vitamin D inactivation in patients with CYP24A1 mutations [26].

Despite initial response to medical management with intravenous hydration, diuretics, calcitonin, bisphosphonate, and corticosteroid therapy and notwithstanding adherence to a calcium restricted diet provided through the assistance of the dietary and nutritional services, our patient experienced rebound hypercalcemia at every interruption in management. After almost a month, our focus shifted to efforts to eliminate vitamin D from his serum. Peritoneal dialysis is established to cause vitamin D deficiency. Alwakeel et al. presented data from 27 patients who had been on peritoneal dialysis for more than six months. Blood was sampled for 25-hydroxyvitamin D levels. The majority of patients (59.2%) had levels below 15 nmol/L (6 ng/mL) [27]. Literature review yielded a sole case report from 1966 presented at the Third International Congress of Nephrology, in which peritoneal dialysis was used to clear vitamin D and calcium in the case of a 54-year-old woman with hypercalcemia secondary to hypervitaminosis D. This latter patient had received more

Table 1: Daily upper limit for vitamin D supplementation (adapted from dietary reference intakes for calcium and vitamin D [14]).

Life stage group	UL
Infant	
0–6 m	1,000 IU (25 μg)
6–12 m	1,500 IU (38 μg)
Children	
1–3 y	2,500 IU (63 μg)
4–8 y	3,000 IU (75 μg)
Male	
9–13 y	4,000 IU (100 μg)
14–18 y	4,000 IU (100 μg)
19–30 y	4,000 IU (100 μg)
31–50 y	4,000 IU (100 μg)
51–70 y	4,000 IU (100 μg)
>70 y	4,000 IU (100 μg)
Female	
9–13 y	4,000 IU (100 μg)
14–18 y	4,000 IU (100 μg)
19–30 y	4,000 IU (100 μg)
31–50 y	4,000 IU (100 μg)
51–70 y	4,000 IU (100 μg)
>70 y	4,000 IU (100 μg)
Pregnancy	
14–18 y	4,000 IU (100 μg)
19–30 y	4,000 IU (100 μg)
31–50 y	4,000 IU (100 μg)
Lactation	
14–18 y	4,000 IU (100 μg)
19–30 y	4,000 IU (100 μg)
31–50 y	4,000 IU (100 μg)

Note: IU, international unit.

than 100 million units of vitamin D orally and intramuscularly over a period of 3 1/2 years for vitamin D resistant rickets [28].

4. Conclusion

Peritoneal dialysis is often used as a means of addressing hypercalcemia; however, since 1966, it has not been used to our knowledge for the treatment of hypervitaminosis D. In the case we presented, we were able to safely use peritoneal dialysis to clear 25-hydroxyvitamin D from the plasma resulting in faster resolution of hypercalcemia.

The increase in our patient's 25-hydroxyvitamin D level after discharge can be explained by the release of vitamin D from adipose tissue stores. Fortunately, his calcium level has remained in the normal range, and he remains on a restricted calcium diet.

This case, in addition to providing an alternative option for the treatment of vitamin D toxicity, raises concern regarding vitamin D reserves in patients who routinely undergo peritoneal dialysis for renal replacement therapy as Alwakeel et al. described in 2014 [27]. According to our calculation, a single cycle of peritoneal dialysis leads to the extraction of approximately 75–90 k ng of vitamin D. This urges the question about the systemic effects of chronic vitamin D losses in this group of patients. More research is needed in this field to study these outcomes.

Sequalae of vitamin D toxicity remain a concern. Nephrocalcinosis defined as a generalized deposition of calcium salts in the kidney is a well-known but rare complication of VDT as seen in a 14-year follow-up report of an 8-month-old child [29]. Vascular calcification, resulting in increased cardiovascular risk, is another complication of hypercalcemia and vitamin D toxicity. Reversal of VDT and hypercalcemia has resulted in resolution of vascular calcifications [30].

References

[1] M. F. Holick, "The vitamin D deficiency pandemic: approaches for diagnosis, treatment and prevention," *Reviews in Endocrine and Metabolic Disorders*, vol. 18, no. 2, pp. 153–165, 2017.

[2] O. Sizar, S. Khare, A. Goyal, P. Bansal, and A. Givler, *Vitamin D Deficiency*, StatPearls, Treasure Island, FL, USA, 2020.

[3] K. Y. Z. Forrest and W. L. Stuhldreher, "Prevalence and correlates of vitamin D deficiency in US adults," *Nutrition Research*, vol. 31, no. 1, pp. 48–54, 2011.

[4] M. R. Rooney, L. Harnack, E. D. Michos, R. P. Ogilvie, C. T. Sempos, and P. L. Lutsey, "Trends in use of high-dose vitamin D supplements exceeding 1000 or 4000 international units daily, 1999–2014," *JAMA*, vol. 317, no. 23, pp. 2448–2450, 2017.

[5] G. Ferrer-Mayorga, M. J. Larriba, P. Crespo, and A. Muñoz, "Mechanisms of action of vitamin D in colon cancer," *The Journal of Steroid Biochemistry and Molecular Biology*, vol. 185, pp. 1–6, 2019.

[6] S. M. Jeon and E. A. Shin, "Exploring vitamin D metabolism and function in cancer," *Experimental & Molecular Medicine*, vol. 50, no. 4, pp. 1–14, 2018.

[7] H. Guo, J. Guo, W. Xie, L. Yuan, and X. Sheng, "The role of vitamin D in ovarian cancer: epidemiology, molecular mechanism and prevention," *Journal of Ovarian Research*, vol. 11, no. 1, p. 71, 2018.

[8] Y. Xu, D. J. Baylink, C.-S. Chen et al., "The importance of vitamin D metabolism as a potential prophylactic, immunoregulatory and neuroprotective treatment for COVID-19," *Journal of Translational Medicine*, vol. 18, no. 1, p. 322, 2020.

[9] W. B. Grant, H. Lahore, S. L. McDonnell et al., "Evidence that vitamin D supplementation could reduce risk of influenza and COVID-19 infections and deaths," *Nutrients*, vol. 12, no. 4, 2020.

[10] N. Ali, "Role of vitamin D in preventing of COVID-19 infection, progression and severity," *Journal of Infection and Public Health*, vol. 13, no. 10, pp. 1373–1380, 2020.

[11] R. P. Heaney, R. L. Horst, D. M. Cullen, and L. A. G. Armas, "Vitamin D3 distribution and status in the body," *Journal of the American College of Nutrition*, vol. 28, no. 3, pp. 252–256, 2009.

[12] M. F. Holick, "Vitamin D: a millenium perspective," *Journal of Cellular Biochemistry*, vol. 88, no. 2, pp. 296–307, 2003.

[13] M. Holick, J. MacLaughlin, and S. Doppelt, "Regulation of cutaneous previtamin D3 photosynthesis in man: skin pigment is not an essential regulator," *Science*, vol. 211, no. 4482, pp. 590–593, 1981.

[14] A. C. Ross, C. L. Taylor, A. L. Yaktine, and H. B. Del Valle,

"Dietary reference intakes for calcium and vitamin D," in *The National Academies Collection*National Academies Press (US), Washington, DC, USA, 2011.
[15] T. P. Griffin, C. M. Joyce, S. Alkanderi et al., "Biallelic CYP24A1 variants presenting during pregnancy: clinical and biochemical phenotypes," *Endocrine Connections*, vol. 9, no. 6, pp. 530–541, 2020.
[16] H. Spiller, T. Good, N. Spiller, and A. Aleguas, "Vitamin D exposures reported to US poison centers 2000–2014," *Human & Experimental Toxicology*, vol. 35, no. 5, pp. 457–461, 2016.
[17] A. Rajadhyaksha, N. Sarate, and P. Kharapkar, "Hypervitaminosis D and cortical venous thrombosis; an unusual presentation," *Journal of the Association of Physicians of India*, vol. 68, no. 9, pp. 72-73, 2020.
[18] M. I. Ghauri, S. B. Bareeqa, A. Riaz, and A. Kumar, "Redundancy is of no good; iatrogenic hypervitaminosis D: a rare case of persistent vomiting due to hypercalcemia," *Clinical Medicine Insights: Case Reports*, vol. 12, 2019.
[19] S. Ellis, G. Tsiopanis, and T. Lad, "Risks of the "sunshine pill"—a case of hypervitaminosis D," *Clinical Medicine*, vol. 18, no. 4, pp. 311–313, 2018.
[20] K. Demir, H. Döneray, C. Kara et al., "Comparison of treatment regimens in management of severe hypercalcemia due to vitamin D intoxication in children," *Journal of Clinical Research in Pediatric Endocrinology*, vol. 11, no. 2, pp. 140–148, 2019.
[21] K. Galior, S. Grebe, and R. Singh, "Development of vitamin D toxicity from overcorrection of vitamin D deficiency: a review of case reports," *Nutrients*, vol. 10, no. 8, 2018.
[22] V. Guerra, O. M. Vieira Neto, A. F. Laurindo, F. J. Paula, and M. Moysés Neto, "Hypercalcemia and renal function impairment associated with vitamin D toxicity: case report," *Brazilian Journal of Nephrology (BJN)*, vol. 38, no. 4, pp. 466–469, 2016.
[23] M. Wani, I. Wani, K. Banday, and M. Ashrafâ, "The other side of vitamin D therapy: a case series of acute kidney injury due to malpractice-related vitamin D intoxication," *Clinical Nephrology*, vol. 86, pp. 236–241, 2016.
[24] E. Marcinowska-Suchowierska, M. Kupisz-Urbańska, J. Łukaszkiewicz, P. Płudowski, and G. Jones, "Vitamin D toxicity-a clinical perspective," *Frontiers in Endocrinology*, vol. 9, p. 550, 2018.
[25] B. L. Auguste, C. Avila-Casado, and J. M. Bargman, "Use of vitamin D drops leading to kidney failure in a 54-year-old man," *Canadian Medical Association Journal*, vol. 191, no. 14, pp. E390–E394, 2019.
[26] Z. Wang, E. G. Schuetz, Y. Xu, and K. E. Thummel, "Interplay between vitamin D and the drug metabolizing enzyme CYP3A4," *The Journal of Steroid Biochemistry and Molecular Biology*, vol. 136, pp. 54–58, 2013.
[27] J. Alwakeel, S. Usama, A. Mitwalli, A. Alsuwaida, and M. Alghonaim, "Prevalence of vitamin D deficiency in peritoneal dialysis patients," *Saudi Journal of Kidney Diseases and Transplantation*, vol. 25, no. 5, pp. 981–985, 2014.
[28] R. I. Henkin, M. Lotz, and F. C. Bartter, "Peritoneal dialysis removes vitamin D," *JAMA: The Journal of the American Medical Association*, vol. 198, no. 3, p. 47, 1966.
[29] A. Goyal, S. H. Rahaman, N. Raizada, D. Kandasamy, A. P. Mehta, and R. Khadgawat, "Bilateral medullary nephrocalcinosis secondary to vitamin D toxicity: a 14-year follow-up report," *Indian Journal of Endocrinology and Metabolism*, vol. 22, no. 6, pp. 853-854, 2018.
[30] M. Cirillo, G. Bilancio, and C. Cirillo, "Reversible vascular calcifications associated with hypervitaminosis D," *Journal of Nephrology*, vol. 29, no. 1, pp. 129–131, 2016.

43

Challenges of Diagnosing Pseudohypoaldosteronism (PHA) in an Infant

Ghufran Saeed Babar[1] **and Minah Tariq**[2]

[1]*Children's Mercy Hospital and Clinics Endocrinology, 3101 Broadway Blvd, Kansas, Missouri 64111, USA*
[2]*Kansas City University, College of Osteopathic Medicine DO Candidate, Class No 2024, Kansas, Missouri 64124, USA*

Correspondence should be addressed to Ghufran Saeed Babar; gbabar@cmh.edu

Academic Editor: Toshihiro Kita

Background. Pseudohypoaldosteronism (PHA) is characterized by renal tubular resistance to aldosterone. As a result, the symptoms typically involve hyperkalemia and hyponatremia. The aim of this clinical case report is to highlight the severe electrolyte imbalance PHA can present within an infant, as well as difficulties in diagnosing the condition. *Case Presentation.* A 5-week-old male arrived at the ER with episodes of emesis, lethargy, and difficulty in feeding. He had significant electrolyte abnormalities and was being treated by his PCP for failure to thrive. He presented with urinary sodium wasting, indicated by hyponatremia, hyperkalemia, low chloride, and hypercalcemia. Patient was treated with IVF and NaCl supplementation to normalize the electrolytes. The patient showed heterozygosity for a variant in the *WNK1* gene, which typically causes Gordon syndrome; however, our patient had a normal blood pressure. The electrolyte imbalance self-resolved during several months of follow-up, and currently, the patient is not on any treatment.

1. Introduction

Pseudohypoaldosteronism is a heterogeneous group of disorders with end organ resistance to aldosterone resulting in hyponatremia, hyperkalemia, and metabolic acidosis. The intravascular volume could be low or normal with a corresponding low or high blood pressure. The various forms of PHA can have elevated, normal, or low levels of renin and aldosterone, in the absence of elevated 17-OHP level [1, 2].

PHA can be further subcategorized into PHA types 1 and 2. PHA1 is a rare autosomal recessive disease caused by impaired transepithelial sodium transport that typically effects children and causes end organ resistance to aldosterone [3]. Patients with this disease do not benefit from mineralocorticoid treatment and must be given large doses of sodium supplementation to correct their symptoms. There are multiple mutations that can result in PHA1, which can either cause inactivation of the human mineralocorticoid receptor (MR, NR3C2 gene) in the kidneys or biallelic inactivation in the genes encoding the α, β, or γ subunits of the epithelial sodium channel (ENaC) [3]. Inactivation of the ENaC channels is typically caused by inactivation of *SCNN1A*, *SCNN1B*, or *SCNN1G* and results in systemic salt loss from the kidneys, salivary glands, colon, and sweat ducts [3]. Most children with the renal form of PHA1 are weaned off sodium supplementation relatively early due to maturation of the handling capacity of the kidneys [3]. However, patients effected by the systemic form of PHA1 often require life-long salt supplementation and have extensive medical needs [4].

There is a second form of PHA known as Gordon syndrome (PHA2) [5]. It characteristically presents as hypertension (HTN) and hyperkalemia with a normal glomerular filtration rate, acidosis, and a low plasma renin level. The aldosterone levels can be low to inappropriately high [6]. Gordon syndrome is predominantly an autosomal dominant condition with four genes that are implicated: *WNK1*, *WNK4*, *KLHL3*, and *CUL3* [7].

Young patients who present with the symptoms of hyponatremia and hyperkalemia are typically screened for congenital adrenal hyperplasia (CAH), as it is associated with PHA like electrolyte imbalance [8, 9].

2. Case Presentation

We report a case of a 5-week-old male presenting with severe salt-wasting, hyperkalemia, and resultant failure to thrive. The patient was born at 36 weeks with an uncomplicated vaginal delivery. The mother had preeclampsia and thus required induction of labor. He had an uncomplicated postnatal course and regained birth weight by 14 days, being fed primarily through breastfeeding. Initially, the patient was feeding well, but for 10 days, leading to his ED visit, he had developed a weight plateau, and he was transitioned to formula feeds. He had nonbloody, nonbilious emesis that was worsening. Patient was taking 3–3.5 ounces per feed every 3-4 h, but then it decreased to 1-2 ounces at a time. He was stooling 1-2/day and urinating 4-5/day. He was being followed by his PCP for failure to thrive. He had been placed on ranitidine to treat his reflux but had no significant improvement. Newborn screening had been done, but parents did not receive any notable results.

The patient was referred to the ED with increased difficulty in feeding, lethargy, and episodes of emesis. In the ED, the child was afebrile and in a compensated shock and had a low normal BP: 76/35, HR: 169/min, and fast breathing R/R; 80/min. Lab work completed for the patient showed Na of 112 mEq/L (132–142) and K of 10.1 mEq/L (3.5–6.2), calcium was 12.3 mg/dl (8.6–10.5), and CRP was normal. The urine test was normal and did not show signs of urinary tract infection (UTI). There is no previous history of UTI. Once endocrinology was consulted, patient was given a normal saline (NS) fluid bolus 20 ml/kg, and a repeat BMP was ordered that showed Na of 110 mEq/L and K of 9.3 mEq/L with normal LFTs (liver function tests). With continued salt imbalance, a second NS bolus was given and a dose of Florinef 0.2 mg was given due to suspicion of CAH. Subsequently, fluids were started with D5NS at 1.5 times maintenance for electrolyte and caloric replenishment. Follow-up electrolytes showed a stable Na of 109 mEq/L, a decreased K of 8.3 mEq/L, and a normal Ca of 10.2 mg/dl. Rest of the labs showed TSH level 5.3 mcIU/mL (0.35–7.60), free T4 2.2 ng/dL (0.8–1.9), random cortisol 20.5 mcg/dL (≥3), and a baseline 17-hydroxyprogesterone level of 99 ng/dl (normal).

The patient was admitted to the pediatric intensive care unit (PICU), was hemodynamically stable, and hydrocortisone was not started. Repeat labs were performed that showed an Na of 133 mEq/L, K of 4.7 mEq/L, Cl of 102 mEq/L, and a glucose level of 90 mg/dL. Considering a strong suspicion for CAH, a high dose ACTH stimulation test was performed. Results of this test showed a stimulated 17 OH-pregnenolone of 88 ng/dL, cortisol of 27.1 mcg/dL, and normal DOC (deoxy-corticosterone). His urine sodium level was elevated at 35 mmol/L (<20). The kidney and urinary system ultrasound were normal. Upon further evaluation, the patient's aldosterone levels were discovered to be elevated at 632 ng/dL (6.5–86) and renin level at 351 ng/dL (1.4–7.8). A diagnosis of PHA was made and the child stopped receiving Florinef, only receiving NaCl supplementation with an eventual dose of 22.5 mEq/kg/day to stabilize his electrolytes and compensate for his salt-wasting. He was discharged from the PICU in 6 days with a sodium level of 139 mEq/L.

Genetic testing was conducted on the patient and was negative for *NR3C2*, *CUL3*, *KLHL3*, *SCNN1A*, *SCNN1B*, *SCNN1G*, and *WNK4*. However, the patient showed heterozygosity for a variant of unknown significance, c.6276 T > A (*p.* Ser2092Arg) in the *WNK1* gene. Patient currently has normal electrolytes with salt supplementation and was gradually weaned off with PHA that has self resolved.

3. Discussion

Salt-wasting crisis presenting as a severe hyponatremia, hyperkalemia, and dehydration is life-threatening in an infant and requires urgent treatment. It could be caused by CAH (congenital adrenal hyperplasia), hypoadrenalism, congenital adrenal hypoplasia, isolated aldosterone deficiency, nephrotoxic medications (e.g., ACE inhibitors, nonsteroidal anti-inflammatory drugs) and pseudohypoaldosteronism [10, 11]. Like our patient, PHA can present as failure to thrive with symptoms of poor feeding, reduced weight gain, and vomiting [12]. However, infants can deteriorate and present with hypovolemic shock and life-threatening hyperkalemia, which can cause ventricular flutter [13, 14]. Our patient had elevated urine sodium level which indicated aldosterone deficiency or resistance; however, definitive diagnosis of PHA is made after the results of aldosterone levels and genetic tests.

Our patient showed elevated aldosterone level and a gene heterozygosity for *WNK1*, which is typically implicated in Gordon syndrome (PHA2) [2]. PHA2 is caused by molecular abnormalities in two *WNK* genes, including *WNK1* and *WNK4* [15]. Genetic defects in Kelch-like 3 (*KLHL3*) or Cullin 3 (*CUL3*) can also cause PHA2 [16]. However, our patient did not present with the typical hypertension which is present in Gordon syndrome due to an imbalance in electrolyte and acid–base equilibrium with increased circulating blood volume. Analysis of the patient's genetic study did not indicate any abnormalities in the genes that typically cause PHA1. Thus, the phenotype and genotype of this patient's transient illness did not correspond to the known presentations of PHA1 or 2, further making his case unique [17].

The patient's initial presentation to the ED of severe salt-wasting did not have any known precipitating events. There have been multiple accounts of pediatric PHA patients who show salt-wasting crisis after contracting a urinary tract infection (UTI) and is associated with obstructive uropathologies [18, 19]. These forms of PHA are frequently transient, like our patient's presentation, and present with a decreased glomerular filtration rate [20]. However, our patient did not have any known UTI prior to the onset of his weight loss and salt-wasting symptoms nor did he have a congenital obstructive uropathology.

4. Conclusions

There are several very interesting aspects about this case of transient PHA. First, it indicates that pseudohypoaldosteronism should be considered in any infant presenting with hyponatremia and hyperkalemia after the first few weeks of life, since congenital adrenal hyperplasia usually gets diagnosed by this time either by the results of the newborn screening or because the newborn has already presented with salt-wasting crisis. Second, our patient had a non-apparent cause of his symptoms and there were no obvious precipitating factors such as UTI or obstructive uropathies. Determining the exact cause of the onset of this patient's severe symptoms was difficult because the many subtypes of PHA have different presentations and genetic mutations. His genetic testing showed that he does not have any mutations in the genes that cause PHA1 specifically, yet he showed the corresponding symptoms of hyperkalemia, hyponatremia, and failure to thrive. Third, our patient showed the transient form of aldosterone resistance, distinguishing this condition from the known genetic causes of pseudohypoaldosteronism. The patient gradually recovered from the electrolyte imbalance and all medications, and later, salt supplementation was also discontinued. The child continues to have normal sodium, potassium, anion gap, and glucose levels. Furthermore, although the child does display heterozygosity for the *WNK1* gene which is typically implicated in Gordon syndrome (PHA2), he did not present with the characteristic hypertension of Gordon syndrome as well. Long term clinical follow-up will be required to determine if there any changes in electrolyte balance.

References

[1] F. G. Riepe, "Pseudohypoaldosteronism," *Endocrine Development*, vol. 24, pp. 86–95, 2013.

[2] H. Mabillard and J. A. Sayer, "The molecular genetics of Gordon syndrome," *Genes*, vol. 10, no. 12, p. 986, 2019.

[3] A. Cayir, I. Sahin, and T. Guran, "Diagnosis and management of pseudohypoaldosteronism type 1 in children," *Internal Medicine Review*, vol. 4, no. 12, 2018.

[4] D. B. Cheek and J. W. Perry, "A salt wasting syndrome in infancy," *Archives of Disease in Childhood*, vol. 33, no. 169, pp. 252–256, 1958.

[5] W. K. A. Paver and G. J. Pauline, "Hypertension and hyperpotassæmia without renal disease in a young male," *Medical Journal of Australia*, vol. 2, no. 8, pp. 305-306, 1964.

[6] J. E. Arnold and J. K. Healy, "Hyperkalemia, hypertension and systemic acidosis without renal failure associated with a tubular defect in potassium excretion," *The American Journal of Medicine*, vol. 47, no. 3, pp. 461–472, 1969.

[7] J. S. Park, E. Park, H. S. Hyun et al., "Three cases of gordon syndrome with dominant KLHL3 mutations.KLHL3 mutations," *Journal of Pediatric Endocrinology & Metabolism: Journal of Pediatric Endocrinology & Metabolism*, vol. 30, no. 3, pp. 361-364, 2017.

[8] L. Manikam, M. P. Cornes, D. Kalra, C. Ford, and R. Gama, "Transient pseudohypoaldosteronism masquerading as congenital adrenal hyperplasia," *Annals of Clinical Biochemistry: International Journal of Laboratory Medicine*, vol. 48, no. 4, pp. 380–382, 2011.

[9] M. De Clerck, J. Vande Walle, E. Dhont, J. Dehoorne, and W. Keenswijk, "An infant presenting with failure to thrive and hyperkalaemia owing to transient pseudohypoaldosteronism: case report," *Paediatrics and International Child Health*, vol. 38, no. 4, pp. 277–280, 2018.

[10] J. Zieg, "Evaluation and management of hyponatraemia in children," *Acta Paediatrica*, vol. 103, no. 10, pp. 1027–1034, 2014.

[11] R. Bogdanovic, N. Stajic, J. Putnik, and A. Paripovic, "Transient type 1 - pseudo-hypoaldosteronism: report on an eight-patient series and literature review," *Pediatric Nephrology*, vol. 24, no. 11, pp. 2167–2175, 2009.

[12] M. A. Ruiz Gines, J. A. Ruiz Gines, J. Saura Montalban, R. Fontelles Alcover, and A. N. Piqueras Martinez, "Pseudohypoaldosteronism type 1 secondary to vesicoureteral reflux: an endocrinologic emergency," *Endocrinología y Nutrición*, vol. 61, no. 9, pp. 495–497, 2014.

[13] K.-C. Thies, K. Boos, K. Müller-Deile, W. Ohrdorf, T. Beushausen, and P. Townsend, "Ventricular flutter in a neonate—severe electrolyte imbalance caused by urinary tract infection in the presence of urinary tract malformation," *Journal of Emergency Medicine*, vol. 18, no. 1, pp. 47–50, 2000.

[14] S. S. Yang, T. Morimoto, T. Rai et al., "Molecular pathogenesis of pseudohypoaldosteronism type II: generation and analysis of a Wnk4(D561A/+) knockin mouse model," *Cell Metabolism*, vol. 5, no. 5, pp. 331-344, 2007.

[15] L. M. Boyden, M. Choi, K. A. Choate et al., "Mutations in kelch-like 3 and cullin 3 cause hypertension and electrolyte abnormalities," *Nature*, vol. 482, no. 7383, pp. 98–102, 2012.

[16] U. Kuhnle, M. D. Nielsen, H. U. Tietze et al., "Pseudohypoaldosteronism in eight families: different forms of inheritance are evidence for various genetic defects," *The Journal of Clinical Endocrinology & Metabolism*, vol. 70, no. 3, pp. 638–641, 1990.

[17] R. Nandagopal, P. Vaidyanathan, and P. Kaplowitz, "Transient pseudohypoaldosteronism due to urinary tract infection in infancy: a report of 4 cases," *International Journal of Pediatric Endocrinology*, vol. 2009, p. 1, 2009.

[18] F. Tütüncüler, H. Günöz, F. Bas, R. Bundak, N. Saka, and O. Neyzi, "Transient pseudohypoaldosteronism in an infant with urinary tract anomaly," *Pediatrics International*, vol. 46, no. 5, pp. 618–620, 2004.

[19] E. J. Schoen, S. Bhatia, G. T. Ray, W. Clapp, and T. T. To, "Transient pseudohypoaldosteronism with hyponatremia-hyperkalemia in infant urinary tract infection," *The Journal of Urology*, vol. 167, pp. 680–682, 2002.

[20] F. H. Wilson, S. Disse-Nicodeme, K. A. Choate et al., "Human hypertension caused by mutations in WNK kinases," *Science*, vol. 293, no. 5532, pp. 1107-1112, 2001.

44

Bacteremia in a Newborn with Hypocalcemic Seizures and Vitamin D Deficiency

Rebecca L. Moore,[1,2,3] Matthew L. Lorenz,[1,2,3] Meghan E. Fredette,[1,4] and Lisa Swartz Topor[1,4]

[1]*Department of Pediatrics, Brown University, Providence, RI, USA*
[2]*Department of Internal Medicine, Rhode Island Hospital, Providence, RI, USA*
[3]*Department of Internal Medicine, Brown University, Providence, RI, USA*
[4]*Division of Pediatric Endocrinology, Hasbro Children's Hospital, Providence, RI, USA*

Correspondence should be addressed to Lisa Swartz Topor; lisa_swartz_topor@brown.edu

Academic Editor: Osamu Isozaki

Infants with neonatal hypocalcemia often present with seizures, and neonatal hypocalcemia can be due to parathyroid (PTH) insufficiency or resistance. Causes of hypocalcemia with PTH elevation include increased phosphate load, vitamin D deficiency (VDD) or defects in metabolism, renal dysfunction, hypomagnesemia, genetic mutations resulting in end-organ resistance to PTH, or critical illness. Hypocalcemia has also been shown to be associated with Gram-negative bacteremia and sepsis in adults. We present the case of a full-term, formula-fed newborn presenting with late-onset hypocalcemic seizures and VDD in the setting of *Klebsiella pneumoniae* bacteremia. This case highlights that newborns presenting with hypocalcemic seizures should undergo a workup for sepsis.

1. Background

Hypocalcemia in a term infant is defined as a total serum calcium <8 mg/dL or an ionized calcium <4.4 mg/dL. Late-onset hypocalcemia is defined as hypocalcemia that occurs in neonates after the second or third day of life. Most infants with hypocalcemia are asymptomatic; those who present with symptoms most commonly present with increased neuromuscular irritability or seizures [1] and less commonly with stridor, wheezing, or vomiting caused by laryngospasm, bronchospasm, or pylorospasm, respectively [2]. The majority of infants with hypocalcemia have parathyroid hormone (PTH) insufficiency, low vitamin D (25-hydroxy vitamin D), low magnesium, or are formula fed [3]. Treatment of symptomatic hypocalcemia in infants begins with administration of intravenous (IV) calcium gluconate followed by oral calcium for maintenance therapy and identification and treatment of contributing factors such as hypomagnesemia, hyperphosphatemia, and vitamin D deficiency (VDD) [4].

2. Case Report

A 17-day-old full-term formula-fed female infant was admitted to the hospital for seizures. Four days prior to presentation, parents noticed brief episodes of left-sided upper and lower extremity shaking and lip smacking with associated vomiting and decreased oral intake. She was not taking any medications or vitamins at home. Evaluation in the Emergency Department (ED) revealed an afebrile, nondysmorphic female infant with normal vital signs. Shortly after arrival, she had a seizure with upper and lower extremity shaking and increased drooling, which lasted for one minute and resolved without treatment. Initial labs showed total calcium 6.4 mg/dL (reference range 9–10.9), ionized calcium 2.8 mg/dL (4.2–5.2), magnesium 1.3 mEq/L (1.3–1.9), and phosphorus 9 mg/dL (3.4–5.9). Bicarbonate was 17 mEq/L (22–32) with an anion gap of 16 mEq/L. Lactic acid was 2.2 mEq/L (0.2–1.9) with a normal pH. Sodium, potassium, creatinine, liver function tests, complete blood count, urinalysis, and cerebral spinal fluid (CSF) studies were unremarkable. Urine, blood, and CSF cultures were collected. A noncontrast computed tomography scan of the brain was normal. Electrocardiogram (EKG) showed prolongation of the corrected QT interval (QTc) to 468 milliseconds. She received calcium gluconate (1 mL/kg of 10% calcium gluconate) and phenobarbital (20 mg/kg) intravenously. Repeat laboratory studies demonstrated low serum calcium at 6.8 mg/dL (9–10.9) and persistently high phosphorus of 7.9 mg/dL (3.4–5.9). Additional tests showed elevated PTH of 143 pg/mL (18–80), low vitamin D of 7.4 ng/mL (>30), and 1.25(OH)D of 56 pg/mL (31–87). Thyroid-stimulating hormone (TSH) was normal. Maternal labs revealed normocalcemic VDD with a vitamin D of 9.4 ng/mL.

The infant was admitted to the hospital and treated with oral calcium carbonate (100 mg/kg/day of elemental calcium), phenobarbital, and broad-spectrum antimicrobial therapy with acyclovir, ampicillin, and gentamicin.

Blood cultures grew *Klebsiella pneumoniae*, and antimicrobial therapy was changed to cefazolin based on sensitivities. Urine and CSF cultures were negative; repeat blood cultures obtained on the third day of admission were negative. The patient started low-phosphate formula and cholecalciferol on the third day of admission. Serum calcium normalized by day 4 of calcium therapy. Magnetic resonance imaging of the brain, obtained due to concern for focal seizures on presentation, was normal. Repeat EKG showed normalized QTc. After discharge home, laboratory studies were closely monitored, and calcium supplementation and phenobarbital were gradually tapered. At seven weeks of age, she resumed cow's milk infant formula with continued normal calcium, phosphorus, and PTH levels (Figure 1).

3. Discussion

We describe an infant with late-onset hypocalcemia with multiple potential contributing factors including (1) VDD with biochemical findings resembling pseudohypoparathyroidism, (2) use of cow's milk formula, and (3) Gram-negative rod bacteremia. While the association between bacteremia and hypocalcemia has been described in adults, it has not been previously reported in infants or children. Thorough diagnostic evaluation allowed for recognition and treatment of both hypocalcemia and bacteremia.

In a retrospective review, Thomas et al. summarized clinical and laboratory characteristics as well as outcomes of neonates presenting with transient late-onset hypocalcemia. The majority of patients in this study had hypomagnesemia, low vitamin D, and PTH insufficiency with low or inappropriately normal phosphorus; none had bacteremia [1]. In contrast, our patient was found to have normal magnesium level, *Klebsiella* bacteremia, and VDD with elevated PTH and high serum phosphorous.

VDD is consistently reported in neonates with hypocalcemia [1, 3]. However, there are no well-established thresholds for vitamin D levels of clinical significance nor a clear relationship between low vitamin D and symptomatic hypocalcemia. Yilmaz et al. measured vitamin D, calcium, and PTH levels in 750 infants and found significantly lower vitamin D levels in preterm infants with hypocalcemia, but no significant difference in vitamin D levels between hypocalcemia and normocalcemia in term infants [5]. Nevertheless, there are multiple reports of hypocalcemic seizures in infancy attributed to VDD [6, 7]. A population-based study in the United Kingdom estimated the incidence of hypocalcemic seizures due to VDD to be 3.49 per million children 0–15 years of age (95% CI: 2.81–4.26) and 44.36 per million in children 0-1 year of age (95% CI: 35.12–55.28) [8]. The increased incidence of hypocalcemic seizures in infancy may be related to maternal VDD, which leads to inadequate passage of vitamin D across the placenta during pregnancy and predisposes the infant to hypocalcemia. Interestingly, phosphate levels vary in infants with VDD in contrast to older children with VDD, who classically have low-to-normal phosphorus levels due to secondary hyperparathyroidism [3, 6].

The term pseudohypoparathyroidism (PHP) encompasses a heterogeneous group of disorders characterized by end-organ resistance to PTH, which can be accompanied by features of Albright Hereditary Osteodystrophy (AHO) and resistance to other hormones [9]. The AHO phenotype includes short stature, subcutaneous ossifications, obesity, and brachydactyly, among other findings. Type 1 PHP has an impaired 3′,5′-cyclic adenosine monophosphate (cAMP) response to PTH infusion. Type II PHP is characterized by a normal cAMP response to PTH infusion, without a phosphaturic response, and has no AHO phenotype or other hormonal resistances. VDD has been described in previous reports to mimic PHP type II, with a clinical picture of PTH resistance, manifesting biochemically as hypocalcemia, elevated PTH and phosphorous, and low urinary phosphorus excretion despite typical cAMP generation [10]. The PTH resistance in these cases of VDD was responsive to vitamin D supplementation, with re-established phosphaturic response to PTH after vitamin D repletion. Additionally, neonates can have transient PTH resistance that has been proposed as a developmental condition of the kidney that resolves with time [11]. Our patient had a clinical picture resembling PHP type II, which was responsive to treatment with vitamin D, as has been previously reported.

Excess phosphate intake has also been reported as a cause of late-onset hypocalcemia, including in infants fed bovine-milk formula with a high phosphorus concentration [12] and in other forms of phosphate administration, such as with phosphate enema use. Elevated phosphorus results in calcium precipitation, with resultant hypocalcemia and increased PTH. Although excess phosphorus intake from standard infant formula has been described to cause hypocalcemia, it was unlikely the only contributing factor in this case given the use of standard infant formula with age-appropriate volumes.

Klebsiella pneumoniae bacteremia may have also contributed to our patient's hypocalcemia. A review of the adult literature reveals an association between hypocalcemia and sepsis from Gram-negative bacteria. In a study of 60 critically ill patients with bacterial sepsis by Zaloga and Chernow, only those with Gram-negative sepsis developed

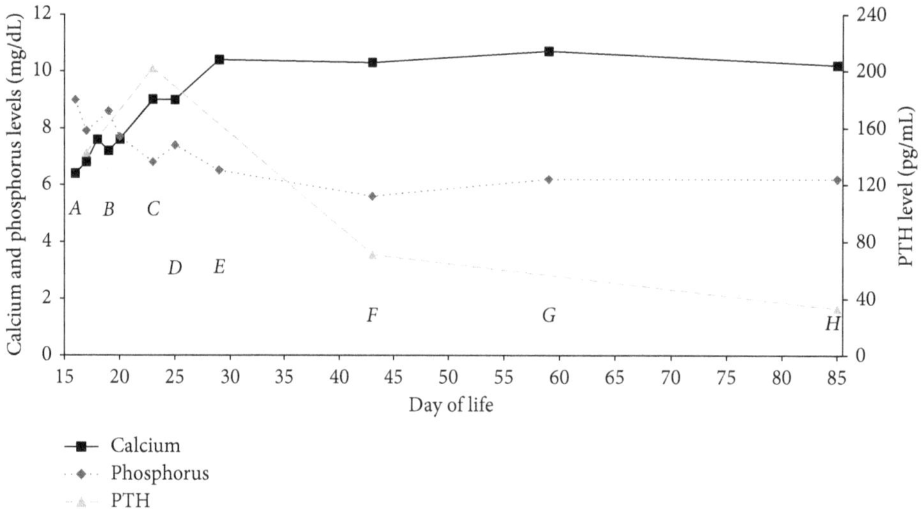

Figure 1: Initiated calcium carbonate at 100 mg/kg/day and low-phosphate formula (A: day of life (DOL) 16) and cholecalciferol at 2000 units/day (B: DOL 19). Weaned calcium carbonate to 75 mg/kg/day (C: DOL 23), 56 mg/kg/day (D: DOL 25), and 26 mg/kg/day (E: DOL 29). Transitioned to regular formula (F: DOL 43). Discontinued calcium carbonate (G: DOL 59). Weaned cholecalciferol to 400 units/day (H: DOL 85).

hypocalcemia, and calcium levels normalized in those patients who survived after treatment for infection [13]. Similarly, a study by Aderka et al. found that 37% of patients with bacteremia had hypocalcemia, compared with 4% of patients without bacteremia; however, the incidence and magnitude of hypocalcemia in Gram-positive and Gram-negative bacteremia were similar. Patients with normocalcemia and hypocalcemia both experienced significant hypoalbuminemia and impaired renal function compared to those without bacteremia [14]. Desai et al. found a strong association between sepsis and hypocalcemia with higher mortality rates in patients with hypocalcemia (44% mortality with hypocalcemia versus 17% without), suggesting calcium dysregulation may be an indicator of disease severity [15]. Although the mechanism for the association between Gram-negative bacteremia and hypocalcemia is not fully elucidated, animal studies have shown that administration of endotoxin induces hypocalcemia most likely by impairing calcium mobilization [16]. Multiple pediatric studies suggest an association between hypocalcemia and sepsis, particularly in neonates; however, these studies largely focused on critically ill children, for whom the etiology of hypocalcemia was often uncertain and potentially multifactorial. These reports did not identify any association between hypocalcemia and bacteremia in children with noncritical illness [17–19].

In addition, immune system activity involves vitamin D metabolism and receptor activation [20]. As such, VDD may increase susceptibility to infection, as suggested by associations of inadequate vitamin "*D*" with confirmed sepsis and worse outcomes compared to controls in an observational study of pediatric patients in an intensive-care unit [21]. VDD in our patient may have placed her at higher risk of developing bacteremia. Further studies are needed to better understand if there is a role for vitamin D supplementation in pediatric infections [22].

4. Conclusions

We describe an infant with late-onset transient neonatal hypocalcemia with VDD who was also found to have Gram-negative bacteremia. The association between hypocalcemia and Gram-negative bacteremia has been reported in adults but has not been described in children outside of the setting of critical illness. Our case suggests that there may be an association between infection and hypocalcemia in a susceptible infant. Based on our case and review of the literature, we suggest that infection be considered as a possible contributing factor in newborns presenting with hypocalcemic seizures.

Abbreviations

AHO: Albright hereditary osteodystrophy
CSF: Cerebrospinal fluid
DOL: Day of life
ED: Emergency department
EKG: Electrocardiogram
IV: Intravenous
PHP: Pseudohypoparathyroidism
PTH: Parathyroid hormone
QTc: Corrected QT
TSH: Thyroid-stimulating hormone
VDD: Vitamin D deficiency.

Authors' Contributions

Dr. Moore performed literature review, drafted the initial manuscript, and reviewed and revised the manuscript. Dr. Lorenz and Dr. Fredette performed literature review and reviewed and revised the manuscript. Dr. Swartz Topor is a guarantor and conceptualized the study, oversaw data collection and interpretation, and critically revised and edited the manuscript. All authors approved the final manuscript as submitted and agree to be accountable for all aspects of the work.

References

[1] T. C. Thomas, J. M. Smith, P. C. White, and S. Adhikari, "Transient neonatal hypocalcemia: presentation and outcomes," *Pediatrics*, vol. 129, no. 6, pp. e1461–e1467, 2012.

[2] L. Rubin, "Disorders of calcium and phosphorus metabolism," in *Avery's Diseases of the Newborn*p. 1189, 7th edition, WB Saunders, Philadelphia, PA, USA, 1998.

[3] W. I. Cho, H. W. Yu, H. R. Chung et al., "Clinical and laboratory characteristics of neonatal hypocalcemia," *Annals of Pediatric Endocrinology and Metabolism*, vol. 20, no. 2, pp. 86–91, 2015.

[4] F. Mimouni and R. C. Tsang, "Neonatal hypocalcemia: to treat or not to treat? (a review)," *Journal of the American College of Nutrition*, vol. 13, no. 5, pp. 408–415, 1994.

[5] B. Yılmaz, C. Aygün, and E. Çetinoğlu, "Vitamin D levels in newborns and association with neonatal hypocalcemia," *The Journal of Maternal-Fetal and Neonatal Medicine*, vol. 31, no. 14, pp. 1889–1893, 2018.

[6] B. W. Jo, Y. J. Shim, J. H. Choi, J. S. Kim, H. J. Lee, and H. S. Kim, "Formula fed twin infants with recurrent hypocalcemic seizures with vitamin D deficient rickets and hyperphosphatemia," *Annals of Pediatric Endocrinology and Metabolism*, vol. 20, no. 2, pp. 102–105, 2015.

[7] C. Pedrosa, N. Ferraria, C. Limbert, and L. Lopes, "Hypovitaminosis D and severe hypocalcaemia: the rebirth of an old disease," *BMJ Case Reports*, vol. 2013, Article ID bcr2012007406, 2013.

[8] E. Basatemur and A. Sutcliffe, "Incidence of hypocalcemic seizures due to vitamin D deficiency in children in the United Kingdom and Ireland," *The Journal of Clinical Endocrinology and Metabolism*, vol. 100, no. 1, pp. E91–E95, 2015.

[9] G. Mantovani, "Pseudohypoparathyroidism: diagnosis and treatment," *The Journal of Clinical Endocrinology and Metabolism*, vol. 96, no. 10, pp. 3020–3030, 2011.

[10] D. S. Rao, A. M. Parfitt, M. Kleerekoper, B. S. Pumo, and B. Frame, "Dissociation between the effects of endogenous parathyroid hormone on adenosine 3′,5′-monophosphate generation and phosphate reabsorption in hypocalcemia due to vitamin D depletion: an acquired disorder resembling pseudohypoparathyroidism type II," *The Journal of Clinical Endocrinology and Metabolism*, vol. 61, no. 2, pp. 285–290, 1985.

[11] M. Minagawa, T. Yasuda, Y. Kobayashi, and H. Niimi, "Transient pseudohypoparathyroidism of the neonate," *European Journal of Endocrinology*, vol. 133, no. 2, pp. 151–155, 1995.

[12] P. S. Venkataraman, R. C. Tsang, F. R. Greer, A. Noguchi, P. Laskarzewski, and J. J. Steichen, "Late infantile tetany and secondary hyperparathyroidism in infants fed humanized cow milk formula," *American Journal of Diseases of Children*, vol. 139, no. 7, pp. 664–668, 1985.

[13] G. P. Zaloga and B. Chernow, "The multifactorial basis for hypocalcemia during sepsis. Studies of the parathyroid hormone-vitamin D axis," *Annals of Internal Medicine*, vol. 107, no. 1, pp. 36–41, 1987.

[14] D. Aderka, D. Schwartz, M. Dan, and Y. Levo, "Bacteremic hypocalcemia. a comparison between the calcium levels of bacteremic and nonbacteremic patients with infection," *Archives of Internal Medicine*, vol. 147, no. 2, pp. 232–236, 1987.

[15] T. K. Desai, R. W. Carlson, and M. A. Geheb, "Prevalence and clinical implications of hypocalcemia in acutely III patients in a medical intensive care setting," *The American Journal of Medicine*, vol. 84, no. 2, pp. 209–214, 1988.

[16] G. P. Zaloga, D. Malcolm, B. Chernow, and J. Holaday, "Endotoxin-induced hypocalcemia results in defective calcium mobilization in rats," *Circulatory Shock*, vol. 24, no. 2, pp. 143–148, 1988.

[17] A. Kelly and M. A. Levine, "Hypocalcemia in the critically ill patient," *Journal of Intensive Care Medicine*, vol. 28, no. 3, pp. 166–177, 2013.

[18] N. Cardenas-Rivero, B. Chernow, M. A. Stoiko, S. R. Nussbaum, and I. D. Todres, "Hypocalcemia in critically ill children," *The Journal of Pediatrics*, vol. 114, no. 6, pp. 946–951, 1989.

[19] C. R. B. Dias, H. P. Leite, P. C. K. Nogueira, and W. Brunow de Carvalho, "Ionized hypocalcemia is an early event and is associated with organ dysfunction in children admitted to the intensive care unit," *Journal of Critical Care*, vol. 28, no. 5, pp. 810–815, 2013.

[20] R. Bouillon, C. Marcocci, G. Carmeliet et al., "Skeletal and extraskeletal actions of vitamin D: current evidence and outstanding questions," *Endocrine Reviews*, vol. 40, no. 4, pp. 1109–1151, 2019.

[21] C. Onwuneme, A. Carroll, D. Doherty et al., "Inadequate vitamin D levels are associated with culture positive sepsis and poor outcomes in paediatric intensive care," *Acta Paediatrica*, vol. 104, no. 10, pp. e433–e438, 2015.

[22] R. R. Das, M. Singh, and S. S. Naik, "Vitamin D as an adjunct to antibiotics for the treatment of acute childhood pneumonia," *Cochrane Database of Systematic Reviews*, vol. 7, no. 7, Article ID CD011597, 2018.

45

Delayed Diagnosis, Difficult Decisions: Novel Gene Deletion Causing X-Linked Hypophosphatemia in a Middle-Aged Man with Achondroplastic Features and Tertiary Hyperparathyroidism

Yun Ann Chin[1] **Yi Zhao**[2] **Gerald Tay**[3] **Weiying Sim**[2] **Chun Yuen Chow**[4] **and Manju Chandran**[5]

[1]*Department of Endocrinology, Singapore General Hospital, Singapore*
[2]*Department of Clinical Translational Research, Singapore General Hospital, Singapore*
[3]*Department of Head and Neck Surgery, Division of Surgery and Surgical Oncology, Singapore General Hospital, Singapore*
[4]*Department of Pathology, Singapore General Hospital, Singapore*
[5]*Complicated Metabolic Bone Disorders Clinic, Osteoporosis and Bone Metabolism Unit, Department of Endocrinology, Singapore General Hospital, Singapore*

Correspondence should be addressed to Manju Chandran; manju.chandran@singhealth.com.sg

Academic Editor: Michaï¿½l R. Laurent

X-linked hypophosphatemia (XLH) is the most prevalent form of hereditary hypophosphatemic rickets associated with phosphate wasting. However, its diagnosis is often missed, resulting in patients presenting late in the course of the disease when complications such as tertiary hyperparathyroidism and renal failure have already set in. Phosphate and calcitriol replacement, both of which have undesirable consequences of their own, have historically been the main stay of therapy. We describe the case of a 57-year-old gentleman with tertiary hyperparathyroidism, who was mislabelled as having achondroplasia for many years before we made a diagnosis of XLH in him. His XLH was found to be due to a hereto unreported deletion of entire exon 14 with partial deletions of introns 13 and 14 of the PHEX gene. Perioperative management in him was fraught with surgical and medical difficulties including an operation that was technically complicated due to his multiple anatomical deformities. Our case also highlights the critical importance of timely recognition and accurate diagnosis of XLH, as well as the long-term multidisciplinary management that is needed for this disorder.

1. Introduction

X-linked hypophosphatemic (XLH) rickets is caused by inactivating mutations of the PHEX (phosphate regulating with homologies to endopeptidases on the X chromosome) gene. Consequently, the circulating humoral phosphaturic factor—fibroblast growth factor 23 (FGF23)—becomes elevated. The resultant hypophosphatemia leads to rickets with skeletal deformities, reduced linear growth, and metabolic bone abnormalities. More than 588 different mutations have been listed in the Human Gene Mutation Database (HGMD, http://www.hgmd.cf.ac.uk/ac/index.php, accessed on January 22, 2021). Despite XLH being the most common form of hereditary renal phosphate-wasting disorder, with an incidence of 1 in 20,000 individuals [1], it is very often under- or misdiagnosed. Though burosumab, a monoclonal antibody directed against FGF23, has recently become available in some parts of the world for the treatment of XLH [2], historically, patients with this disorder have been treated with phosphate and calcitriol replacement—a therapy with several undesirable consequences. Here, we describe the case of a patient with XLH who was misdiagnosed for years as having achondroplasia. His XLH was secondary to a novel, hereto unreported, complete deletion of entire exon 14 and partial deletions of intronic regions 13 and 14 of the PHEX gene. His case was complicated by the severe restrictive anatomical deformities he had, by the development of tertiary hyperparathyroidism and renal failure, all of which necessitated a complex decision-making process and made for a technically challenging parathyroidectomy and complicated postoperative course.

2. Case Presentation

The patient is a 57-year-old Chinese gentleman seen by us in July 2019. He had valgus deformity of bilateral lower limbs requiring bilateral osteotomy of the tibiae and fibulae and corrective osteotomy of the right femur all before he was 24 years old. He also had lumbar spine stenosis that necessitated decompressive spine laminectomy at the age of 51 years. He had decay of multiple teeth since he was young and had also been diagnosed as having sensorineural hearing loss and enthesopathy. On review of his medical records, it was apparent that he had hypophosphatemia since young, and he had been intermittently prescribed oral phosphate and calcitriol. His compliance to oral phosphate was quite limited due to frequent diarrhoea while on it. Compliance to calcitriol also had not been optimal. Due to his short stature of 127 cm and deformed limbs (Figure 1), he had been labelled as having achondroplasia all through his younger years.

There had been no evaluation performed for the aetiology of hypophosphatemia until 6 years ago when he presented initially to our department, whereupon significant phosphaturia was demonstrated with low maximum tubular capacity of phosphate (TmP) per unit volume of glomerular filtrate (TmP/GFR) of 0.24 mmol/L (0.85–1.35) calculated using the nomogram of Walton and Bijvoet [3]. He did not have hypercalciuria, albuminuria, uricosuria, or aminoaciduria. A detailed family history obtained at that time revealed that his parents were of nonconsanguineous marriage, of normal height, and with no obviously stated history of hypophosphatemia. There was a history of short stature and hypophosphatemia in his elder brother (deceased at the age of 50 years due to unknown reasons) and in a sister. This sister had a parathyroidectomy done at the age of 53 years for tertiary hyperparathyroidism. Her operative report stated that just a single adenoma was removed in her. Given this strong family history (Figure 2), the strong possibility that our patient was suffering from a hereditary hypophosphatemic disorder was raised.

Unfortunately, he defaulted subsequent follow-up and did not present to the metabolic bone clinic in the endocrine department till 6 years later at the age of 57 in July 2019. Over the last 6 years, he had developed hypercalcemia with progressively increasing serum intact parathyroid hormone (iPTH) and worsening renal function. He was still intermittently taking oral phosphate and calcitriol. His laboratory values are shown in Table 1. The phosphaturia demonstrated earlier was found to be still present. Serum FGF23 level measured by the immunometric enzyme assay was elevated at 371 RU/ml (≤180 RU/ml).

Due to the severe restrictions in positioning him on the scan table secondary to his anatomical deformities, only a dual-energy X-ray absorptiometry (DXA) scan of the 1/3rd radius could be done, and this showed extremely low BMD with a T-score of −5.2 (ethnic and gender-specific reference). Based on his family history, long-standing hypophosphatemia and skeletal deformities since childhood, and his current clinical, biochemical, and radiological characteristics, the working diagnosis at this point was that he had a hereditary phosphaturic, hypophosphatemic disorder mediated by FGF23 and complicated by tertiary hyperparathyroidism and renal impairment. Whilst admitted for his workup, he had a fall and sustained a low-trauma left fibular fracture. In view of his likely tertiary hyperparathyroidism, compromised skeletal health, and worsening renal impairment, it was decided that the best option for him would be parathyroidectomy. Parathyroid imaging is usually unnecessary in tertiary hyperparathyroidism associated with long-standing renal failure since bilateral neck exploration and total parathyroidectomy with autotransplantation are the recommended operative procedures. The postoperative course after this type of surgery is usually complicated by the development of hypocalcemia that is often accompanied by hypophosphatemia and hypomagnesemia, i.e., hungry bone syndrome (HBS). The latter would be a devastating complication that our patient could ill-afford given his underlying phosphate-losing disorder. As minimally invasive of a surgery as possible was also preferable in him given his severe anatomical deformities that included an extremely short neck and restricted neck movements. Because of these two reasons, we decided to have the patient undergo parathyroid imaging in the hope that if a circumspect parathyroid adenoma could be identified, this could just be removed as had been possible in his sister. However, though parathyroid ultrasound scan showed a hypoechoic nodule at the posterior aspect of the middle third of the right thyroid lobe, the concomitant Tc-99m sestamibi scan did not reveal any hyperfunctioning parathyroid tissue. In view of the discordant imaging, we proceeded with the 4D computed tomography (4D CT) scan of the neck. It showed 3 indeterminate nodules in the visceral space, but none of them demonstrated the classic definite hypervascular pattern of enhancement classically seen with parathyroid adenomas on 4D CT imaging.

Extensive multidisciplinary discussions were held between the metabolic bone specialist, radiologist, and the head and neck surgeons on the best surgical approach and perioperative management for the patient.

He underwent bilateral neck exploration in July 2020. The operation was technically difficult with limited access due to the inability to extend the patient's rigid neck (Figure 3). The metabolic bone specialist was also in attendance in the operating room to help with intraoperative decisions.

During the surgery that lasted 3 hours, three grossly enlarged and abnormal parathyroid glands were identified and removed. After a discussion between the metabolic bone specialist and the surgeon, it was decided that a relatively normal-looking gland would be left in situ to minimize the risk of postoperative hypocalcemia. An intraoperative iPTH assay did show a decrease from a baseline value of 275 pmol/

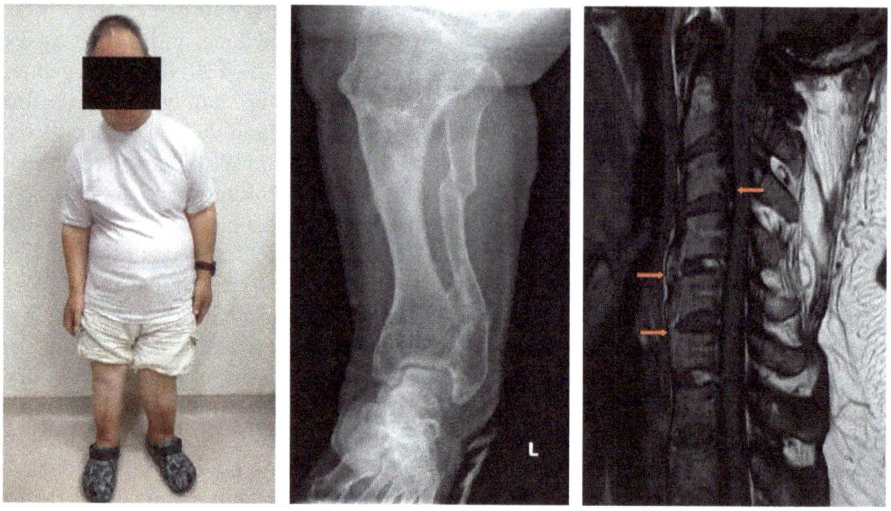

(a) (b) (c)

Figure 1: (a) Short stature, (b) deformities of the lower limb with recent fibular fracture, and (c) MRI cervical spine showing ossification of the anterior longitudinal ligament from C3 to C6 and posterior longitudinal ligaments from C2 to C4 (arrows).

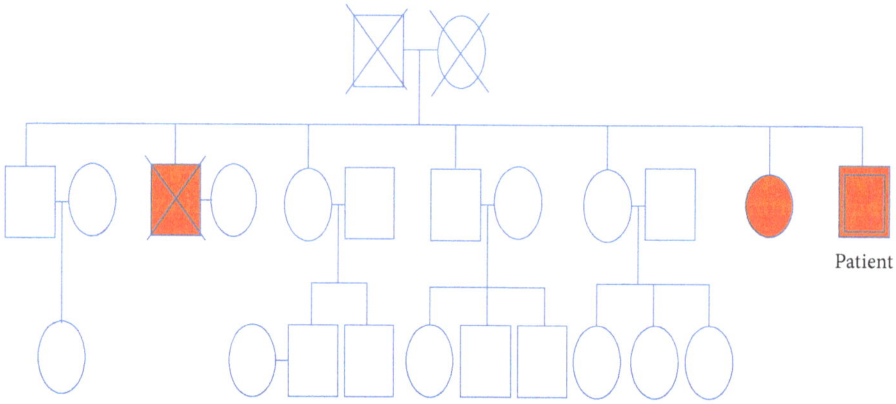

Figure 2: Family pedigree of the patient showing affected individuals.

Table 1: Laboratory values over the years.

	July 2014 (initial consultation with endocrinology)	July 2019 (re-referral to endocrinology)	July 2020 (immediately prior to parathyroidectomy)	Normal range (units)
Serum calcium	2.33	2.67	2.67	2.09–2.46 mmol/L
Serum phosphate	0.39	0.96	1.40	0.94–1.50 mmol/L
Serum iPTH	41.1	117	101	0.9–6.2 pmol/L
Serum creatinine	91	148	180	54–101 umol/L
Serum alkaline phosphatase	140	179	184	9–99 U/L
Serum 1,25-dihydroxyvitamin D	43		30	18–64 pg/ml
Serum 25-hydroxyvitamin D	33.4	11.0	17.5	>30 ng/ml
Serum fibroblast growth factor 23 (FGF23)			371	≤180 RU/ml
24-hour urinary calcium	0.99	0.65		0.82–6.74 mmol/day

L to a level of 154 pmol/l at 10 min. This less than 50% drop at 10 minutes was expected given his significant underlying renal dysfunction. Despite the attempts intraoperatively to minimize it, he did develop HBS postoperatively. He needed continuous intravenous calcium gluconate infusion for 4 days with concurrent high dose of oral calcium carbonate (CaCo3) and calcitriol (Figure 4). His postoperative stay was complicated by respiratory failure and acute on chronic renal failure. He was discharged eventually after 19 days of hospitalisation.

Histology from the parathyroidectomy showed parathyroid hyperplasia in all resected specimens (Figure 5).

For genetic analysis, genomic DNA was extracted from whole EDTA blood via an automated approach using

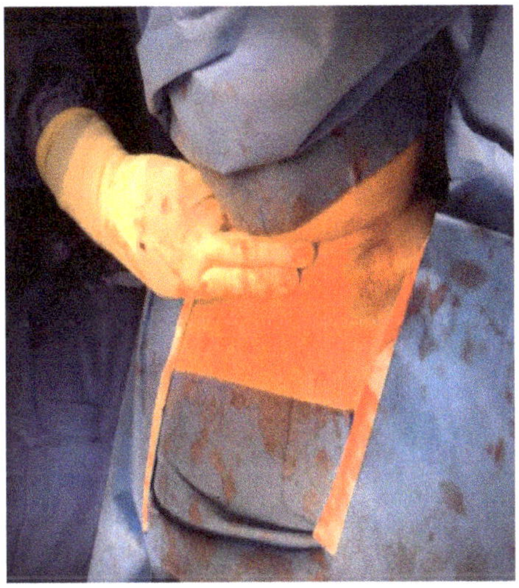

FIGURE 3: The patient's short neck as indicated by the span of <2 fingerbreadths.

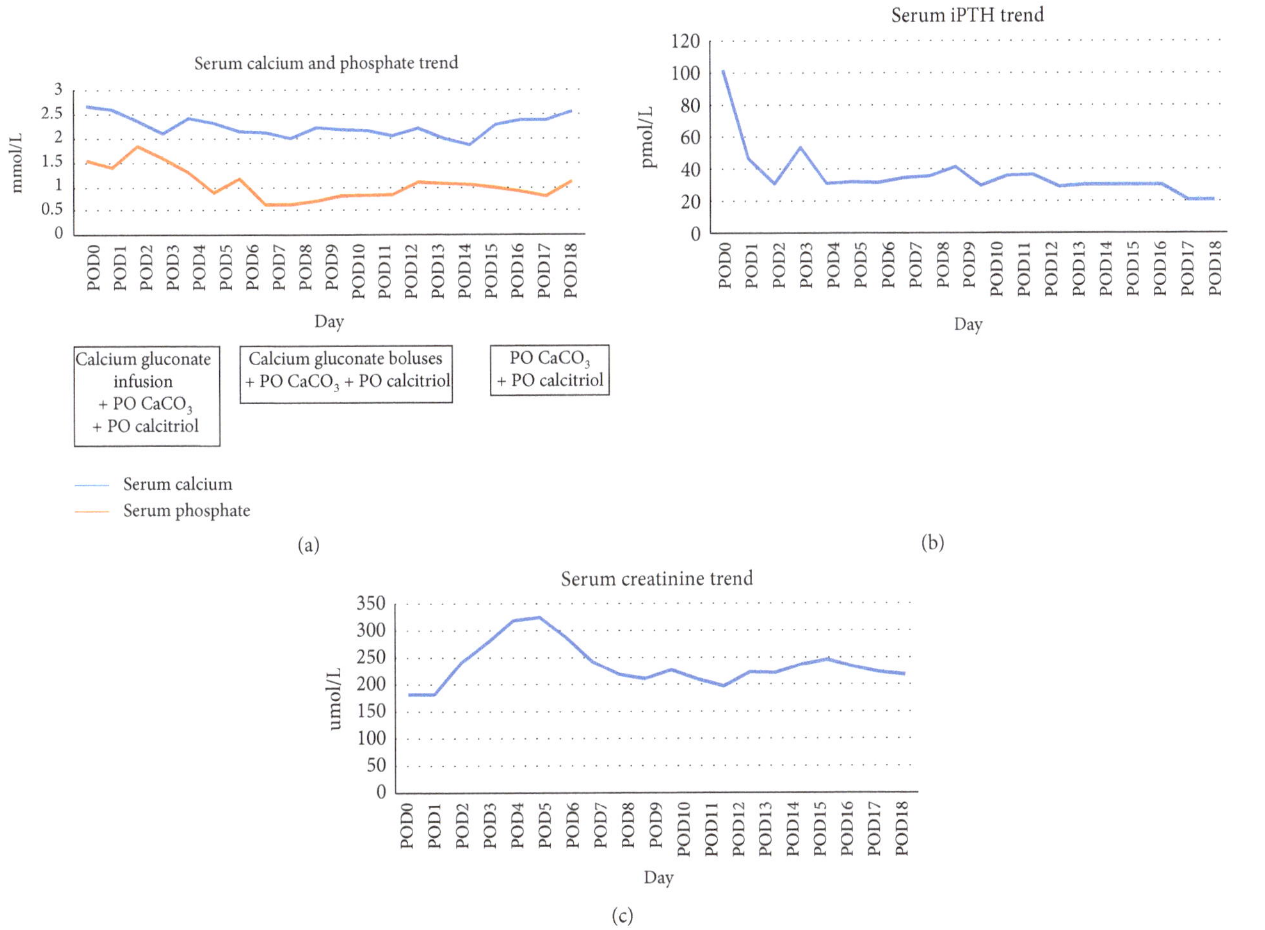

FIGURE 4: Laboratory trend after parathyroidectomy. (a) Serum calcium and phosphate trend. (b) Serum iPTH trend. (c) Serum creatinine trend.

Maxwell® 16 Blood DNA Purification Kit (Promega, USA) in accordance to the manufacturer's protocol. The exons of the PHEX gene of interest were amplified by polymerase chain reaction (PCR) using specific design primers and DNA polymerase kit (Thermo Scientific) under the conditions as illustrated in Table 2. The PCR mix had a total volume of 25 ul, containing 1x Taq PCR buffer, 20 ng of genomic DNA, 0.4 uM of each specific forward and reverse primer, 8% DMSO, and 0.2 mM dNTP, as well as 1.5 mM MgCl. PCR products were purified using Exonuclease I and FastAP

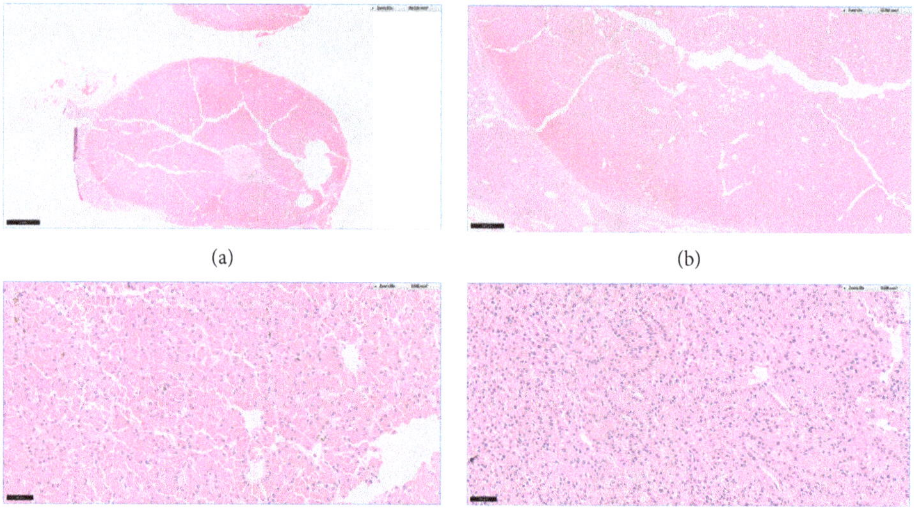

(a) (b) (c) (d)

Figure 5: Section showing nodular proliferation of chief cells and oxyphilic cells. The component cells show a palisaded arrangement around blood vessels. (a) Low power. (b) Medium power. (c) High power (H&E, ×20): oxyphilic cells show round-to-ovoid nuclei with abundant granular eosinophilic cytoplasm. (d) Chief cells (H&E, ×20): chief cells show round nuclei and amphophilic cytoplasm. No nuclear pleomorphism or increased mitotic activity is seen.

Table 2: Genomic DNA isolation and mutation screening, DNA extraction, and amplification of PHEX exons by PCR.

PCR thermocycling conditions for amplifying the PHEX gene		Forward and reverse primer sequences for screening exon 14 [4]	
Steps	Conditions		
Initial denaturation	95°C for 3 minutes	Forward primer	CAACA AGTAGGTGAC TGTCGAGCC (NG_007563.2, 144846–144869)
35 cycles		Reverse primer	GCTAAG CTATGAGGAC ACAAAGGC (NG_007563.2, 147203–147226)
Denaturation	95°C for 30 seconds		
*Annealing	60°C for 45 seconds		
Extension	72°C for 60 seconds		
Final extension	72°C for 10 minutes		
Hold	4°C		

*Annealing temperature is specific to each primer set; 60°C for screening exon 14 of PHEX.

Alkaline Phosphatase (Thermo Scientific) according to the manufacturer's protocol. These purified PCR products were then ready to be sequenced using BigDye® Direct Sanger Cycle Sequencing Kit (Applied Biosystems, Foster City, Calif., USA) with post-cleanup. The specific sequences were obtained through the Sanger sequencing approach using the ABI PRISM 3500 genetic analyser (Applied Biosystems, Foster City, Calif., USA) and compared against the NCBI Nucleotide Bank (NCBI reference sequence: NG_007563.2, 144846–144869) using sequence alignment. To confirm the PCR conditions in amplifying the interests, a normal healthy individual was included in the screening. Primers were redesigned in the case of no amplification of interest. Under the same PCR conditions, for PHEX exon 14, PCR product was present in the healthy individual but not in the patient. Therefore, the screening region revolving PHEX exon 14 was expanded. The primers for PHEX exon 14 were redesigned at a position further upstream and downstream of PHEX IVS 13 and 14 regions. The final sequences of the designed primers to screen for PHEX exon 14 are shown in Table 2. A novel, previously unreported pathogenic deletion of entire exon 14 (104 bp) as well as partial deletions of IVS13 and IVS14 of the PHEX gene was observed, confirming XLH (Figure 6).

FGFR3 gene analysis did not show any mutation, indicating that he had no genetic mutation suggestive of achondroplasia.

After discharge, he continued to require $CaCO_3$ and calcitriol supplementation to maintain serum calcium at low-normal levels. Phosphate supplementation had to be restarted. His kidney function stabilised. Though his serum iPTH remains elevated at 46.4 pmol/l, it has improved significantly from his baseline levels.

3. Discussion

The PHEX gene, which is located on X chromosome Xp22.1, is composed of 22 exons spanning 243 kb and encodes for

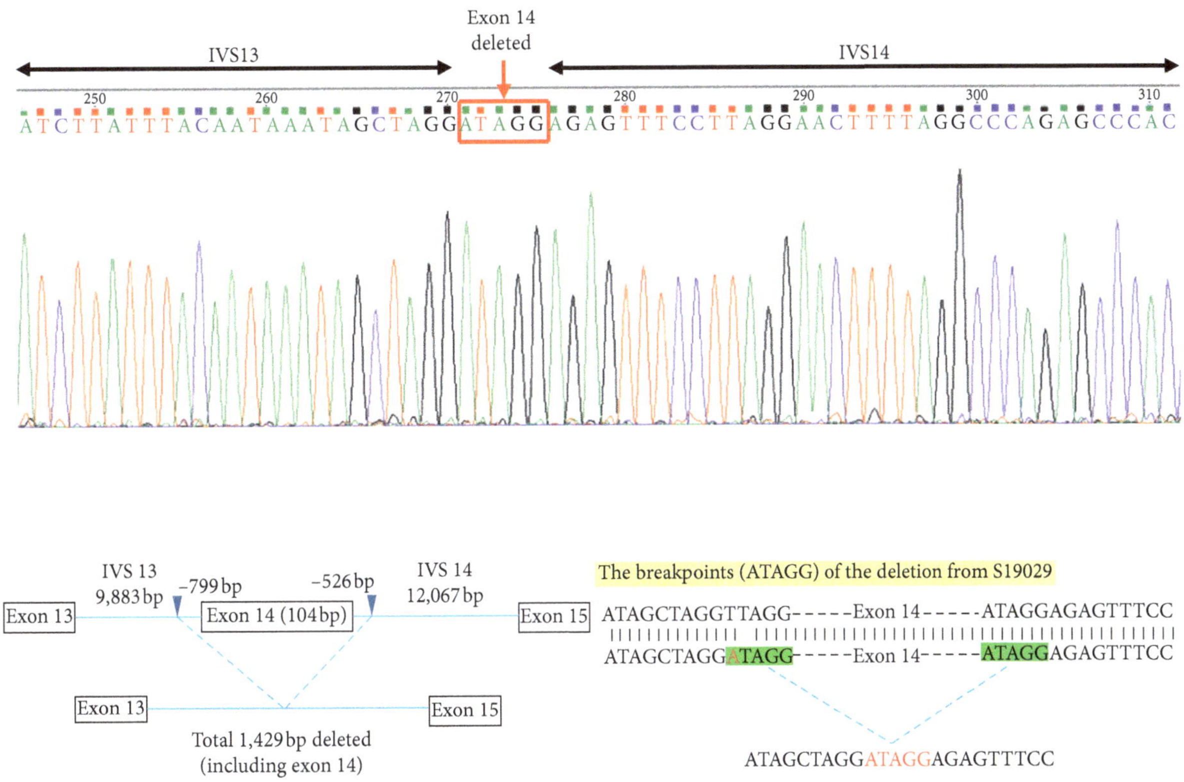

Figure 6: PHEX gene deletion around exon 14 and the breakpoint (ATAGG) of the deletion.

749 amino acid proteins [5]. PHEX mutations can be in the form of nonsense, deletions, duplications, insertions, deletional insertions, splice site, and missense mutations [6, 7]. In our patient, a single nucleotide substitute at intron 13 of the PHEX gene (position IVS13, c.1483-804T >A) was seen. The variant created an upstream breakpoint ATAGG, the pentanucleotide then likely interacted with the same pentanucleotide ATAGG downstream at IVS 14, c.1586 + 521 that then elicited abnormal splicing causing a long nucleotide deletion. This deletion involved 1,429 bp including entire exon 14 (104 bp) as well as part of IVS13 and IVS14 (Figure 5). This deletion resulted in amino acid coding frameshift starting from exon 15. This deletion has not been reported previously.

XLH usually presents in infancy or early childhood. Relative unawareness of the disease amongst physicians and orthopaedic surgeons has resulted in patients often being misdiagnosed as having achondroplasia, an autosomal dominant form of short-limbed dwarfism due to mutations of the FGFR3 gene. Other causes of hereditary hypophosphatemia such as autosomal dominant hypophosphatemia, hypophosphatemic rickets with hypercalciuria, Dent's disease, and Fanconi's syndrome were obviously unlikely in our patient with his genetic and clinical features that were typical of XLH [8].

Management of XLH has traditionally included phosphate and calcitriol replacement [9]. Diarrhoea is a common limiting factor to adequate phosphate replacement and compliance, as was evident in our patient's case. Phosphate replacement in XLH is associated with increases in PTH levels. It is postulated that high oral phosphate doses lower ionised calcium thereby stimulating PTH release through activation of the parathyroid gland calcium-sensing receptor [10, 11]. However, hyperparathyroidism is sometimes seen even before the onset of medical therapy. The pathophysiologic mechanism behind this occurrence is still poorly understood. It is also speculated that hyperparathyroidism in untreated or partially treated XLH could be a secondary event that compensates for impaired skeletal calcium mobilization, a probable feature of the underlying osteomalacia [12]. Elevated levels of FGF23 have also been linked to hyperparathyroidism in patients with XLH [13]. These two phenomena could explain the hyperparathyroidism that was seen in our patient who could be only considered as partially replaced with phosphate since he was noncompliant with his supplements. The insufficient and erratic calcitriol replacement that he was on also likely contributed to inadequate suppression of PTH and secondary hyperparathyroidism with subsequent quasi-autonomous functioning of the parathyroid glands, i.e., tertiary hyperparathyroidism [14].

The calcimimetic cinacalcet may have a beneficial role in XLH, and some reports have shown it to normalize calcium and to reduce PTH concentrations in patients with XLH [15, 16] with possible resultant amelioration of PTH-induced phosphaturia. Long-term cinacalcet is a costly proposition, and hence, our patient declined it. In addition, this is only a temporizing measure, and hypercalcemia and hypophosphatemia usually recur when it is stopped. Therefore, this was not really a viable option for our patient in whom the deleterious effects of tertiary hyperparathyroidism were already manifest with bone loss, fractures, and renal failure and in whom surgery was the only definitive therapy that could be offered.

The paradigm of treatment of XLH will likely undergo a dramatic shift with the widespread use of burosumab [2]. However, no long-term data currently exist regarding the effect of burosumab on hyperparathyroidism. Burosumab is not currently available or approved in Singapore, and therefore, this was not a therapeutic option in our patient.

Parathyroidectomy in patients with XLH is technically challenging. The operative field may be extremely limited due to anatomical deformities. Rigidity of the cervical spine caused by enthesopathy with resultant inability to extend the neck can make intubation and exploration of the thyroid bed difficult. This was the case with our patient too. Parathyroidectomy in XLH is associated with a high rate of recurrence or persistence of tertiary hyperparathyroidism postoperatively [17], and it is likely that many patients may need a repeat surgery over their lifetimes.

4. Conclusion

Our patient, who has XLH due to a novel, hereto unreported gene deletion, is an unfortunate example of how a diagnosis of a devastating phosphate-wasting disorder is often missed resulting in a presentation of the disease when it is already beset with complications. The pathogenesis of relentless continued elevations of PTH in this disorder remains largely unknown. Surgery for secondary and tertiary hyperparathyroidism in patients with skeletal, cartilage, and joint sequelae of this disease remains one of the most challenging operations for the head and neck surgeon. The management of metabolic derangements including that of hypocalcemia after parathyroidectomy in these patients with ongoing concurrent phosphate losses from the underlying disorder needs to be carefully planned and thought out. This is one situation where a close synergy between the metabolic bone specialist and the surgeon is imperative.

Consent was obtained from the patient for both obtaining photographs as well as for the case write-up.

Authors' Contributions

All authors contributed equally to the manuscript.

References

[1] S. S. Beck-Nielsen, B. Brock-Jacobsen, J. Gram, K. Brixen, and T. K. Jensen, "Incidence and prevalence of nutritional and hereditary rickets in southern Denmark," *European Journal of Endocrinology*, vol. 160, no. 3, pp. 491–497, 2009.

[2] S. Fukumoto, "FGF23-related hypophosphatemic rickets/osteomalacia: diagnosis and new treatment," *Journal of Molecular Endocrinology*, vol. 66, no. 2, pp. R57–R65, 2020.

[3] R. J. Walton and O. L. M. Bijvoet, "Nomogram for derivation of renal threshold phosphate concentration," *The Lancet*, vol. 306, no. 7929, pp. 309-310, 1975.

[4] P. Rowe, C. L. Oudet, F. Francis, C. Sinding, S. Pannetier et al., "Distribution of mutations in the PEX gene in families with X-linked hypophosphataemic rickets (HYP)," *Human Molecular Genetics*, vol. 6, no. 4, pp. 539–549, 1997.

[5] L. D. Quarles, "FGF23, PHEX, and MEPE regulation of phosphate homeostasis and skeletal mineralization," *American Journal of Physiology-Endocrinology and Metabolism*, vol. 285, no. 1, pp. E1–E9, 2003.

[6] C. Zhang, Z. Zhao, Y. Sun et al., "Clinical and genetic analysis in a large Chinese Cohort of patients with X-linked hypophosphatemia," *Bone*, vol. 121, pp. 212–220, 2019.

[7] S. Acar, H. A. BinEssa, K. Demir et al., "Clinical and genetic characteristic of 15 families with hereditary hypophosphatemia: novel mutations in PHEX and SLC34A3," *PLoS One*, vol. 13, no. 3, p. e0193388, 2018.

[8] Y. Kinoshita and S. Fukumoto, "X-linked hypophosphatemia and FGF23-related hypophosphatemic diseases: prospect for new treatment," *Endocrine Reviews*, vol. 39, no. 3, pp. 274–291, 2018.

[9] D. Haffner, F. Emma, D. M. Eastwood et al., "Clinical practice recommendations for the diagnosis and management of X-linked hypophosphataemia," *Nature Reviews Nephrology*, vol. 15, no. 7, pp. 435–455, 2019.

[10] Y. Almaden, A. Hernandez, V. Torregrosa et al., "High phosphate level directly stimulates parathyroid hormone secretion and synthesis by human parathyroid tissue in vitro," *Journal of the American Society of Nephrology: JASN*, vol. 9, no. 10, pp. 1845–1852, 1998.

[11] C. R. McHenry, K. Mostafavi, and T. A. Murphy, "Tertiary hyperparathyroidism attributable to long-term oral phosphate therapy," *Endocrine Practice*, vol. 12, no. 3, pp. 294–298, 2006.

[12] T. O. Carpenter, M. A. Mitnick, A. Ellison, C. Smith, and K. L. Insogna, "Nocturnal hyperparathyroidism: a frequent feature of X-linked hypophosphatemia," *The Journal of Clinical Endocrinology & Metabolism*, vol. 78, no. 6, pp. 1378–1383, 1994.

[13] T. O. Carpenter, K. L. Insogna, J. H. Zhang et al., "Circulating levels of soluble klotho and FGF23 in X-linked hypophosphatemia: circadian variance, effects of treatment, and relationship to parathyroid status," *The Journal of Clinical Endocrinology & Metabolism*, vol. 95, no. 11, pp. E352–E357, 2010.

[14] R. M. Savio, J. E. Gosnell, S. Posen, T. S. Reeve, and L. W. Delbridge, "Parathyroidectomy for tertiary hyperparathyroidism associated with X-linked dominant hypophosphatemic rickets," *Archives of Surgery*, vol. 139, no. 2, pp. 218–222, 2004.

[15] M. Yavropoulou, K. Kotsa, A. Gotzamani Psarrakou et al., "Cinacalcet in hyperparathyroidism secondary to X-linked hypophosphatemic rickets: case report and brief literature review," *Hormones*, vol. 9, no. 3, pp. 274–278, 2010.

[16] H. Raeder, N. Shaw, C. Netelenbos, and R. Bjerknes, "A case of X-linked hypophosphatemic rickets: complications and the therapeutic use of cinacalcet," *European Journal of Endocrinology*, vol. 159, no. Suppl 1, pp. S101–S105, 2008.

[17] S. DeLacey, Z. Liu, A. Broyles et al., "Hyperparathyroidism and parathyroidectomy in X-linked hypophosphatemia patients," *Bone*, vol. 127, pp. 386–392, 2019.

Permissions

All chapters in this book were first published by Hindawi Publishing Corporation; hereby published with permission under the Creative Commons Attribution License or equivalent. Every chapter published in this book has been scrutinized by our experts. Their significance has been extensively debated. The topics covered herein carry significant findings which will fuel the growth of the discipline. They may even be implemented as practical applications or may be referred to as a beginning point for another development.

The contributors of this book come from diverse backgrounds, making this book a truly international effort. This book will bring forth new frontiers with its revolutionizing research information and detailed analysis of the nascent developments around the world.

We would like to thank all the contributing authors for lending their expertise to make the book truly unique. They have played a crucial role in the development of this book. Without their invaluable contributions this book wouldn't have been possible. They have made vital efforts to compile up to date information on the varied aspects of this subject to make this book a valuable addition to the collection of many professionals and students.

This book was conceptualized with the vision of imparting up-to-date information and advanced data in this field. To ensure the same, a matchless editorial board was set up. Every individual on the board went through rigorous rounds of assessment to prove their worth. After which they invested a large part of their time researching and compiling the most relevant data for our readers.

The editorial board has been involved in producing this book since its inception. They have spent rigorous hours researching and exploring the diverse topics which have resulted in the successful publishing of this book. They have passed on their knowledge of decades through this book. To expedite this challenging task, the publisher supported the team at every step. A small team of assistant editors was also appointed to further simplify the editing procedure and attain best results for the readers.

Apart from the editorial board, the designing team has also invested a significant amount of their time in understanding the subject and creating the most relevant covers. They scrutinized every image to scout for the most suitable representation of the subject and create an appropriate cover for the book.

The publishing team has been an ardent support to the editorial, designing and production team. Their endless efforts to recruit the best for this project, has resulted in the accomplishment of this book. They are a veteran in the field of academics and their pool of knowledge is as vast as their experience in printing. Their expertise and guidance has proved useful at every step. Their uncompromising quality standards have made this book an exceptional effort. Their encouragement from time to time has been an inspiration for everyone.

The publisher and the editorial board hope that this book will prove to be a valuable piece of knowledge for researchers, students, practitioners and scholars across the globe.

List of Contributors

Juan M. Colazo
Department of Biomedical Engineering, Vanderbilt University, Nashville, TN, USA
Medical Scientist Training Program, Vanderbilt University School of Medicine, Nashville, TN, USA

Seth A. Reasoner
Medical Scientist Training Program, Vanderbilt University School of Medicine, Nashville, TN, USA
Department of Pathology, Microbiology and Immunology, Vanderbilt University Medical Center, Nashville, TN, USA

Ginger Holt
Department of Orthopedics, Vanderbilt University Medical Center, Nashville, TN, USA

Marie C. M. Faugere
Division of Nephrology, Bone and Mineral Metabolism, University of Kentucky, Albert B. Chandler Medical Center, Lexington, KY, USA

Kathryn M. Dahir
Division of Diabetes, Endocrinology and Metabolism, Vanderbilt University Medical Center, Nashville, TN, USA

Ravali Nallu, Parvathy Madhavan and Pooja Luthra
Department of Medicine, Division of Endocrinology and Metabolism, University of Connecticut, School of Medicine, Farmington, CT, USA

Lisa Chirch
Department of Medicine, Division of Infectious Diseases, University of Connecticut, School of Medicine, Farmington, CT, USA

Aurore Catteau
Laboratoire de biochimie, Institut de Biologie, CHU de Nantes, Nantes, France

Kalyane Bach-Ngohou, Justine Blin and Damien Masson
Laboratoire de biochimie, Institut de Biologie, CHU de Nantes, Nantes, France
Faculté de médecine, Université de Nantes, Nantes, France

Paul Barrière and Thomas Fréour
Faculté de médecine, Université de Nantes, Nantes, France
Service de médecine et biologie du développement et de la reproduction, CHU de Nantes, Nantes, France

Davida A. Robinson, Margaret Kemeny, Juliana E. Muchinyi, Hanna Jang and Nilda I. Montes
Icahn School of Medicine at Mount Sinai, Queens Hospital Center, Department of Surgery, 82-68 164th Street, New York, NY 11432, USA

Madiha Yasin, Radhika Jaiswal, Amanda Carter and Michal-Ann Derezil
Zucker School of Medicine at Hofstra and Northwell, Northwell Health-North Shore University Hospital, Department of Medicine, Division of Endocrinology, 500 Hofstra University Hempstead, New York, NY 11549, USA

Sandeep Tuli
Ichahn School of Medicine at Mount Sinai- Queens Hospital Center, Department of Radiology, 82-68 164th Street, New York, NewYork 11432, USA

David Reich
Ichahn School of Medicine at Mount Sinai- Queens Hospital Center, Department of Medicine, Division of Endocrinology, 82-68 164th Street, New York, New York 11432, USA

Ambreen Sonawalla
Pediatric Residency Program, University of Arkansas for Medical Sciences, Little Rock, AR, USA

Vildan Tas
Department of Pediatrics, University of Arkansas for Medical Sciences, Little Rock, AR, USA

Manish Raisingani and Emir Tas
Department of Pediatrics, Division of Endocrinology and Diabetes, University of Arkansas forMedical Sciences, Little Rock, AR, USA

Claudia Ramirez-Rentería and Moises Mercado
Endocrinology Service, UIM Enfermedades Endocrinas, Hospital de Especialidades, Centro M´edico Nacional, S.XXI, Instituto Mexicano del Seguro Social, Av Cuauhtemoc 330, Col. Doctores, CP 06720, Mexico City, Mexico
UIM Enfermedades Endocrinas, Hospital de Especialidades, 23 Centro M´edico Nacional, S.XXI, Instituto Mexicano del Seguro Social, Mexico City, Mexico

Ana-Laura Espinosa-de-Los-Monteros and Etual Espinosa-Cardenas
Endocrinology Service, UIM Enfermedades Endocrinas, Hospital de Especialidades, Centro M´edico Nacional, S.XXI, Instituto Mexicano del Seguro Social, Av Cuauhtemoc 330, Col. Doctores, CP 06720, Mexico City, Mexico

Daniel Marrero-Rodriguez
UIM Enfermedades Endocrinas, Hospital de Especialidades, 23 Centro M´edico Nacional, S.XXI, Instituto Mexicano del Seguro Social, Mexico City, Mexico
Molecular Biomedicine Department, Center for Research and Advanced Studies, Instituto Polit´ecnico Nacional, Av Cuauhtemoc 330, Col. Doctores, CP 06720, Mexico City, Mexico

Guillermo Castellanos and Rocio Arreola-Rosales
Pathology Department, Hospital de Especialidades, Centro M´edico Nacional, S.XXI, Instituto Mexicano del Seguro Social, City. Av Cuauhtemoc 330, Col. Doctores, CP 06720, Mexico City, Mexico

Guillermo Montoya-Martinez
Urology Department, Hospital de Especialidades, Centro M´edico Nacional, S.XXI, Instituto Mexicano del Seguro Social, Av Cuauht´emoc 330, Col. Doctores, CP 06720, Mexico City, Mexico

Keiko Taniguchi-Ponciano
Laboratorio de Neuroendocrinolog´ıa Comparada, Departamento de Ecolog´ıa y Recursos Naturales, Biolog´ıa, Facultad de Ciencias, Universidad Nacional Aut´onoma de M´exico, Exterior Circuit S / N, C.U. Coyoac´an 04510, Mexico City, Mexico

Paola Briseño-Diaz
Pathology Department, Hospital de Especialidades, Centro M´edico Nacional, S.XXI, Instituto Mexicano del Seguro Social, City. Av Cuauhtemoc 330, Col. Doctores, CP 06720, Mexico City, Mexico

Mayte-Lizeth Padilla-Cristerna and Maria-Del-Pilar Figueroa-Corona
Departamento de Biomedicina Molecular Centro de Investigacion y 49 Estudios Avanzados, Av Instituto Polit´ecnico Nacional 2508, San Pedro Zacatenco, Gustavo A. Madero, 07360 Ciudad de M´exico, Mexico City, Mexico

Jia Wei Tan
Department of Internal Medicine, Bridgeport Hospital, Yale New Haven Health System, Bridgeport, Connecticut, USA

Sachin K. Majumdar
Department of Endocrinology, Bridgeport Hospital, Yale New Haven Health System, Bridgeport, Connecticut, USA
Department of Endocrinology, Bridgeport Hospital, Yale New Haven Health System, Bridgeport, CT, USA

Kenneth Sluis, Hyon Kim, Yuling He, Beatrice Wong and Xiangbing Wang
Division of Endocrinology, Metabolism, and Nutrition, Department of Medicine, Rutgers University-Robert Wood Johnson Medical School, New Jersey, NJ 08903, USA

W. G. P. Kanchana, V. Pinto, K. B. Galketiya and D. D. Karunasagara
Department of Surgery, Teaching Hospital Peradeniya, Kandy, Sri Lanka

P. A. D. M. Kumarathunga, Gajawathana Shakthilingham, Charles Antonypillai and Sonali Gunatilake
Diabetes and Endocrine Clinic, National Hospital Kandy, Kandy, Sri Lanka

T. Jayasingharachchi
Department of Anaesthesiology, Teaching Hospital Peradeniya, Kandy, Sri Lanka

Sungeeta Agrawal
Division of Pediatric Endocrinology, Tufts Children's Hospital, Boston, MA, USA

Serife Uysal
Division of Pediatric Endocrinology, Texas Children's Hospital, Houston, TX, USA

Meghan Fredette, Jose Bernardo Quintos and Shara R. Bialo
Division of Pediatric Endocrinology and Diabetes, Rhode Island Hospital, Providence, RI, USA

Lisa Swartz Topor
Division of Pediatric Endocrinology and Diabetes, Rhode Island Hospital, Providence, RI, USA
Department of Pediatrics, Brown University, Providence, RI, USA
Division of Pediatric Endocrinology, Hasbro Children's Hospital, Providence, RI, USA

Michael Herzlinger and Jason Shapiro
Division of Pediatric Gastroenterology, Rhode Island Hospital, Providence, RI, USA

Linda K. Snelling
Division of Critical Care, Rhode Island Hospital, Providence, RI, USA

Charlotte M. Boney
Department of Pediatrics, Baystate Children's Hospital, Springfield, MA, USA

Nthabiseng Ellen Mothata and Moshawa Calvin Khaba
Department of Anatomical Pathology, Dr George Mukhari Academic Laboratory, National Health Laboratory Services, Sefako Makgatho Health Sciences University, Ga-Rankuwa, South Africa

Takalani Gidion Morulana and Nyaweleni Tshifularo
Department of Paediatric Surgery, Dr George Mukhari Academic Hospital, Sefako Makgatho Health Sciences University, Ga-Rankuwa, South Africa

Phumudzo Bridgett Nemutaduni and Nozipho Elizabeth Nyakale
Department of Nuclear Medicine, Dr George Mukhari Academic Hospital, Sefako Makgatho Health Sciences University, Ga-Rankuwa, South Africa

Ibrahim Al Alwan and Amir Babiker
College of Medicine, King Saud Bin Abdulaziz University for Health Sciences, Riyadh, Saudi Arabia
Endocrine Division, Department of Pediatrics, King Abdullah Specialized Children Hospital, Riyadh, Saudi Arabia
King Abdullah International Medical Research Centre, Ministry of the National Guard Health Affairs, Riyadh, Saudi Arabia

Nouf Al Issa
Endocrine Division, Department of Pediatrics, King Abdullah Specialized Children Hospital, Riyadh, Saudi Arabia

Yousef Al Anazi
Endocrine Division, Department of Pediatrics, King Abdullah Specialized Children Hospital, Riyadh, Saudi Arabia
Department of Pediatrics, College of Medicine, Majmaah University, Majmaah, Saudi Arabia

Khalid Al Noaim
Endocrine Division, Department of Pediatrics, King Abdullah Specialized Children Hospital, Riyadh, Saudi Arabia
Department of Pediatrics, College of Medicine, King Faisal University, Al-Ahsa, Saudi Arabia

M. Zulf Mughal
Department of Paediatric Endocrinology, Royal Manchester Children's Hospital, Manchester University NHS Foundation Trust, Manchester, UK
Faculty of Biology, Medicine and Health, University of Manchester, Manchester, UK

Ni Wayan Wina Dharmesti
Resident: Internal Medicine Department, Faculty of Medicine Udayana University, Sanglah Hospital, Denpasar, Bali, Indonesia

Made Ratna Saraswati, Ketut Suastika, Wira Gotera, and I Made Pande Dwipayana
Endocrine and Metabolism Division, Internal Medicine Department, Faculty of Medicine Udayana University, Sanglah Hospital, Denpasar, Bali, Indonesia

Cathy Zhou and Ghaneh Fananapazir
Department of Radiology, University of California, Davis Medical Center, Sacramento, CA, USA

Michael J. Campbell
Department of Surgery, University of California, Davis Medical Center, Sacramento, CA, USA

S. B. Smedegaard
Department of Internal Medicine, Horsens Regional Hospital, Sundvej 30, 8700 Horsens, Denmark J. O. Jørgensen
Department of Diabetes and Hormone Diseases (DoH), Aarhus University Hospital, Palle Juul-Jensens Blvd 99, 8200 Aarhus N, Denmark

N. Rittig
Department of Internal Medicine, Horsens Regional Hospital, Sundvej 30, 8700 Horsens, Denmark
Department of Diabetes and Hormone Diseases (DoH), Aarhus University Hospital, Palle Juul-Jensens Blvd 99, 8200 Aarhus N, Denmark
Steno Diabetes Center Aarhus, Aarhus University Hospital, Palle Juul-Jensens Blvd 99, 8200 Aarhus N, Denmark

Luis Tolento Cortes, Jessica Trinh, Mimi Le and and Lisa Hong
Loma Linda University Health, School of Pharmacy, 24745 Stewart St, Loma Linda, CA, USA

Philip Papayanis and Leah Tudtud-Hans
Loma Linda University Health, School of Medicine, 11175 Campus St, Loma Linda, CA, USA

Sandip Kuikel, Sunil Aryal and Rupesh Shingh Basnyat
Shishuwa Hospital, 33700 Pokhara, Nepal

Suman Rimal
Department of Internal Medicine, Tribhuvan University Institute of Medicine, 44600 Kathmandu, Nepal

Ravi Upadhyay, Claire Ruane, Rachel Umans and Kristin Wong
Departments of Medicine and Pediatrics, Rutgers University New Jersey Medical School, Newark, NJ, USA

Beth A. Pletcher and Aditi Khokhar
Department of Pediatrics, Rutgers University New Jersey Medical School, Newark, NJ, USA

Kimya Hassani-Ardakania
Department of Medicine, Jewish General Hospital, McGill University, Montreal, H3T IE2, Canada

Mark L. Lipman
Division of Nephrology, Department of Medicine, Jewish General Hospital, Montreal, H3T IE2, Canada

Denny Laporta
Division of Adult Critical Care, Department of Medicine, Jewish General Hospital, Montreal, H3T IE2, Canada

Oriana Hoi Yun Yu
Centre for Clinical Epidemiology, Lady Davis Institute, Jewish General Hospital, Montreal, H3T IE2, Canada
Division of Endocrinology, Department of Medicine, Jewish General Hospital, Montreal, H3T IE2, Canada

Tess Jacob and Jeffrey Kwon
Department of Internal Medicine, Bridgeport Hospital, Yale New Haven Health System, Bridgeport, CT, USA

Allen Bale, Allison Bailey, Andrea L. Barbieri, William Laskin and Paul Cohen
Department of Pathology, Yale University School of Medicine, New Haven, CT, USA

Terence Hughes
Department of Radiology, Bridgeport Hospital, Yale New Haven Health System, Bridgeport, CT, USA

Tobias John Eric Carling
Section of Endocrine Surgery, Department of Surgery, Yale University School of Medicine, New Haven, CT, USA

S. D. N. De Silva and M. Sumanatilleke
Diabetes and Endocrinology Unit, National Hospital of Sri Lanka, Colombo, Sri Lanka

D. Lokuhetty and U. V. V. Ranathunga
Department of Pathology, Faculty of Medicine, University of Colombo, Colombo, Sri Lanka

Giuseppe S. Sica, Leandro Siragusa, Bruno Sensi and Vittoria Bellato
Department of Surgery, University of Rome "Tor Vergata", 00133 Rome, Italy

Pierangela Floris, Valentina Rovella, Valerio Ciavoni, Nicola Di Daniele and Manfredi Tesauro
Department of Systems Medicine, University of Rome "Tor Vergata", 00133 Rome, Italy

Alessandro Mauriello, Monia Di Prete and Rossana Telesca
Department of Experimental Medicine, University of Rome "Tor Vergata", 00133 Rome, Italy

Carmine Cardillo
Department of Internal Medicine, Universit´a Cattolica del Sacro Cuore, Rome 00168, Italy

Rym Belaid, Ibtissem Oueslati , Melika Chihaoui, Meriem Yazidi, Wafa Grira, and Fatma Chaker
Department of Endocrinology, La Rabta University Hospital, Faculty of Medicine, University of Tunis El Manar, Tunis, Tunisia

Somayyeh Hashemian, Rahim Vakili, Siroos Karimdadi, Nosrat Ghaemi and Peyman Eshraghi
Department of Pediatric Diseases, Akbar Hospital, Faculty of Medicine, Mashhad University of Medical Sciences, Mashhad, Iran

Reza Jafarzadeh Esfehani
Department of Medical Genetics, Faculty of Medicine, Mashhad University of Medical Sciences, Mashhad, Iran

Najmeh Malekzadeh Gonabadi
Faculty of Sciences, Sistan and Baluchestan University, Zahedan, Iran

Amirhossein Sahebkar
Biotechnology Research Center, Pharmaceutical Technology Institute, Mashhad University of Medical Sciences, Mashhad, Iran
Applied Biomedical Research Center, Mashhad University of Medical Sciences, Mashhad, Iran
School of Pharmacy, Mashhad University of Medical Sciences, Mashhad, Iran

Mohammad Reza Abbaszadegan
Medical Genetic Research Center, Medical School, Mashhad University of Medical Sciences, Mashhad, Iran

Luca Foppiani
Internal Medicine, Galliera Hospital, Genoa, Italy

Simona Sola
Department of Pathology, Galliera Hospital, Genoa, Italy

Manlio Cabria, Gianluca Bottoni and Arnoldo Piccardo
Nuclear Medicine, Galliera Hospital, Genoa, Italy

Nipun Lakshitha de Silva and Noel Somasundaram
Diabetes and Endocrine Unit, National Hospital of Sri Lanka, Colombo 10, Sri Lanka

Janith Galhenage and Madhubhashinee Dayabandara
University Psychiatry Unit, National Hospital of Sri Lanka, Colombo 10, Sri Lanka

Samar Malaeb
Division of Diabetes, Endocrinology and Metabolism, Department of Medicine, University of Minnesota, Minneapolis, MN 55407, USA

Christopher Spoke
Department of Medical Education, Abbott Northwestern Hospital, Minneapolis, MN 55455, USA

Andrew Spiro, Aqueel Usman, Asif Ajmal, Thanh D. Hoang and Mohamed K. M. Shakir
Division of Endocrinology, Walter Reed National Military Medical Center, 8901 Wisconsin Ave., Bethesda, MD 20889, USA

Takaaki Sakaue, Yosuke Okuno, Kosuke Mukai, Shingo Fujita, Junji Kozawa, Michio Otsuki, Iichiro Shimomura, Hitoshi Nishizawa and Taka-Aki Matsuoka
Department of Metabolic Medicine, Osaka University Graduate School of Medicine, Osaka 565-0871, Japan

Hiromi Iwahashi
Department of Metabolic Medicine, Osaka University Graduate School of Medicine, Osaka 565-0871, Japan
Department of Diabetes Care Medicine, Osaka University Graduate School of Medicine, Osaka 565-0871, Japan

Maeda Norikazu
Department of Metabolic Medicine, Osaka University Graduate School of Medicine, Osaka 565-0871, Japan
Department of Metabolism and Atherosclerosis, Osaka University Graduate School of Medicine, Osaka 565-0871, Japan

Yuto Yamazaki and Hironobu Sasano
Department of Pathology, Tohoku University Graduate School of Medicine, Sendai 980-8574, Japan

Moon Kyung Choi and Prapaipan Putthapiban
Department of Internal Medicine, Einstein Medical Center Philadelphia, 5501 Old York Road, Philadelphia, PA 19141, USA

Patamaporn Lekprasert
Department of Endocrinology, Einstein Endocrine Associates, 50 East Township Line Road Medical Arts Building, Suite G01, Elkins Park, PA 19027, USA

Gerry Samantha Eichelberger
Florida State University College of Medicine, 1115 W. Call Street, Tallahassee, FL, USA 32304

Jordan Carbono and Zachary Field
Department of Internal Medicine, Orlando Regional Healthcare, 21 W. Columbia St., Orlando, FL, USA 32806

KanwarAnoop Kainaur
Department of Pathology, Orlando Regional Healthcare, 52 W. Underwood St., Orlando, FL, USA 32806

Federico Montalvo
Florida State University College of Medicine, 1115 W. Call Street, Tallahassee, FL, USA 32304
Department of Internal Medicine, Orlando Regional Healthcare, 21 W. Columbia St., Orlando, FL, USA 32806

Igor Alexander Harsch
Department of Internal Medicine II, Division of Endocrinology and Metabolism, Rainweg 68, Saalfeld 07318, Germany

Anders Boisen Jensen and Vojtech Pavlicek
Department of Endocrinology, Kantonsspital Münsterlingen, Spitalcampus 1, 8596 Münsterlingen, Switzerland

Elise Durand
Department of Radiology, Kantonsspital Münsterlingen, Spitalcampus 1, 8596 Münsterlingen, Switzerland

S. Pathmanathan
Diabetes and Endocrinology Unit, District General Hospital-Kaluthara, Kaluthara, Sri Lanka
Diabetes and Endocrinology Unit, National Hospital of Sri Lanka, Colombo, Sri Lanka

I. Ranathunga and N. P. Somasundaram
Diabetes and Endocrinology Unit, National Hospital of Sri Lanka, Colombo, Sri Lanka

Francesca Galbiati
Department of Medicine, University of Pittsburgh Medical Center, 200 Lothrop Street, Suite N715, Pittsburgh, PA 15213, USA

Maria M. Pineyro, Leonardo Diaz, Macarena Guzzetti, Mariana Risso and Jimena Pereda
Clinica de Endocrinología y Metabolismo, Hospital de Clínicas, Facultad de Medicina, Universidad de la Republica, Montevideo, Uruguay

Elin Rebecka Carlsson, Anne Mette Høgh, Mogens Fenger and Louise Ambye
Department of Clinical Biochemistry, Copenhagen University Hospital Hvidovre, Denmark

Mai-Britt Toft Nielsen
Department of Endocrinology, Copenhagen University Hospital Hvidovre, Denmark

Rikke Veggerby Grønlund
Gubra, Hørsholm, Denmark

Wann Jia Loh and Linsey Gani
Department of Endocrinology, Changi General Hospital, 2 Simei Street, Singapore

Louise Hughes
Department of Anatomical Pathology, Concord Hospital, Hospital Road, Concord West, New South Wales 2139, Australia

David Thai Chong Chua
Department of Orthopaedics, Changi General Hospital, 2 Simei Street, Singapore

Analía Verónica Yamaguchi and Verónica Andrea Peuchot
Clinical Medicine Department, Metabolism and Nuclear Medicine, Hospital Italiano de Buenos Aires, Buenos Aires, Argentina

Pablo René Costanzo and Pablo Knoblovits
Department of Endocrinology, Metabolism and Nuclear Medicine, Hospital Italiano de Buenos Aires, Buenos Aires, Argentina

Krystel Feghali, Neha Malhotra and Ibitoro Osakwe
Department of Endocrinology, Diabetes and Metabolism, University of Massachusetts Medical School, Baystate Medical Center, Springfield, MA, USA

Kostas Papamarkakis
Division of Nephrology, University of Massachusetts Medical School, Baystate Medical Center, Springfield, MA, USA

Jackson Clark
Division of Internal Medicine, University of Massachusetts Medical School, Baystate Medical Center, Springfield, MA, USA

Lanu Stoddart
Division of Pathology, University of Massachusetts Medical School, Baystate Medical Center, Springfield, MA, USA

Ghufran Saeed Babar
Children's Mercy Hospital and Clinics Endocrinology, 3101 Broadway Blvd, Kansas, Missouri 64111, USA

Minah Tariq
Kansas City University, College of Osteopathic Medicine DO Candidate, Class No 2024, Kansas, Missouri 64124, USA

Rebecca L. Moore and Matthew L. Lorenz
Department of Pediatrics, Brown University, Providence, RI, USA
Department of Internal Medicine, Rhode Island Hospital, Providence, RI, USA
Department of Internal Medicine, Brown University, Providence, RI, USA

Meghan E. Fredette
Department of Pediatrics, Brown University, Providence, RI, USA
Division of Pediatric Endocrinology, Hasbro Children's Hospital, Providence, RI, USA

Yun Ann Chin
Department of Endocrinology, Singapore General Hospital, Singapore

Yi Zhao and Weiying Sim
Department of Clinical Translational Research, Singapore General Hospital, Singapore

Gerald Tay
Department of Head and Neck Surgery, Division of Surgery and Surgical Oncology, Singapore General Hospital, Singapore

Chun Yuen Chow
Department of Pathology, Singapore General Hospital, Singapore

Manju Chandran
Complicated Metabolic Bone Disorders Clinic, Osteoporosis and Bone Metabolism Unit, Department of Endocrinology, Singapore General Hospital, Singapore

Index

www.ingramcontent.com/pod-product-compliance
Lightning Source LLC
LaVergne TN
LVHW082128200926
848484LV00008B/2026